NINTH EDITION

ADVANCED TRAUMA LIFE SUPPORT®

ATLS®

STUDENT COURSE MANUAL

American College of Surgeons
Committee on Trauma

Chair of Committee on Trauma: Michael F. Rotondo, MD, FACS
Medical Director of Trauma Program: John Fildes, MD, FACS
ATLS Committee Chair: Karen J. Brasel, MD, MPH, FACS
ATLS Program Manager: Will Chapleau, EMT-P, RN, TNS
Project Manager: Claire Merrick
Development Editor: Nancy Peterson
Production Services: Anne Seitz and Laura Horowitz, Hearthside Publishing Services
Media Services: Steve Kidd and Alex Menendez, Delve Productions
Designer: Terri Wright Design
Artist: Dragonfly Media Group
Book Layout and Composition: Greg Johnson/Textbook Perfect

Ninth Edition

Advanced Trauma Life Support® Student Course Manual
Library of Congress Control Number: 2012941519
ISBN 13: 978-1-880696-02-6

Dedication

To Paul "Skip" Collicott, MD, FACS

We all leave tracks in the sand as we pass through life. Occasionally we pause and look back at those tracks. This Ninth Edition of the ATLS® manual is truly the sum of the contributions of many who have made tracks, directly and indirectly. But there are no tracks wider or more firmly planted than those made by Paul E. "Skip" Collicott, MD, FACS.

It's hard to remember the "bad ol' days" when an injured patient was evaluated in the Emergency Department by an intern or medical student. The evaluation started with a complete history and physical. Unless the patient was crashing, the ABCs were not given any particular priority. Imagine an intern questioning the family of a patient with a gunshot wound to the chest about childhood illnesses as the patient was in significant respiratory distress! Yet, it happened. How differently such a patient is managed today.

Today, as the news media broadcasts various conflicts and other traumatic events from around the world, one thing that becomes obvious is that first responders and physicians caring for the injured are using the principles and methods of ATLS. Why? Because the principles and methods work.

We and the injured patients we treat owe you a debt of gratitude, Skip—you and your small group of original authors. If we were to be so lucky to have the opportunity to touch as many lives around the world as your vision and effort have through the birth, adolescence and now maturity of ATLS®, then we could feel justifiably proud of our accomplishments. It seems inadequate to say but... thank you for your vision. ATLS works!

This tribute to Skip and the legacy he will leave goes far beyond the dedication of this edition of the manual to him. Well done, my Friend.

Max L. Ramenofsky, MD, FACS
Professor of Surgery
Robert Wood Johnson College of Medicine
New Brunswick, NJ

Richard M. Bell, MD, FACS
Professor, Department of Surgery
University of South Carolina
Columbia, SC

Brief Contents

Foreword

My first exposure with ATLS was in San Diego in 1980 while I was a resident. The instructor course was conducted by Paul E. "Skip" Collicott, MD, FACS, and fellow students included a young surgeon in San Diego, A. Brent Eastman, MD, FACS, and one from San Francisco, Donald D. Trunkey, MD, FACS. Over the next year or two, we trained everyone in San Diego, and this became the language and glue for the San Diego Trauma System. The experience was enlightening, inspiring, and deeply personal. In a weekend, I was educated and had my confidence established: I was adept and skilled in something that had previously been a cause of anxiety and confusion. For the first time, I had been introduced to an "organized course," standards for quality, validated education and skills training, and verification of these skills. It was a life-transforming experience and I chose a career in trauma in part as a result. During that weekend, I also was introduced to the American College of Surgeons—at its very best.

The tradition of ATLS and the newest course—the Ninth Edition—carry on this powerful tradition. This type of education fulfills our responsibility with our patients and the public at large—we are committed to consistency in practice and excellence in delivery above all else.

The fellow creators of the Ninth Edition under the leadership of Dr. Karen Brasel, MD, FACS, Will Chapleau, EMT-P, RN, TNS, and the wonderful College staff have furthered the tradition, the experience, and broadened the global impact. ATLS has been and remains one of the finest achievements of the American College of Surgeons and its Fellows. The Ninth Edition takes this achievement to an even higher level.

David B. Hoyt, MD, FACS
Executive Director
American College of Surgeons
Chicago, Illinois
United States

Remember and Celebrate!

The Advanced Trauma Life Support (ATLS) Course arose from the zeal and passion of a small group of surgeons intent on improving patient care. In 1976, when orthopedic surgeon Dr. James Styner encountered a woefully inadequate response to the needs of his children injured in a light plane crash in rural Nebraska, he was compelled to take action. He spurred the development of an organized systematic approach to the evaluation and care of the injured patient. Recently retired Director of Member Services for the American College of Surgeons, Paul "Skip" Collicott MD, FACS, joined forces with his then-colleague Dr. Styner and the movement called "Advanced Trauma Life Support" was born. In short order, it was adopted by the Committee on Trauma and since then, the course has been developed and refined year after year, decade after decade, in that same spirit of dedication kindled by its founders. Since its inception, ATLS has trained more than one million physicians in 63 countries and no doubt has saved countless lives. In recent years, several individuals central to the development and promulgation of ATLS have been lost. While we miss them, their spirit lives on as we celebrate the launch of the Ninth Edition of ATLS.

The Ninth Edition represents the latest in evidence-based care for the injured. The course materials were thoroughly vetted by a group of international experts and the content was vigorously debated for both its scientific merit and practical application. The result is a vibrant offering for health care providers across the world who seek an easily remembered framework to care for patients with complex injures. The new edition has many changes including the latest techniques in initial assessment, a balanced strategy for resuscitation, and an interactive approach to learning.

So then, on the occasion of this, the Ninth Edition of ATLS, we remember the spirit in which it was founded and we celebrate our work as we carry out the mission of the Committee on Trauma. We hope you will find the course stimulating and interesting. Above all, we hope it will help you save a life.

Michael F. Rotondo, MD, FACS
Chair, Committee on Trauma
American College of Surgeons
Chicago, Illinois
United States

Preface

Role of the American College of Surgeons Committee on Trauma

The American College of Surgeons (ACS) was founded to improve the care of surgical patients, and it has long been a leader in establishing and maintaining the high quality of surgical practice in North America. In accordance with that role, the ACS Committee on Trauma (COT) has worked to establish guidelines for the care of injured patients.

Accordingly, the COT sponsors and contributes to the continued development of the Advanced Trauma Life Support (ATLS) Program. The ATLS Student Course does not present new concepts in the field of trauma care; rather, it teaches established treatment methods. A systematic, concise approach to the early care of trauma patients is the hallmark of the ATLS Program.

This Ninth Edition was developed for the ACS by members of the ATLS Committee and the ACS COT, other individual Fellows of the College, members of the international ATLS community, and nonsurgical consultants to the Committee who were selected for their special competence in trauma care and their expertise in medical education. (Please see the listing at the end of the Preface and the Acknowledgements section for names and affiliations of these individuals.) The COT believes that those individuals who are responsible for caring for injured patients will find the information extremely valuable. The principles of patient care presented in this manual may also be beneficial for the care of patients with nontrauma-related diseases.

Injured patients present a wide range of complex problems. The ATLS Student Course presents a concise approach to assessing and managing multiply injured patients. The course presents providers with knowledge and techniques that are comprehensive and easily adapted to fit their needs. The skills described in this manual represent one safe way to perform each technique. The ACS recognizes that there are other acceptable approaches. However, the knowledge and skills taught in the course are easily adapted to all venues for the care of these patients.

The ATLS Program is revised by the ATLS Committee approximately every four years to respond to changes in available knowledge and incorporate newer and perhaps even safer skills. ATLS Committees in other countries and regions where the Program has been introduced have participated in the revision process, and the ATLS Committee appreciates their outstanding contributions. National and international educators review the educational materials to ensure that the course is conducted in a manner that facilitates learning. All of the course content is available in other resources, such as textbooks and journals. However, the ATLS Course is a specific entity, and the manuals, slide presentations, skill procedures, and other resources are used for the entire course only and cannot be fragmented into separate, freestanding lectures or practical sessions. Members of the ACS COT and the ACS Regional and State/Provincial Committees, as well as the ACS ATLS Program Office staff members, are responsible for maintaining the high quality of the program. By introducing this course and maintaining its high quality, the COT hopes to provide another instrument by which to reduce the mortality and morbidity related to trauma. The COT recommends that providers participating in the ATLS Student Course reverify their status every four years to maintain both their current status in the program and their knowledge of current ATLS core content.

New to this Edition

This Ninth Edition of the *Advanced Trauma Life Support Student Course Manual* reflects several changes designed to enhance the educational content and its visual presentation.

Content Updates

All chapters were rewritten and revised to ensure clear coverage of the most up-to-date technical content, which is also represented in updated references. New to this edition are:

▶▶ Concept of balanced resuscitation
▶▶ Emphasis on the pelvis as a source of blood loss
▶▶ Use of more advanced airway techniques for the difficult airway
▶▶ Optional DPL and pericardiocentesis
▶▶ New FAST Skill Station
▶▶ New multiple-choice questions for pre-test and post-test
▶▶ Optional expanded content on heat injury
▶▶ New initial assessment scenarios
▶▶ Many new images
▶▶ New Instructor Course Content
▶▶ New Skills Videos
▶▶ New ATLS App

Mobile Application

We are pleased to offer a mobile application with both Universal iOS and Android compatibility that is full of useful reference content for retrieval at the bedside and for review at your leisure. Content includes:

- Interactive visuals, such as treatment algorithms and x-ray identification
- Just in Time video segments capturing key skills
- Calculators, such as pediatric burn calculator and the Parkland Formula to determine fluid administration
- Animations, such as airway management and surgical cricothyroidotomy

Students, instructors, coordinators, and educators can access the app through the MyATLS.com website.

Skills Video

As part of the course, video is provided via the MyATLS.com website to show critical skills that providers should be familiar with before taking the course. Skill Stations during the course will allow providers the opportunity to fine tune skill performance in preparation for the practical assessment. Review of the demonstrated skills prior to participating in the skills stations will enhance the learner's experience.

> ### Editorial Notes

The ACS Committee on Trauma is referred to as the ACS COT or *the Committee,* and the State/Provincial Chair(s) is referred to as *S/P Chair(s).*

The international nature of this edition of the ATLS Student Manual may necessitate changes in commonly used terms to facilitate understanding by all students and teachers of the Program.

Advanced Trauma Life Support® and ATLS® are proprietary trademarks and service marks owned by the American College of Surgeons and cannot be used by individuals or entities outside the ACS COT organization for their goods and services without ACS approval. Accordingly, any reproduction of either or both marks in direct conjunction with the ACS ATLS Program within the ACS Committee on Trauma organization must be accompanied by the common law symbol of trademark ownership.

Textbook Features

The pedagogical features of the textbook help to improve student comprehension and knowledge retention. Look for the following features:

Chapter Statement

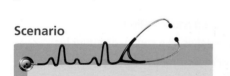

New to this edition, the Chapter Statement capsulizes the overall learning goal of the chapter.

Scenario

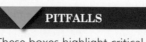

Also new to this edition, each chapter opens with a Scenario that progresses throughout the chapter and concludes at the end. Follow the initial assessment and treatment of each patient, and learn the final outcome. This feature showcases the practical application of chapter content.

Chapter Outline

Outline

This feature provides a "road map" to the chapter content.

Key Questions

? These questions are aligned with the instructor's PowerPoint presentations to prepare students for key discussions during lectures.

Key Points

Sentences appear in red font to attract the reader's attention to key points of information.

Pitfalls

PITFALLS

These boxes highlight critical pitfalls to avoid while caring for trauma patients.

Links

See Skill Station IV: Shock Assessment and Management.

Cross-references to other chapters, Skill Stations, and additional resources help to pull all of the information together. These cross-references are hotlinks in the interactive textbook PDF, which is available at MyATLS.com.

Summary

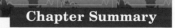

Chapter Summary

Chapter summaries tie back to the Chapter Objectives to ensure understanding of the most pertinent chapter content.

American College of Surgeons Committee on Trauma

Michael F. Rotondo, MD, FACS
Committee on Trauma, Chair
Professor of Surgery, Chair of Department of Surgery, East Carolina University
Chief of Surgery, Director of Center of Excellence for Trauma and Surgical Critical Care
Pitt County Memorial Hospital University Health Systems of Eastern Carolina
Greenville, North Carolina
United States

John Fildes, MD, FACS
Trauma Program, Medical Director
Professor of Surgery, Vice Chair Department of Surgery, Program Director, General Surgery Residency Chief Division of Trauma & Critical Care
University of Nevada School of Medicine
Las Vegas, Nevada
United States

Committee on Advanced Trauma Life Support of the American College of Surgeons Committee on Trauma

Karen Brasel, MD, MPH, FACS
ATLS Committee, Chair
Professor Trauma Surgery & Critical Care
Froedtert Hospital & Medical College of Wisconsin, Trauma Surgery Division
Milwaukee, Wisconsin
United States

John B. Kortbeek, MD, FRCSC, FACS
ATLS Committee, International Course Director
Professor Departments of Surgery and Critical Care
University of Calgary and Calgary Health Region
Calgary, Alberta
Canada

Saud Al Turki, MD, FRCS, ODTS, FACA, FACS
Chief, COT Region 17
Director, Trauma Courses Office, Postgraduate Education & Academic Affairs
King Abdulaziz Medical City
Riyadh
Kingdom of Saudi Arabia

John L.D. Atkinson, MD, FACS
Department of Neurosurgery
Mayo Clinic
Rochester, Minnesota
United States

Raphael Bonvin, MD, PhD
Chair, ATLS Senior Educator Advisory Group
Faculté de biologie et de médecine, Unité de Pédagogie médicale, Lausanne
Switzerland

Mark W. Bowyer, MD, FACS, DMCC
Col (Ret), USAF, MC
Professor of Surgery
Chief, Division of Trauma and Combat Surgery
Director of Surgical Simulation
The Norman M. Rich Dept of Surgery
Uniformed Services University
Bethesda, Maryland
United States

Mary-Margaret Brandt, MD, FACS
Assistant Professor
General Surgery, Division of Trauma, Burn and Emergency Surgery
University of Michigan
Ann Arbor, Michigan
United States

Reginald A. Burton, MD, FACS
Director, Trauma and Surgical Critical Care
Bryan LGH Medical Center
Lincoln, Nebraska
United States

Julie A. Dunn, MD, FACS
Medical Director- Research and Education
Trauma and Acute Care Surgical Services
Poudre Valley Health System
Loveland, Colorado
United States

Lesley Dunstall
EMST/ATLS National Coordinator, Australia
Royal Australasian College of Surgeons
North Adelaide, South Australia
Australia

Gregory M. Georgiadis, MD, FACS
Orthopaedic Trauma Service
The Toledo Hospital
Toledo, Ohio
United States

Sharon M. Henry, MD, FACS
Anne Scalea Professor of Trauma
University of Maryland School of Medicine
Director Wound Healing and Metabolism Service
R Adams Cowley Shock Trauma Center
Baltimore, Maryland
United States

Michael Hollands, MB BS, FRACS, FACS
Head of Hepatobiliary and Gastro-oesophageal Surgery
Westmead Hospital
Sydney, New South Wales
Australia

Claus Falck Larsen, MD, dr.med., MPA, FACS
Medical Director
The Abdominal Centre, University of Copenhagen,
  Rigshopitalet Denmark
Copenhagen
Denmark

Douglas W. Lundy, MD, FACS
Orthopaedic Trauma Surgery
Resurgens Orthopaedics
Marietta, Georgia
United States

R. Todd Maxson, MD, FACS
Chief , Trauma Program
Dell Children's Medical Center
Little Rock, Arkansas
United States

Daniel B. Michael MD, PhD, FACS
Chief, Neurotrauma and Critical Care
Beaumont Hospital
Royal Oak, Michigan
United States

Kimberly K. Nagy, MD, FACS
Vice-Chairman, Department of Trauma
Cook County Trauma Unit
Chicago, Illinois
United States

Renato Sergio Poggetti, MD, FACS
Director of Emergency Surgical Service
Hospital das Clinicas Universidad de São Paulo
Brazil

Raymond R. Price, MD, FACS
Adjunct Clinical Assistant Professor
University of Utah
Murray, Utah
United States

Jeffrey P. Salomone, MD, FACS
*Associate Professor of Surgery, Division of Trauma/Surgical
  Critical Care*
Emory University School of Medicine
Atlanta, Georgia
United States

R. Stephen Smith, MD, RDMS, FACS
System Chief, Acute Care Surgery
West Penn Allegheny Health SystemPittsburgh, Pennsylvania
United States

Robert J. Winchell, MD, FACS
Head, Trauma and Burn Surgery
Maine Medical Center
Portland, Maine
United States

Jay A. Yelon, MD, FACS
Chairman, Department of Surgery
Lincoln Medical Center
Professor of Clinical Surgery
Weill Cornell Medical College
Bronx, New York
United States

Associate Members to the Committee on Advanced Trauma Life Support of the American College of Surgeons Committee on Trauma

Guy F. Brisseau, MD, FACS
Assistant Dean, Post Graduate Medical Education
Dalhousie University
Halifax, Nova Scotia
Canada

Regina Sutton Chennault, MD, FACS
Trauma Medical Director
Alaska Regional Hospital
Anchorage, Alaska
United States

Kimberly A. Davis, MD, FACS
Trauma Medical Director
Surgical Director, Quality and Performance Improvement
Yale-New Haven Hospital
New Haven, Connecticut
United States

Glen A. Franklin, MD, FACS
Associate Program Director, General Surgery
Program Director, Surgical Critical Care
University of Louisville Department of Surgery
Louisville, Kentucky
United States

Lewis E. Jacobson, MB, CHB, FACS
Medical Director, Trauma Program
St. Vincent Indianapolis Hospital
Indianapolis, Indiana
United States

Sarvesh Logsetty, MD, FACS
Director of Manitoba Firefighters Burn Unit
Associate Professor
Department of Surgery and Children's Health
  University of Manitoba
Winnipeg, Manitoba
Canada

George E. McGee, MD, FACS
Forrest General Hospital
Trauma Surgery Clinic
Hattiesburg, Mississippi
United States

Drew W. McRoberts, MD, FACS
General Surgeon
Portneuf Medical Center
Pocatello, Idaho
United States

Charles E. Morrow, Jr, MD, FACS
Program Director, General Surgery
Medical Director, Trauma Surgery
Department of Trauma, Spartanburg Regional Medical Center
Spartanburg, South Carolina
United States

Neil G. Parry, MD, FRCSC, FACS
Associate Professor
Victoria Hospital
London, Ontario
Canada

Martin A. Schreiber, MD, FACS
Professor of Surgery
Director, Trauma Service
Oregon Health & Science University, Trauma & Critical Care
  Section
Portland, Oregon
United States

Gustavo J. Tisminetzky, MD, MAAC, FACS
ATLS Program Director
Jefe Unidad Urgencia Hospital J.A. Fernández
Buenos Aires
Argentina

Special Members to the Committee on Advanced Trauma Life Support of the American College of Surgeons Committee on Trauma

Jameel Ali, MD, M.Med.Ed, FRCS, FACS
Professor of Surgery
University of Toronto
St. Michael's Hospital, Division of General Surgery/Trauma
Toronto, Ontario
Canada

Christoph R. Kaufmann, MD, FACS
Medical Director, Trauma Services
Forbes Regional Hospital
Monroeville, Pennsylvania
United States

Consultant to the Committee on Advanced Trauma Life Support of the American College of Surgeons Committee on Trauma

Arthur Cooper, MD, MS, FACS, FAAP, FCCM
Professor of Surgery
Columbia University Medical Center
Affiliation at Harlem Hospital

American Society of Anesthesiology Liaison to the Committee on Advanced Trauma Life Support of the American College of Surgeons Committee on Trauma

Peter J. Dunbar, MD
Associate Professor, Anesthesiology
Harborview Medical Center
Seattle, Washington
United States

American College of Emergency Physicians Liaison to the Committee on Advanced Trauma Life Support of the American College of Surgeons Committee on Trauma

Robert R. Bass, MD, FACEP
Executive Director
Maryland Institute for Emergency Medical Services Systems
Baltimore, Maryland
United States

Robert E. O' Connor, MD, FACEP
Professor and Chair
Department of Emergency Medicine
University of Virginia School of Medicine
Charlottesville, Virginia
United States

ATLS Senior Educator Advisory Group

Raphael Bonvin, MD, PhD
Faculté de biologie et de médecine, Unité de Pédagogie médicale
Lausanne
Switzerland

Wesam Abuznadah, MD, Med, FRCS(C), RPVI
Assistant Professor, Consultant Vascular & Endovascular
  Surgery
Medical Educator In-Charge, Department of Medical Education
King Saud Bin Abdulaziz University For Health Sciences
Jeddah
Kingdom of Saudi Arabia

Joe Acker, III, MS, MPH, EMT-P
Executive Director
Birmingham Regional EMS
Birmingham, Alabama
United States

Peggy Chehardy, EdD, CHES
New Orleans, Louisiana
United States

Debbie Paltridge
Confederation of Postgraduate Medical Education Councils
Member, ATLS Senior Educator Advisory Group
Victoria
Australia

Elizabeth de las Mercedes Vallejo de Solezio, MA, PhD
Member, ATLS Senior Educator Advisory Group
Consultora Internacional en Educación, Evaluación y
  Capacitación
Quito, Pichincha
Ecuador

Claus Dieter Strobaus
Member, ATLS Senior Educator Advisory Group
Departamento de Pós-Graduação em Educação
Pontifícia Universidade Católica do Rio Grande do Sul
Porto Allegre
Brazil

Kum Ying Tham, MBBS, FRCS (Edin), FAMS
Member, ATLS Senior Educator Advisory Group
Senior Consultant, Clinical Associate Professor
Tan Tock Seng Hospital
Singapore City
Singapore

ATLS Regional Coordinator Representatives

Donna Allerton, RN
Critical Care, Coordinator, ATLS Program
McMaster University Medical Centre
Hamilton, Ontario
Canada

Vilma Cabading
ATLS National Coordinator, Saudi Arabia
Academic Affairs Department
King Abdulaziz Medical City-NGHA
Riyadh
Kingdom of Saudi Arabia

Cristiane de Alencar Domingues, RN
Coordenadora Nacional ATLS/PHTLS/ATOM
Diretora Nacional ATCN
University of São Paulo
São Paulo
Brazil

Lesley Dunstall
EMST/ATLS National Coordinator, Australia
Royal Australasian College of Surgeons
North Adelaide, South Australia
Australia

Ruth Dyson, BA (hons)
External Programmes Coordinator, Education Department
The Royal College of Surgeons of England
London
United Kingdom

Chad McIntyre, NREMT-P, FP-C
ATLS Coordinator
Shands Jacksonville Medical Center
Jacksonville, Florida
United States

Acknowledgments

ATLS Program Office Staff

While it is clear that there are many people responsible for the Ninth Edition, the outstanding staff in the ATLS Program Office deserves special mention. It is their dedication and hard work that not only produces the new edition while ensuring that each one is better than the last, but facilitates its use in hundreds of courses around the world each and every year.

Will Chapleau, EMT-P, RN, TNS
ATLS Program Manager
American College of Surgeons ATLS
  Program Office
Chicago, Illinois
United States

Bill Jenkins
Administrative Supervisor
American College of Surgeons ATLS
  Program Office
Chicago, Illinois
United States

Jasmine Alkhatib
*COT Regional Program Coordinator
  (14, 15, 16, 17)*
American College of Surgeons
Chicago, Illinois
United States

Sharon E. Borum
COT Regional Program Coordinator (3, 9)
American College of Surgeons
Chicago, Illinois
United States

Gerardo Cuauhtémoc Alvizo Cárdenas
*COT Administrative Assistant and
  Special Projects Coordinator*
American College of Surgeons
Chicago, Illinois
United States

Danielle S. Haskin, MSW
*COT CME & Course Development
  Specialist*
American College of Surgeons
Chicago, Illinois
United States

Pascale Leblanc
COT Regional Program Coordinator (6, 13)
American College of Surgeons
Chicago, Illinois
United States

Richard H. Sallee
COT Regional Program Coordinator (4, 10)
American College of Surgeons
Chicago, Illinois
United States

Freddie L. Scruggs
*COT Regional Program Coordinator
  (2, 5, 8)*
American College of Surgeons ATLS
  Program Office
Chicago, Illinois
United States

Natalie M. Torres
*COT Regional Program Coordinator
  (1, 7, 11, 12)*
American College of Surgeons
Chicago, Illinois
United States

Contributors

During development of this revision, we received a great deal of assistance from many individuals—whether reviewing information at meetings, submitting images, or evaluating research. ATLS thanks the following contributors for their time and effort in the development of the Ninth Edition:

Georges Abi Saad
ATLS Program Director
Beirut
Lebanon

Omar Al Ghanimi
ATLS Educator
Taif
Kingdom of Saudi Arabia

Abdullah Al-Harthy
*Consultant, Trauma Surgeon, and
  Intensivist*
Sultan Qaboos University Hospital
Al Khod
Oman

**Saud Al Turki, MD, FRCS, ODTS,
  FACA, FACS**
*Director, Trauma Courses Office,
  Postgraduate Education & Academic
  Affairs*
King Abdulaziz Medical City
Riyadh
Kingdom of Saudi Arabia

Celia Aldana
ATLS Coordinator
Santiago
Chile

**Jameel Ali, MD, M.Med.Ed, FRCS,
  FACS**
Professor of Surgery
University of Toronto
St. Michael's Hospital, Division of
  General Surgery/Trauma
Toronto, Ontario
Canada

Donna Allerton, RN
*Critical Care, Coordinator, ATLS
  Program*
McMaster University Medical Centre
Hamilton, Ontario
Canada

John A. Androulakis, MD, FACS
Emeritus Professor of Surgery
University Hospital of Patras
Patras
Greece

Marjorie J. Arca, MD, FACS
Assistant Professor
Children's Hospital of Wisconsin
Milwaukee, Wisconsin
United States

John H. Armstrong, MD, FACS
Medical Director
Center for Advanced Medical Learning
  and Simulation, University of South
  Florida
Tampa, Florida
United States

John L.D. Atkinson, MD, FACS
Department of Neurosurgery
Mayo Clinic
Rochester, Minnesota
United States

Mahmood Ayyaz, MD
Professor of Surgery
Lehore, Punjab
Pakistan

Andrew Baker, MD
ATLS Program Director
Durban
South Africa

David P. Blake, MD, FACS
Col, USAF, MC, FS
*Commander, 88th Surgical Operations
  Squadron*
Wright Patterson Air Force Base, Ohio
United States

Mark W. Bowyer, MD, FACS, DMCC
Col (Ret), USAF, MC
Professor of Surgery
Chief, Division of Trauma and Combat Surgery
Director of Surgical Simulation
The Norman M. Rich Dept of Surgery
Uniformed Services University
Bethesda, Maryland
United States

Mary-Margaret Brandt, MD, FACS
Assistant Professor
General Surgery, Division of Trauma, Burn and Emergency Surgery
University of Michigan
Ann Arbor, Michigan
United States

Frank J. Branicki, MBBS, DM, FRCS, FRACS, FCS(HK), FHKAM(Surg)
Professor and Chair of Surgery
UAE University, Al-Ain Faculty of Medicine & Health Services
Al-Ain
United Arab Emirates

Karen Brasel, MPH, MD, FACS
ATLS Committee, Chair
Professor Trauma Surgery & Critical Care
Froedtert Hospital & Medical College of Wisconsin, Trauma Surgery Division
Milwaukee, Wisconsin
United States

George Brighton, MD
Core Surgical Trainee
Trauma and Orthopaedics
North Devon District Hospital
Barnstaple
United Kingdom

James Brown, MA
ATLS Educator
Maryland Institute for Emergency Medical Services System
Baltimore, Maryland
United States

Laura Bruna, RN
Italian National Coordinator
Assitrauma
Torino
Italy

Reginald A. Burton MD, FACS
Director, Trauma and Surgical Critical Care
Bryan LGH Medical Center
Lincoln, Nebraska
United States

Jacqueline Bustraan, MSc
Educational Consultant and Researcher
PLATO, Centre for Research and Development of Education and Training, Leiden University
Leiden
Netherlands

Vilma Cabading
ATLS National Coordinator, Saudi Arabia
Academic Affairs Department
King Abdulaziz Medical City-NGHA
Riyadh
Kingdom of Saudi Arabia

Carlos Carvajal Hafemann, MD, FACS
Chairperson, Chile Committee on Trauma
Professor of Surgery
Director of Surgery of the East Campus
Universidad de Chile
Santiago
Chile

Gustavo H. Castagneto, MD, FACS
Professor of Surgery
Buenos Aires British Hospital, Department of Surgery
Buenos Aires
Argentina

Candice L. Castro, MD, FACS
COL, MC, USA
ATLS Course Director
San Antonio, Texas
United States

Zafar Ullah Chaudhry, MD, FRCS, FCPS, FACS
Professor of Surgery
National Hospital and Medical Center
President
College of Physicians and Surgeons Pakistan
Karachi
Pakistan

Peggy Chehardy, EdD, CHES
New Orleans, Louisiana
United States

Regina Sutton Chennault, MD, FACS
Trauma Medical Director
Alaska Regional Hospital
Anchorage, Alaska
United States

Wei Chong CHUA, MD
Chief Army Medical Officer
Singapore Armed Forces
Singapore City
Singapore

Emmanuel Chrysos, MD, PhD, FACS
Associate Professor of Surgery
Department of General Surgery, University Hospital of Crete
Heraklion, Crete
Greece

Raul Coimbra, MD, PhD, FACS
Chief of Trauma/Burn/Surgical Critical Care Division
Department of Surgery
University of California, San Diego Medical Center
San Diego, California
United States

Francisco Collet e Silva, MD, FACS, PhD (med)
Medical Doctor-Emergency Surgical Services
Hospital das Clinicas of the University of São Paulo
São Paulo
Brazil

Arthur Cooper, MD, MS, FACS, FAAP, FCCM
Professor of Surgery
Columbia University Medical Center
Affiliation at Harlem Hospital
New York, New York
United States

Jaime Cortes Ojeda, MD
Chief, General Surgery
National Children's Hospital
Professor
University of Costa Rica
San Jose
Costa Rica

Clay Cothren Burlew MD, FACS
Director, Surgical Intensive Care Unit
Program Director, Trauma and Acute Care Surgery Fellowship
Denver Health Medical Center
Denver, Colorado
United States

Diane Chetty
ATLS Coordinator
Tawam Hospital
Al Ain, Abu Dhabi
United Arab Emirates

Kimberly A. Davis, MD, FACS
Trauma Medical Director
Surgical Director, Quality and Performance Improvement
Yale-New Haven Hospital
New Haven, Connecticut
United States

Cristiane de Alencar Domingues, RN
*Coordenadora Nacional ATLS/PHTLS/
  ATOM*
Diretora Nacional ATCN
University of São Paulo
São Paulo
Brazil

Mauricio Di Silvio-Lopez, MD, FACS
Chair, Mexico Committee on Trauma
Hospital Regional 20 de Noviembre,
  ISSSTE Mexico City, Districto Federal
Mexico

Jay J. Doucet, MD, FACS
Director, Surgical Intensive Care Unit
University of California, San Diego
  Medical Center
San Diego, California
United States

**Hermanus Jacobus Christoffel
  Du Plessis, MB, ChB, MMed(Surg),
  FCS(SA), FACS**
Chief Surgeon, Colonel
SAMHS (South African Military Health
  Services)
*Head of the Department of Surgery and
  Intensive Care*
1 Military Hospital
Adjunct Professor of Surgery
University of Pretoria
Pretoria
South Africa

Julie A. Dunn, MD, FACS
*Medical Director- Research and
  Education*
Trauma and Acute Care Surgical Services
Poudre Valley Health System
Loveland, Colorado
United States

Ruth Dyson, BA (hons)
*External Programmes Coordinator -
  Education Department The Royal
  College of Surgeons of England*
London
United Kingdom

Martin Eason MD, JD
Assistant Professor
East Tennessee State University
Johnson City, Tennessee
United States

A. Brent Eastman, MD, FACS
*President, American College of Surgeons
Chief Medical Officer
N. Paul Whittier Chair of Trauma,
  Scripps Memorial Hospital, La Jolla*
Scripps Health
San Diego, California
United States

Abdelhakim Talaat Elkholy, MBBCh
ATLS Program Director
Cairo
Egypt

**Claus Falck Larsen, MD, dr.med.,
  MPA, FACS**
*Chief, Committee on Trauma Region 15
Medical Director*
The Abdominal Centre, University of
  Copenhagen, Rigshopitalet Denmark
Copenhagen
Denmark

Froilan A. Fernandez, MD
ATLS Program Director
Medical Director Emergency Service
Hospital del Trabajador
Santiago
Chile

Esteban Foianini, MD, FACS
General Surgeon
Director
Foianini Clinic
Santa Cruz
Bolivia

Joan Foerster
ATLS Coordinator
UBC Health Sciences Hospital
Vancouver, British Columbia
Canada

Heidi Frankel, MD, FACS
Assistant Professor of Surgery
University of Maryland Medical Center
Baltimore, Maryland
United States

**Subash C. Gautam, MD, MBBS,
  FRCS, FACS**
ATLS Program Director
Senior Consultant and Head of
  Department of Surgery
Fujairah Hospital
Fujairah
United Arab Emirates

Gerardo A. Gomez, MD, FACS
Medical Director
IU/Wishard Level I Trauma Center
Indianapolis, Indiana
United States

**Hugo Alfredo Gomez Fernandez,
  MD, FACS**
ATLS Program Director
Sociedad Paraguaya de Cirugía
Asuncion
Paraguay

Oscar D. Guillamondegu, MD, FACS
*Associate Professor of Surgery, Division
  of Trauma & Surgical Critical Care*
Vanderbilt University Medical Center
Nashville, Tennessee
United States

**Enrique A. Guzman Cottallat, MD,
  FACS**
*Chair, Ecuador Committee on
  TraumaDiplomat in Public Health*
Director, Neurosurgery Services
Guayaquil Hospital
Guayaquil, Guayas
Ecuador

Betty Jean Hancock, MD, FACS
Section Head, Pediatric General Surgery
University of Manitoba
Winnipeg, Manitoba
Canada

Richard Henn, RN, BSN, M.ED
Director, Education Department
Northern Arizona Healthcare
Flagstaff, Arizona
United States

Walter Henny, MD
Formerly of Erasmus Medical Center
Rotterdam
Netherlands

Sharon M. Henry, MD, FACS
Anne Scalea Professor of Trauma
University of Maryland School of
  Medicine
*Director Wound Healing and Metabolism
  Service*
R A Cowley Shock Trauma Center
Baltimore, Maryland
United States

Grace Herrera-Fernandez
ATLS Coordinator
College of Physicians and Surgeons of
  Costa Rica
San Jose
Costa Rica

**Michael Hollands, MB BS, FRACS,
  FACS**
*Head of Hepatobiliary and Gastro
  oesophageal Surgery*
Westmead Hospital
Sydney, New South Wales
Australia

Roxolana Horbowyj, MD, FACS
ATLS Instructor
Holmes, Pennsylvania
United States

Christopher M. Hults, MD, FACS
CDR, USN
Trauma and Surgical Critical Care
University of South Florida
Tampa, Florida
United States

Randeep S. Jawa, MD, FACS
Assistant Professor of Surgery
University of Nebraska Medical Center
Omaha, Nebraska
United States

Jose María Jover Navalon, MD, FACS
ATLS Program Director
Hospital Universitario de Getafe,
  Department of General Surgery
Madrid
Spain

Gregory J. Jurkovich MD, FACS
Professor of Surgery
Harborview Medical Center
Seattle, Washington
United States

Christoph R. Kaufmann, MD, FACS
Medical Director, Trauma Services
Forbes Regional Hospital
Monroeville, Pennsylvania
United States

Peggy Knudson, MD, FACS
Professor of Surgery
University of California, San Francisco
  General Hospital, Department of
  Surgery
San Francisco, California
United States

John B. Kortbeek, MD, FRCSC, FACS
*ATLS Committee, International Course
  Director*
*Professor Departments of Surgery and
  Critical Care*
University of Calgary and Calgary Health
  Region
Calgary, Alberta
Canada

Roman Kosir, MD
ATLS Program Director
Assistant of Surgery
University Clinical Center Maribor,
  Department of Traumatology
Maribor
Slovenia

Eric J. Kuncir, MD, FACS
University of California, San Diego
San Diego, California
United States

Roslyn Ladner
ATLS Coordinator
British Columbia
Canada

Chong-Jeh Lo, MD, FACS
Associate Dean for Student Affairs
National Chen Kung University College
  of Medicine
Tainan
Taiwan

Sarvesh Logsetty, MD, FACS
*Director of Manitoba Firefighters Burn
  Unit*
Associate Professor
Department of Surgery and Children's
  Health
University of Manitoba
Winnipeg, Manitoba
Canada

Ka Ka Lui
ATLS Coordinator
Department of Neurosurgery, Queen
  Mary Hospital
Hong Kong
China

Siew-Kheong Lum
ATLS Program Director
Sungai Buloh Hospital
Kuala Lumpur
Malaysia

Douglas W. Lundy, MD, FACS
Orthopaedic Trauma Surgery
Resurgens Orthopaedics
Marietta, Georgia
United States

Fernando Machado, MD
Universidad de la Republica
Montevideo
Uruguay

Patrizio Mao, MD, FACS
Responsabile Urgenze Chirurgiche
Chirurgia Generale Universitaria, A.S.O.
  San Luigi Gonzaga di Orbassano
Torino
Italy

Khalid Masood Gondal
ATLS Instructor
Lahore
Pakistan

R. Todd Maxson, MD, FACS
Chief, Trauma Program
Dell Children's Medical Center
Little Rock, Arkansas
United States

Chad McIntyre, NREMT-P, FP-C
ATLS Coordinator
Shands Jacksonville Medical Center
Jacksonville, Florida
United States

Daniel B. Michael, MD, PhD, FACS
Chief, Neurotrauma and Critical Care
Beaumont Hospital
Royal Oak, Michigan
United States

Mahesh C. Misra, MD, FACS
ATLS Program Director
All India Institute of Medical Sciences,
  New Delhi
India

Forrest O. Moore, MD, FACS
Trauma Surgeon
St. Joseph's Hospital and Medical Center
Phoenix, Arizona
United States

Newton Djin Mori, MD
General Surgeon
Emergency Surgical Services,
Hospital das Clinicas Universidad de São
  Paulo
São Paulo
Brazil

Charles E. Morrow, Jr, MD, FACS
Program Director, General Surgery
Medical Director, Trauma Surgery
Department of Trauma, Spartanburg
  Regional Medical Center
Spartanburg, South Carolina
United States

Stephen G. Murphy, MD
Division of Pediatric General Surgery
Wilmington, Delaware
United States

Kimberly K. Nagy, MD, FACS
Vice-Chairman, Department of Trauma
Cook County Trauma Unit
Chicago, Illinois
United States

Nicolaos Nicolau, MD, FACS
ATLS Instructor
Larnaca
Cyprus

Han Boon Oh
ATLS Instructor
Singapore City
Singapore

Osama Ali Omari, MD
ATLS Instructor
Saudi ARAMCO Medical Services
  Organization
Dhahran
Kingdom of Saudi Arabia

Hock Soo Ong, MD, FACS
Senior Consultant in General Surgery
Singapore General Hospital
Singapore City
Singapore

Giorgio Olivero, MD, FACS
Professor of Surgery
University of Torino, Department of
  Medicine and Surgery, St. John the
  Baptist Hospital
Torino
Italy

Gonzalo Ostria, MD
ATLS-Bolivia Chair
Bolivia
Chile

Rattaplee Pak-Art, MD
ATLS Program Director
Bangkok
Thailand

Neil G. Parry, MD, FRCSC, FACS
Associate Professor
Victoria Hospital
London, Ontario
Canada

BiPinchandra R. Patel, MD, FACS
ATLS Course Director
Vestal, New York
United States

Jasmeet S. Paul, MD
ATLS Instructor
Medical College of Wisconsin
Milwaukee, Wisconsin
United States

Pedro Moniz Pereira, MD
ATLS Program Director
General Surgeon
Lisboa Portugal

Renato Sergio Poggetti, MD, FACS
Chief, COT Region 14
Director of Emergency Surgical Service
Hospital das Clinicas Universidad de São
  Paulo
Brazil

Alex Poole, MD, FACS
ATLS Course Director
Nelson, British Columbia
Canada

Marcelo Recalde Hidrobo, MD, FACS
ATLS Course Director
Universidad San Francisco de Quito
Quito
Ecuador

Raymond R. Price, MD, FACS
Adjunct Clinical Assistant Professor
University of Utah
Murray, Utah
United States

Sonia Primeau
ATLS Coordinator
Montreal General Hospital
Montreal, Quebec
Canada

Cristina Quintana
ATLS Coordinator
Sociedad Paraguaya de Cirugía
Asuncion
Paraguay

Tarek S. A. Razek, MD, FACS
Director, Trauma Unit
Montreal General Hospital
Montreal, Quebec
Canada

Rosalind Roden, FFAEM
Chair, ATLS Steering Group
The Royal College of Surgeons
London
United Kingdom

Jakob Roed, MD
ATLS Program Director
Copenhagen
Denmark

Martha Romero
ATLS Coordinator
AMDA Bolivia
Santa Cruz
Bolivia

Michael F. Rotondo, MD, FACS
Committee on Trauma, Chair
*Professor of Surgery, Chair of Department
  of Surgery, East Carolina University*
*Chief of Surgery, Director of Center of
  Excellence for Trauma and Surgical
  Critical Care*
Pitt County Memorial Hospital, Univer-
  sity Health Systems of Eastern Carolina
Greenville, North Carolina
United States

Majid Sabahi, MD
ATLS Instructor
Tehran
Iran

Nicole Schaapveld, RN
*Managing Director / National
  Coordinator ATLS NL*
Advanced Life Support Group–NL
Riel
The Netherlands

Inger B. Schipper, MD, PhD, FACS
Program Director, ATLS Netherlands
Head, Department of Trauma surgery
Leiden University Medical Center
Leiden The Netherlands

Patrick Schoettker, MD, M.E.R.
ATLS Instructor
Responsable Anesthésie Neurochirurgicale,
  ORL et UrgenceService
  d'Anesthésiologie
Lausanne
Switzerland

Martin A. Schreiber, MD, FACS
Professor of Surgery
Director, Trauma Service
Oregon Health & Science University,
  Trauma & Critical Care Section
Portland, Oregon
United States

Estrellita C. Serafico
ATLS Coordinator
King Abdulaziz Medical City
Riyadh
Kingdom of Saudi Arabia

Juan Carlos Serrano, MD, FACS
ATLS Course Director
Director, Department of Trauma
Hospital Santa Inés
Cuenca
Ecuador

Brian Siegel, MD, FACS
ATLS Course Director
Staff Physician
Department of Surgery
Morristown Memorial Hospital
Morristown, New Jersey
United States

Preecha Siritongtaworn, MD, FACS
Chief, Division of Trauma Surgery
Department of Surgery, Faculty of
  Medicine Siriraj Hospital, Mahidol
  University
Bangkok
Thailand

Diana Skaff
ATLS Coordinator
American University of Beirut Medical
  Centre
Beirut
Lebanon

R. Stephen Smith, MD, RDMS, FACS
System Chief, Acute Care Surgery
West Penn Allegheny Health System
Pittsburgh, Pennsylvania
United States

Ricardo M. Sonneborn, MD, FACS
Santiago
Chile

Anne Sorvari
ATLS Coordinator
St. Michael's Hospital
Toronto, Ontario
Canada

Paul-Martin Sutter, MD
Department of Surgery, Spitalzentrum
Biel
Switzerland

John Sutyak, MD, FACS
Associate Director
Southern Illinois Trauma Center
Springfield, Illinois
United States

Lars Bo Svendsen, MD, DMSci
Associate Professor Surgery
Copenhagen University, Department
   of Abdominal Surgery and
   Transplantation, Rigshospitalet
Copenhagen
Denmark

Wa' el S. Taha, MD
Assistant Professor of Surgery
King Abdulaziz Medical City
National Guard Health Affairs
Riyadh
Kingdom of Saudi Arabia

Kathryn Tchorz, MD, FACS
Associate Professor
Wright State University School of Medicine
Dayton, Ohio
United States

Wei Ting Lee
ATLS Instructor
Singapore City
Singapore

**Gustavo Tisminetzky, MD, FACS,
   MAAC**
ATLS Program Director
Professor of Surgery
Universidad de Buenos Aires
Buenos Aires
Argentina

Julio L. Trostchansky, MD, FACS
ATLS Program Director
Sociedad de Cirugía del Uruguay
Montevideo
Uruguay

Philip Truskett, MB BS, FRACS
The University of New South Wales
Prince of Wales Hospital, Randwick
Cronulla, New South Wales
Australia

Jeffrey Upperman, MD, FACS
Assistant Professor
Children's Hospital of Los Angeles
Los Angeles, California
United States

Yvonne van den Ende
Office Manager
Stichting Advanced Life Support Group
Riel
The Netherlands

Allan Vennike
ATLS National Educator
Næstved
Denmark

Tore Vikström, MD, PhD
*Director and Head Consultant, General
   Surgery Professor of Disaster Medicine
   & Traumatology*
Centre for Teaching & Research in
   Disaster Medicine and Traumatology
University Hospital
Linköping
Sweden

Eric Voiglio, MD, PhD, FACS, FRCS
Senior Lecturer, Consultant Surgeon
Department of Emergency Surgery,
University Hospitals of Lyon
Centre Hospitalier Lyon-Sud
Pierre-Bénite
France

Leonard J. Weireter Jr., MD, FACS
Professor of Surgery
Eastern Virginia Medical School
Norfolk, Virginia
United States

Nicholas M. Wetjen, MD
*Assistant Professor of Neurosurgery and
   Pediatrics*
Mayo Clinic
Rochester, Minnesota
United States

Richard L. Wigle, MD, FACS
Assistant Professor
LSU Health Sciences Center
Shreveport, Louisiana
United States

**Stephen Wilkinson, MBBS, MD,
   FRACS**
General Surgeon
Tasmania Antiobesity Surgery Centre
Hobart
Australia

Robert J. Winchell, MD, FACS
Head, Trauma and Burn Surgery
Maine Medical Center
Portland, Maine
United States

Robert Winter, FRCP, FRCA, DM
Consultant in Critical Care Medicine
Mid Trent Critical Care Network and
   Nottingham University Hospitals
Nottingham
United Kingdom

Jay A. Yelon, MD, FACS
Chairman, Department of Surgery
Lincoln Medical Center
Professor of Clinical Surgery
Weill Cornell Medical College
Bronx, New York
United States

Ahmad M. Zarour, MD, FACS
Department of Surgery
Hamad General Hospital
Doha
Qatar

Honor Roll

Over the past 30 years, ATLS has grown from a local course training Nebraska doctors to care for trauma patients to a family of trauma specialists from more than 60 countries who volunteer their time to ensure that our materials reflect the most current research and that our course is designed to improve patient outcomes. The Ninth Edition of ATLS reflects the efforts of the following individuals who contributed to the first eight editions, and we honor them here.

Honor Roll Members

Sabas F. Abuabara, MD, FACS
Joe E. Acker, II, MS, MPH, EMT
Raymond H. Alexander, MD, FACS
Fatimah Albarracin, RN
Jameel Ali, MD, MMed Ed, FRCS (C), FACS
Heri Aminuddin, MD
Charles Aprahamian, MD, FACS
Guillermo Arana, MD, FACS
Ana Luisa Argomedo Manrique
Ivar Austlid
Gonzalo Avilés
Richard Baillot, MD
Barbara A. Barlow, MA, MD, FACS
James Barone, MD, FACS
John Barrett, MD, FACS
Pierre Beaumont, MD
Margareta Behrbohm Fallsberg, PhD, BSc
Richard M. Bell, MD, FACS
Eugene E. Berg, MD, FACS
Richard Bergeron, MD
François Bertrand, MD
Renato Bessa de Melo, MD
Mike Betzner, MD
Emidio Bianco, MD, JD
Ken Boffard, MB BCh, FRCS, FRCS (Ed), FACS
Bertil Bouillon, MD
Don E. Boyle, MD, FACS
Marianne Brandt
Fred Brenneman, MD, FRCSC, FACS
Susan M. Briggs, MD, FACS
Åse Brinchmann-Hansen, PhD
Peter Brink, MD, PhD
Karim Brohi, MD
Rea Brown, MD, FACS
Allen F. Browne, MD, FACS
Gerry Bunting, MD
Andrew R. Burgess, MD, FACS
Richard E. Burney, MD, FACS
David Burris, MD, FACS
Sylvia Campbell, MD, FACS
C. James Carrico, MD, FACS
C. Gene Cayten, MD, FACS
June Sau-Hung Chan

Robert A. Cherry, MD, FACS
Chin-Hung Chung, MB BS, FACS
David E. Clark, MD, FACS
Paul E. Collicott, MD, FACS
Arthur Cooper, MD, FACS
Ronald D. Craig, MD
Doug Davey, MD
Elizabeth de Solezio, PhD
Subrato J. Deb, MD
Alejandro De Gracia, MD, FACS, MAAC
Laura Lee Demmons, RN, MBA
Ronald Denis, MD
Jesus Díaz Portocarrero, MD, FACS
Frank X. Doto, MS
Anne-Michéle Droux
Marguerite Dupré, MD
Candida Durão
Brent Eastman, MD, FACS
Frank E. Ehrlich, MD, FACS
Martin R. Eichelberger, MD, FACS
David Eduardo Eskenazi, MD, FACS
Vagn Norgaard Eskesen, MD
Denis Evoy, MCH, FRCSI
William F. Fallon, Jr, MD, FACS
David V. Feliciano, MD, FACS
Froilan Fernandez, MD
Carlos Fernandez-Bueno, MD
John Fildes, MD, FACS
Ronald P. Fischer, MD, FACS
Stevenson Flanigan, MD, FACS
Lewis M. Flint, Jr, MD, FACS
Cornelia Rita Maria Getruda Fluit, MD, MEdSci
Jorge E. Foianini, MD, FACS
Susanne Fristeen, RN
Knut Fredriksen, MD, PhD
Richard Fuehling, MD
Christine Gaarder, MD
Sylvain Gagnon, MD
Richard Gamelli, MD, FACS
Paul Gebhard
James A. Geiling, MD, FCCP
Thomas A. Gennarelli, MD, FACS
John H. George, MD
Aggelos Geranios, MD
Michael Gerazounis, MD
Roger Gilbertson, MD
Robert W. Gillespie, MD, FACS
Marc Giroux, MD
Javier González-Uriarte, MD, PhD, EBSQ, FSpCS
John Greenwood
Russell L. Gruen, MBBS, PhD, FRACS
Niels Gudmundsen-Vestre
J. Alex Haller, Jr., MD, FACS
Burton H. Harris, MD, FACS
Michael L. Hawkins, MD, FACS
Ian Haywood, FRCS (Eng), MRCS, LRCP
James D. Heckman, MD, FACS
June E. Heilman, MD, FACS
David M. Heimbach, MD, FACS
David N. Herndon, MD, FACS
Fergal Hickey, FRCS, FRCS Ed.(A&E), DA(UK), FCEM
Erwin F. Hirsch, MD, FACS
Francisco Holguin, MD

Scott Holmes
David B. Hoyt, MD, FACS
Arthur Hsieh, MA, NREMT-P
Irvene K. Hughes, RN
Richard C. Hunt, MD, FACEP
John E. Hutton, Jr, MD, FACS
Miles H. Irving, FRCS (Ed), FRCS (Eng)
José María Jover Navalon, MD, FACS
Richard Judd, PhD, EMSI
Gregory J. Jurkovich, MD, FACS
Aage W. Karlsen
Christoph R. Kaufmann, MD, FACS
Howard B. Keith, MD, FACS
James F. Kellam, MD, FRCS, FACS
Steven J. Kilkenny, MD, FACS
Darren Kilroy, FRCSEd, FCEM, M.Ed
Lena Klarin, RN
Amy Koestner, RN, MSN
Radko Komadina , MD, PhD
Digna R. Kool, MD
John B. Kortbeek, MD, FACS
Brent Krantz, MD, FACS
Jon R. Krohmer, MD, FACEP
Ada Lai Yin Kwok
Maria Lampi, BSc, RN
Katherine Lane, PhD
Francis G. Lapiana, MD, FACS
Pedro Larios Aznar
Anna M. Ledgerwood, MD, FACS
Dennis G. Leland, MD, FACS
Frank Lewis, MD, FACS
Wilson Li, MD
Helen Livanios, RN
Nur Rachmat Lubis, MD
Edward B. Lucci, MD, FACEP
Eduardo Luck, MD, FACS
Thomas G. Luerssen, MD, FACS
J.S.K. Luitse, MD
Arnold Luterman, MD, FACS
LAM Suk-Ching, BN, MHM
LEO Pien Ming, MBBS, MRCS (Edin), M.Med (Orthopaedics)
Jaime Manzano, MD, FACS
Fernando Magallanes Negrete, MD
Donald W. Marion, MD, FACS
Michael R. Marohn, DO, FACS
Barry D. Martin, MD
Salvador Martín Mandujano, MD, FACS
Kimball I. Maull, MD, FACS
Mary C. McCarthy, MD, FACS
Gerald McCullough, MD, FACS
John E. McDermott, MD, FACS
James A. McGehee, DVM, MS
William F. McManus, MD, FACS
Norman E. McSwain, Jr., MD, FACS
Philip S. Metz, MD, FACS
Cynthia L. Meyer, MD
Salvijus Milašius, MD
Frank B. Miller, MD, FACS
Sidney F. Miller, MD, FACS
Soledad Monton, MD
Ernest E. Moore, MD, FACS
Johanne Morin, MD
David Mulder, MD, FACS
Raj K. Narayan, MD, FACS
James B. Nichols, DVM, MS

Martín Odriozola, MD, FACS
Franklin C. Olson, EdD
Steve A. Olson, MD, FACS
Gonzalo Ostria P., MD, FACS
Arthur Pagé, MD
José Paiz Tejada
Fatima Pardo, MD
Steven N. Parks, MD, FACS
Chester (Chet) Paul, MD
Andrew Pearce, BScHons, MBBS,
  FACEM PG Cert Aeromed retrieval
Mark D. Pearlman, MD
Andrew B. Peitzman, MD, FACS
Nicolas Peloponissios, MD
Jean Péloquin, MD
Philip W. Perdue, MD, FACS
J.W. Rodney Peyton, FRCS (Ed), MRCP
Lawrence H. Pitts, MD, FACS
Galen V. Poole, MD, FACS
Danielle Poretti, RN
Ernest Prégent, MD
Richard R. Price, MD, FACS
Herbert Proctor, MD, FACS
Jacques Provost, MD
Paul Pudimat, MD
Max L. Ramenofsky, MD, FACS
Jesper Ravn, MD
Marcelo Recalde, MD, FACS
John Reed, MD
Marleta Reynolds, MD, FACS
Stuart A. Reynolds, MD, FACS
Peter Rhee, MD, MPH, FACS, FCCM,
  DMCC
Bernard Riley, FFARCS
Martin Richardson
Bo Richter
Charles Rinker, MD, FACS
Avraham Rivkind, MD

Diego Rodriguez, MD
Vicente Rodriguez, MD
Olav Røise, MD, PhD
Ronald E. Rosenthal, MD, FACS
Grace Rozycki, MD, FACS
Daniel Ruiz, MD, FACS
J. Octavio Ruiz Speare, MD, MS, FACS
James M. Ryan, MCh, FRCS (Eng),
  RAMC
James M. Salander, MD, FACS
Gueider Salas, MD
Jeffrey P. Salomone, MD, FACS
Rocio Sanchez-Aedo Linares, RN
Mårtin Sandberg, MD, PhD
Thomas G. Saul, MD, FACS
Domenic Scharplatz, MD, FACS
William P. Schecter, MD, FACS
Kari Schrøder Hansen, MD
Thomas E. Scott, MD, FACS
Stuart R. Seiff, MD, FACS
Bolivar Serrano, MD, FACS
Steven R. Shackford, MD, FACS
Marc J. Shapiro, MD, FACS
Thomas E. Shaver, MD, FACS
Mark Sheridan, MBBS, MMedSc, FRACS
Richard C. Simmonds, DVM, MS
Richard K. Simons, MB, BChir, FRCS,
  FRCSC, FACS
Nils Oddvar Skaga, MD
Peter Skippen, MBBS, FRCPC, FJFICM,
  MHA
David V. Skinner, FRCS (Ed), FRCS
  (Eng)
Arnold Sladen, MD, FACS
Tone Slåke
Birgitte Soehus
Ricardo Sonneborn, MD, FACS
Michael Stavropoulos, MD, FACS

Spyridon Stergiopoulos, MD
Gerald O. Strauch, MD, FACS
Luther M. Strayer, III, MD
James K. Styner, MD
Vasso Tagkalakis
Joseph J. Tepas, III, MD, FACS
Stéphane Tétraeault, MD
Gregory A. Timberlake, MD, FACS
Peter G. Trafton, MD, FACS
Stanley Trooksin, MD, FACS
David Tuggle, MD, FACS
Wolfgang Ummenhofer, MD, DEAA
Jay Upright
Armand Robert van Kanten, MD
Endre Varga, MD, PhD
Edina Várkonyi
Panteleimon Vassiliu, MD, PhD
Eugenia Vassilopoulou, MD
Antigoni Vavarouta
Antonio Vera Bolea
Alan Verdant, MD
J. Leonel Villavicencio, MD, FACS
Eric Voiglio, MD, PhD, FACS, FRCS
Franklin C. Wagner, MD, FACS
Raymond L. Warpeha, MD, FACS
Clark Watts, MD, FACS
John A. Weigelt, MD, FACS
John West, MD, FACS
Robert J. White, MD, FACS
Daryl Williams, MBBS, FANZCA,
  GDipBusAd, GdipCR
Fremont P. Wirth, MD, FACS
Bradley D. Wong, MD, FACS
Nopadol Wora-Urai, MD, FACS
Peter H. Worlock, DM, FRCS (Ed), FRCS
  (Eng)
Bang Wai-Key Yuen, MB BS, FRCS,
  FRACS, FACS

Course Overview: The Purpose, History, and Concepts of the ATLS Program

Program Goals

The Advanced Trauma Life Support (ATLS) course provides its participants with a safe and reliable method for the immediate treatment of injured patients and the basic knowledge necessary to:

1. Assess a patient's condition rapidly and accurately.

2. Resuscitate and stabilize patients according to priority.

3. Determine whether a patient's needs exceed a facility's resources and/or a provider's capabilities.

4. Arrange appropriately for a patient's interhospital or intrahospital transfer (what, who, when, and how).

5. Ensure that optimal care is provided and that the level of care does not deteriorate at any point during the evaluation, resuscitation, or transfer processes.

Course Objectives

The content and skills presented in this course are designed to assist doctors in providing emergency care for trauma patients. The concept of the "golden hour" emphasizes the urgency necessary for successful treatment of injured patients and is not intended to represent a "fixed" time period of 60 minutes. Rather, it is the window of opportunity during which providers can have a positive impact on the morbidity and mortality associated with injury. The ATLS course provides the essential information and skills for providers to identify and treat life-threatening and potentially life-threatening injuries under the extreme pressures associated with the care of these patients in the fast-paced environment and anxiety of a trauma room. The ATLS course is applicable to clinicians in a variety of clinical situations. It is just as relevant to providers in a large teaching facility in North America or Europe as it is in a developing nation with rudimentary facilities.

Upon completion of the ATLS student course, the participant will be able to:

1. Demonstrate the concepts and principles of the primary and secondary patient assessments.

2. Establish management priorities in a trauma situation.

3. Initiate primary and secondary management necessary within the golden hour for the emergency management of acute life-threatening conditions.

4. In a given simulated clinical and surgical skills practicum, demonstrate the following skills, which are often required in the initial assessment and treatment of patients with multiple injuries:

   a. Primary and secondary assessment of a patient with simulated, multiple injuries

   b. Establishment of a patent airway and initiation of assisted ventilations.

   c. Orotracheal intubation on adult and infant manikins

   d. Pulse oximetry and carbon dioxide detection in exhaled gas

   e. Cricothyroidotomy

   f. Assessment and treatment of a patient in shock, particularly recognition of life-threatening hemorrhage

   g. Venous and intraosseous access

   h. Pleural decompression via needle thoracentesis and chest tube insertion

   i. Recognition of cardiac tamponade and appropriate treatment

   j. Clinical and radiographic identification of thoracic injuries

   k. Use of peritoneal lavage, ultrasound (FAST), and computed tomography (CT) in abdominal evaluation

   l. Evaluation and treatment of a patient with brain injury, including use of the Glasgow Coma Scale score and CT of the brain

   m. Assessment of head and facial trauma by physical examination

   n. Protection of the spinal cord, and radiographic and clinical evaluation of spine injuries

   o. Musculoskeletal trauma assessment and management

p. Estimation of the size and depth of burn injury and volume resuscitation

q. Recognition of the special problems of injuries in infants, the elderly, and pregnant women

r. Understanding of the principles of disaster management

The Need

According to the latest information from the WHO and CDC, more than nine people die every minute from injuries or violence, and 5.8 million people of all ages and economic groups die every year from unintentional injuries and violence (Figure 1). The burden of injury is even more significant, accounting for 12% of the world's burden of disease. Motor vehicle crashes (road traffic injuries, in Figure 2) alone cause more than 1 million deaths annually and an estimated 20 million to 50 million significant injuries; they are the leading cause of death due to injury worldwide. Improvements in injury control efforts are having an impact in most developed countries, where trauma remains the leading cause of death in persons 1 through 44 years of age. Significantly, more than 90% of motor vehicle crashes occur in the developing world. Injury-related deaths are expected to rise dramatically by 2020, with deaths due to motor vehicle crashes projected to increase by 80% from current rates in low- and middle-

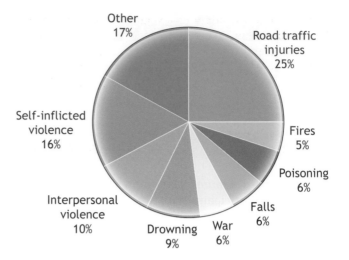

■ FIGURE 2 Distribution of Global Injury Mortality by Cause.

Reproduced with permission from *The Injury Chart Book: a Graphical Overview of the Global Burden of Injuries.* Geneva: World Health Organization Department of Injuries and Violence Prevention. Noncommunicable Diseases and Mental Health Cluster; 2002.

income countries. By 2020 it is estimated that more than 1 in 10 people will die from injuries.

Global trauma-related costs are estimated to exceed $500 billion annually. These costs are much

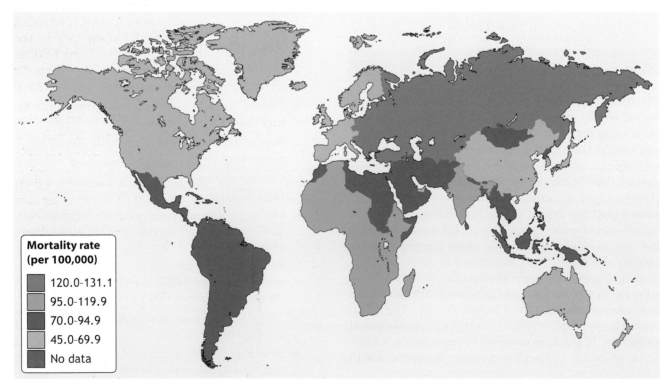

■ FIGURE 1 Global Injury-Related Mortality.

Reproduced with permission from *The Injury Chart Book: a Graphical Overview of the Global Burden of Injuries.* Geneva: World Health Organization Department of Injuries and Violence Prevention. Noncommunicable Diseases and Mental Health Cluster; 2002.

higher if one considers lost wages, medical expenses, insurance administration costs, property damage, fire loss, employer costs, and indirect loss from work-related injuries. Despite these staggering costs, less than 4 cents of each federal research dollar in the United States are spent on trauma research. As monumental as these data are, the true cost can be measured only when it is realized that trauma strikes down a society's youngest and potentially most productive members. Research dollars spent on communicable diseases such as polio and diphtheria have nearly eliminated the incidence of these diseases in the United States. Unfortunately the disease of trauma has not captured the public attention in the same way.

Injury is a disease. It has a host (the patient) and it has a vector of transmission (eg, motor vehicle, firearm, etc). Many significant changes have improved the care of the injured patient since the first edition of the ATLS Program appeared in 1980. The need for the program and for sustained, aggressive efforts to prevent injuries is as great now as it has ever been.

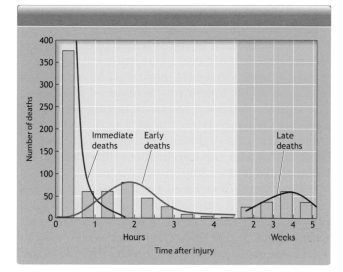

■ **FIGURE 3 Trimodal Death Distribution.**

Trimodal Death Distribution

First described in 1982, the trimodal distribution of deaths implies that death due to injury occurs in one of three periods, or peaks (Figure 3). *The first peak* occurs within seconds to minutes of injury. During this early period, deaths generally result from apnea due to severe brain or high spinal cord injury or rupture of the heart, aorta, or other large blood vessels. Very few of these patients can be saved because of the severity of their injuries. Only prevention can significantly reduce this peak of trauma-related deaths.

The *second peak* occurs within minutes to several hours following injury. Deaths that occur during this period are usually due to subdural and epidural hematomas, hemopneumothorax, ruptured spleen, lacerations of the liver, pelvic fractures, and/or multiple other injuries associated with significant blood loss. The golden hour of care after injury is characterized by the need for rapid assessment and resuscitation, which are the fundamental principles of Advanced Trauma Life Support.

The *third peak*, which occurs several days to weeks after the initial injury, is most often due to sepsis and multiple organ system dysfunction. Care provided during each of the preceding periods impacts on outcomes during this stage. The first and every subsequent person to care for the injured patient has a direct effect on long-term outcome.

The temporal distribution of deaths reflects local advances and capabilities of trauma systems. The development of standardized trauma training, better prehos-

pital care, and the development of trauma centers with dedicated trauma teams and established protocols to care for injured patients has altered the picture.

History

The delivery of trauma care in the United States before 1980 was at best inconsistent. A tragedy occurred in February 1976 that changed trauma care in the "first hour" for injured patients in the United States and in much of the rest of the world. An orthopedic surgeon was piloting his plane and crashed in a rural Nebraska cornfield. The surgeon sustained serious injuries, three of his children sustained critical injuries, and one child sustained minor injuries. His wife was killed instantly. The care that he and his family subsequently received was inadequate by the day's standards. The surgeon, recognizing how inadequate their treatment was, stated: "When I can provide better care in the field with limited resources than what my children and I received at the primary care facility, there is something wrong with the system, and the system has to be changed."

A group of private-practice surgeons and doctors in Nebraska, the Lincoln Medical Education Foundation, and the Lincoln-area Mobile Heart Team Nurses, with the help of the University of Nebraska Medical Center, the Nebraska State Committee on Trauma (COT) of the American College of Surgeons (ACS), and the Southeast Nebraska Emergency Medical Services identified the need for training in advanced trauma life support. A combined educational format of lectures, lifesaving skill demonstrations, and practical laboratory experiences formed the first prototype ATLS course.

A new approach to the provision of care for individuals who suffer major, life-threatening injury premiered in 1978, the year of the first ATLS course. This prototype ATLS course was field-tested in conjunction with the Southeast Nebraska Emergency Medical Services. One year later, the ACS COT, recognizing trauma as a surgical disease, enthusiastically adopted the course under the imprimatur of the College and incorporated it as an educational program.

This course was based on the assumption that appropriate and timely care could significantly improve the outcome of injured patients. The original intent of the ATLS Program was to train doctors who do not manage major trauma on a daily basis, and the primary audience for the course has not changed. However, today the ATLS method is accepted as a standard for the "first hour" of trauma care by many who provide care for the injured, whether the patient is treated in an isolated rural area or a state-of the-art trauma center.

Course Development and Dissemination

The ATLS course was conducted nationally for the first time under the auspices of the American College of Surgeons in January 1980. International promulgation of the course began in 1980.

The program has grown each year in the number of both courses and participants. To date, the course had trained more than 1.5 million participants in more than 75,000 courses around the world. Currently, an average of 50,000 clinicians are trained each year in over 3,000 courses. The greatest growth in recent years has been in the international community, and this group currently represents approximately more than half of all ATLS activity.

The text for the course is revised approximately every 4 years and incorporates new methods of evaluation and treatment that have become accepted parts of the armamentarium of providers who treat trauma patients. Course revisions incorporate suggestions from members of the Subcommittee on ATLS; members of the ACS COT; members of the international ATLS family; representatives to the ATLS Subcommittee from the American College of Emergency Physicians and the American College of Anesthesiologists; and course instructors, coordinators, educators, and participants. Changes that are made to the program reflect accepted, verified practice patterns, not "cutting edge" technology or experimental methods. The international nature

of the program mandates that the course be adaptable to a variety of geographic, economic, social, and medical practice situations. To retain a current status in the ATLS Program, an individual must reverify with the latest edition of the materials.

A parallel course to the ATLS course is the Prehospital Trauma Life Support (PHTLS) course, which is sponsored by the National Association of Emergency Medical Technicians (NAEMT). The PHTLS course, developed in cooperation with the ACS COT, is based on the concepts of the ACS ATLS Program and is conducted for emergency medical technicians, paramedics, and nurses who are providers of prehospital trauma care. Other courses have been developed with similar concepts and philosophies. For example, the Society of Trauma Nurses offers the Advanced Trauma Care for Nurses (ATCN), which is also developed in cooperation with the ACS COT. The ATCN and ATLS courses are conducted parallel to each other with the nurses auditing the ATLS lectures and then participating in skill stations separate from the ATLS skill stations conducted for doctors. The benefits of having both prehospital and in-hospital trauma personnel speaking the same "language" are apparent.

International Dissemination

As a pilot project, the ATLS Program was exported outside of North America in 1986 to the Republic of Trinidad and Tobago. The ACS Board of Regents gave permission in 1987 for promulgation of the ATLS Program in other countries. The ATLS Program may be requested by a recognized surgical organization or ACS Chapter in another country by corresponding with the ATLS Subcommittee Chairperson, care of the ACS ATLS Program Office, Chicago, IL. At the time of publication, 63 countries were actively providing the ATLS course to their trauma providers. These countries include:

1. Argentina (ACS Chapter and Committee on Trauma)

2. Australia (Royal Australasian College of Surgeons)

3. Bahrain (Kingdom of Saudi Arabia ACS Chapter and Committee on Trauma)

4. Bolivia (Bolivian Surgeons Society)

5. Brazil (ACS Chapter and Committee on Trauma)

6. Canada (ACS Chapters and Provincial Committees on Trauma)

7. Chile (ACS Chapter and Committee on Trauma)

8. Colombia (ACS Chapter and Committee on Trauma)

9. Costa Rica (College of Physicians and Surgeons of Costa Rica)

10. Cyprus (ACS Chapter and Committee on Trauma, Greece)

11. Czech Republic (Czech Trauma Society)

12. Denmark (Danish Trauma Society)

13. Ecuador (ACS Chapter and Committee on Trauma)

14. Egypt (Egyptian Society of Plastic and Reconstructive Surgeons)

15. Fiji and the nations of the Southwest Pacific (Royal Australasian College of Surgeons)

16. France (Societe Francaise de Chirurgie d'Urgence)

17. Germany (German Society for Trauma Surgery and Task Force for Early Trauma Care)

18. Greece (ACS Chapter and Committee on Trauma)

19. Greenland (Danish Trauma Society)

20. Grenada (Society of Surgeons of Trinidad and Tobago)

21. Hong Kong (ACS Chapter and Committee on Trauma)

22. Hungary (Hungarian Trauma Society)

23. India (Association for Trauma Care of India)

24. Indonesia (Indonesian Surgeons Association)

25. Iran (Persian Orthopedic and Trauma Association)

26. Ireland (Royal College of Surgeons in Ireland)

27. Israel (Israel Surgical Society)

28. Italy (ACS Chapter and Committee on Trauma)

29. Jamaica (ACS Chapter and Committee on Trauma)

30. Kingdom of Saudi Arabia (ACS Chapter and Committee on Trauma)

31. Kuwait (Kingdom of Saudi Arabia ACS Chapter and Committee on Trauma)

32. Lebanon (Lebanese Chapter of the American College of Surgeons)

33. Lithuania (Lithuanian Society of Traumatology and Orthopaedics)

34. Malaysia (College of Surgeons, Malaysia)

35. Mexico (ACS Chapter and Committee on Trauma)

36. Netherlands, The (Dutch Trauma Society)

37. New Zealand (Royal Australasian College of Surgeons)

38. Nigeria (Nigerian Orthopaedic Association)

39. Norway (Norwegian Surgical Society)

40. Oman (Oman Surgical Society)

41. Pakistan (College of Physicians and Surgeons Pakistan)

42. Panama (ACS Chapter and Committee on Trauma)

43. Papua New Guinea (Royal Australasian College of Surgeons)

44. Paraguay (Sociedad Paraguaya de Cirugía)

45. Peru (ACS Chapter and Committee on Trauma)

46. Portugal (Portuguese Society of Surgeons)

47. Qatar (Kingdom of Saudi Arabia ACS Chapter and Committee on Trauma)

48. Republic of China, Taiwan (Surgical Association of the Republic of China, Taiwan)

49. Republic of Singapore (Chapter of Surgeons, Academy of Medicine)

50. Samoa (Royal Australasian College of Surgeons)

51. Slovenia (Slovenian Society of Trauma Surgeons)

52. Republic of South Africa (South African Trauma Society)

53. Spain (Spanish Society of Surgeons)

54. Sweden (Swedish Society of Surgeons)

55. Switzerland (Swiss Society of Surgeons)

56. Syria (Center for Continuing Medical and Health Education)

57. Thailand (Royal College of Surgeons of Thailand)

58. Trinidad and Tobago (Society of Surgeons of Trinidad and Tobago)

59. United Arab Emirates (Surgical Advisory Committee)

60. United Kingdom (Royal College of Surgeons of England)

61. United States, U.S. territories (ACS Chapters and State Committees on Trauma)

62. Uruguay (Uruguay Society of Surgery)

63. Venezuela (ACS Chapter and Committee on Trauma)

The Concept

The concept behind the ATLS course has remained simple. Historically, the approach to treating injured patients, as taught in medical schools, was the same as that for patients with a previously undiagnosed medical condition: an extensive history including past medical history, a physical examination starting at the top of the head and progressing down the body, the development of a differential diagnosis, and a list of adjuncts to confirm the diagnosis. Although this approach was adequate for a patient with diabetes mellitus and many acute surgical illnesses, it did not satisfy the needs of patients suffering life-threatening injuries. The approach required change.

Three underlying concepts of the ATLS Program were initially difficult to accept:

1. Treat the greatest threat to life first.

2. The lack of a definitive diagnosis should never impede the application of an indicated treatment.

3. A detailed history is not essential to begin the evaluation of a patient with acute injuries.

The result was the development of the ABCDE approach to the evaluation and treatment of injured patients. These concepts are also in keeping with the observation that the care of injured patients in many circumstances is a team effort, allowing medical personnel with special skills and expertise to provide care simultaneously with surgical leadership of the process.

The ATLS course emphasizes that injury kills in certain reproducible time frames. For example, the loss of an airway kills more quickly than does the loss of the ability to breathe. The latter kills more quickly than loss of circulating blood volume. The presence of an expanding intracranial mass lesion is the next most lethal problem. Thus, the mnemonic ABCDE defines the specific, ordered evaluations and interventions that should be followed in all injured patients:

> **A**irway with cervical spine protection
> **B**reathing
> **C**irculation, stop the bleeding
> **D**isability or neurologic status
> **E**xposure (undress) and **E**nvironment (temperature control)

The Course

The ATLS course emphasizes the rapid initial assessment and primary treatment of injured patients, starting at the time of injury and continuing through initial assessment, lifesaving intervention, reevaluation, stabilization, and, when needed, transfer to a trauma center. The course consists of precourse and postcourse tests, core content lectures, interactive case presentations, discussions, development of lifesaving skills, practical laboratory experiences, and a final performance proficiency evaluation. Upon completion of the course, participants should feel confident in implementing the skills taught in the ATLS course.

The Impact

ATLS training in a developing country has resulted in a decrease in injury mortality. Lower per capita rates of deaths from injuries are observed in areas where providers have ATLS training. In one study, a small trauma team led by a clinician with ATLS experience had equivalent patient survival when compared with a larger team with more providers in an urban setting. In addition, there were more unexpected survivors than fatalities. There is abundant evidence that ATLS training improves the knowledge base, the psychomotor skills and their use in resuscitation, and the confidence and performance of participants who have taken part in the program. The organization and procedural skills taught in the course are retained by course participants for at least 6 years, which may be the most significant impact of all.

Acknowledgments

The COT of the ACS and the ATLS Subcommittee gratefully acknowledge the following organizations for their time and efforts in developing and field testing the Advanced Trauma Life Support concept: The Lincoln Medical Education Foundation, Southeast Nebraska Emergency Medical Services, the University of Nebraska College of Medicine, and the Nebraska State Committee on Trauma of the ACS. The committee also is indebted to the Nebraska doctors who supported the development of this course and to the Lincoln Area Mobile Heart Team Nurses who shared their time and ideas to help build it. Appreciation is extended to the organizations identified previously in this overview for their support of the worldwide promulgation of the course. Special recognition is given to the spouses, significant others, children, and practice partners of the ATLS instructors and students. The time that providers spend away from their homes and practices and effort afforded to this voluntary program are essential components for the existence and success of the ATLS Program.

Summary

The ATLS course provides an easily remembered approach to the evaluation and treatment of injured patients for any provider, irrespective of practice specialty, even under the stress, anxiety, and intensity that accompanies the resuscitation process. In addition, the program provides a common language for all providers who care for injured patients. The ATLS course provides a foundation for evaluation, treatment, education, and quality assurance—in short, a system of trauma care that is measurable, reproducible, and comprehensive.

The ATLS Program has had a positive impact on the care provided to injured patients worldwide. This has resulted from the improved skills and knowledge of the doctors and other health care providers who have been course participants. The ATLS course establishes an organized and systematic approach for the evaluation and treatment of patients, promotes minimum standards of care, and recognizes injury as a world health care issue. Morbidity and mortality have been reduced, but the need to eradicate injury remains. The ATLS Program has changed and will continue to change as advances occur in medicine and the needs and expectations of our societies change.

Bibliography

1. Ali J, Adam R, Butler AK, et al. Trauma outcome improves following the Advanced Trauma Life Support program in a developing country. *J Trauma* 1993;34:890-899.

2. Ali J, Adam R, Josa D, et al. Comparison of interns completing the old (1993) and new interactive (1997) Advanced Trauma Life Support courses. *J Trauma* 1999;46:80-86.

3. Ali J, Adam R, Stedman M, et al. Advanced Trauma Life Support program increases emergency room application of trauma resuscitative procedures in a developing country. *J Trauma* 1994;36:391-394.

4. Ali J, Adam R, Stedman M, et al. Cognitive and attitudinal impact of the Advanced Trauma Life Support Course in a developing country. *J Trauma* 1994;36:695-702.

5. Ali J, Cohen R, Adam R, et al. Teaching effectiveness of the Advanced Trauma Life Support program as demonstrated by an objective structured clinical examination for practicing physicians. *World J Surg* 1996;20:1121-1125.

6. Ali J, Cohen R, Adams R, et al. Attrition of cognitive and trauma skills after the Advanced Trauma Life Support (ATLS) course. *J Trauma* 1996;40:860-866.

7. Ali J, Howard M. The Advanced Trauma Life Support Program in Manitoba: a 5-year review. *Can J Surg* 1993;36:181-183.

8. Anderson ID, Anderson IW, Clifford P, et al. Advanced Trauma Life Support in the UK: 8 years on. *Br J Hosp Med* 1997;57:272-273.

9. Aprahamian C, Nelson KT, Thompson BM, et al. The relationship of the level of training and area of medical specialization with registrant performance in the Advanced Trauma Life Support course. *J Emerg Med* 1984;2:137-140.

10. Ben Abraham R, Stein M, Kluger Y, et al. ATLS course in emergency medicine for physicians. *Harefuah* 1997;132:695-697, 743.

11. Ben Abraham R, Stein M, Kluger Y, et al. The impact of Advanced Trauma Life Support Course on graduates with non-surgical medical background. *Eur J Emerg Med* 1997;4:11-14.

12. Berger LR, Mohan D: *Injury Control: A Global View.* Delhi, India: Oxford University Press; 1996.

13. Blumenfield A, Ben Abraham R, Stein M, et al. Cognitive knowledge decline after Advanced Trauma Life Support courses. *J Trauma* 1998;44:513-516.

14. Burt CW. Injury-related visits to hospital emergency departments: United States, 1992. *Adv Data* 1995;261:1-20.

15. Demetriades D, Kimbrell B, Salim A, et al. Trauma deaths in a mature urban trauma system: is "trimodal" distribution a valid concept? *J Am Coll Surg* 2005;201:343-348.

16. Deo SD, Knottenbelt JD, Peden MM. Evaluation of a small trauma team for major resuscitation. *Injury* 1997;28:633-637.

17. Direccao Geral de Vicao, Lisboa, Portugal, data provided by Pedro Ferreira Moniz Pereira, MD, FACS.

18. Fingerhut LA, Cox CS, Warner M, et al. International comparative analysis of injury mortality: findings from the ICE on injury statistics. *Adv Data* 1998;303:1-20.

19. Firdley FM, Cohen DJ, Bienbaum ML, et al. Advanced Trauma Life Support: Assessment of cognitive achievement. *Milit Med* 1993;158:623-627.

20. Gautam V, Heyworth J. A method to measure the value of formal training in trauma management: comparison between ATLS and induction courses. *Injury* 1995;26:253-255.

21. Greenslade GL, Taylor RH. Advanced Trauma Life Support aboard RFA Argus. *J R Nav Med Serv* 1992;78:23-26.

22. Leibovici D, Fedman B, Gofrit ON, et al. Prehospital cricothyroidotomy by physicians. *Am J Emerg Med* 1997;15:91-93.

23. Mock CJ. International approaches to trauma care. *Trauma Q* 1998;14:191-348.

24. Murray CJ, Lopez A. *The global burden of disease: I. A comprehensive assessment of mortality and disability from diseases, and injuries and risk factors in 1990 and projected to 2020.* Cambridge, MA: Harvard University Press; 1996.

25. National Center for Health Statistics: Injury visits to emergency departments.

26. National Safety Council. *Injury Facts* (1999). Itasca, IL: National Safety Council.

27. Nourjah P. National hospital ambulatory medical care survey: 1997 emergency department summary. *Adv Data* 1999;304:1-24.

28. Olden van GDJ, Meeuwis JD, Bolhuis HW, et al. Clinical impact of advanced trauma life support. *Am J Emerg Med* 2004;22;522-525.

29. Rutledge R, Fakhry SM, Baker CC, et al. A population-based study of the association of medical manpower with county trauma death rates in the United States. *Ann Surg* 1994;219:547-563.

30. Walsh DP, Lammert GR, Devoll J. The effectiveness of the advanced trauma life support system in a mass casualty situation by non-trauma experienced physicians: Grenada 1983. *J Emerg Med* 1989;7:175-180.

31. Williams MJ, Lockey AS, Culshaw MC. Improved trauma management with Advanced Trauma Life Support (ATLS) training. *J Accident Emerg Med* 1997;14:81-83.

32. World Health Organization. *The Injury Chart Book: a Graphical Overview of the Global Burden of Injuries.* Geneva: World Health Organization Department of Injuries and Violence Prevention. Noncommunicable Diseases and Mental Health Cluster; 2002.

33. World Health Organization. *Violence and Injury Prevention and Disability (VIP).* http://www.who.int/violence_injury_prevention/publications/other_injury/chartb/en/index.html. Accessed January 9, 2008.

34. World Health Organization. *World Report on Road Traffic Injury Prevention.* Geneva: World Health Organization.

35. World Health Organization (WHO). *Injuries and violence: the facts.* Geneva, Switzerland: WHO; 2010.

36. World Health Organization (WHO). *The global burden of disease: 2004 update.* Geneva, Switzerland: WHO; 2008.

Contents

ADVANCED TRAUMA LIFE SUPPORT®

ATLS®

STUDENT COURSE MANUAL

1 Initial Assessment and Management

The primary survey should be repeated frequently to identify any deterioration in the patient's status that indicates the need for additional intervention.

Scenario A 44-year-old male driver crashed head-on into a wall. The patient was found unresponsive at the scene. He arrives at the hospital via basic life support with a cervical collar in place and strapped to a backboard; technicians are assisting ventilations with a bag-mask.

Outline

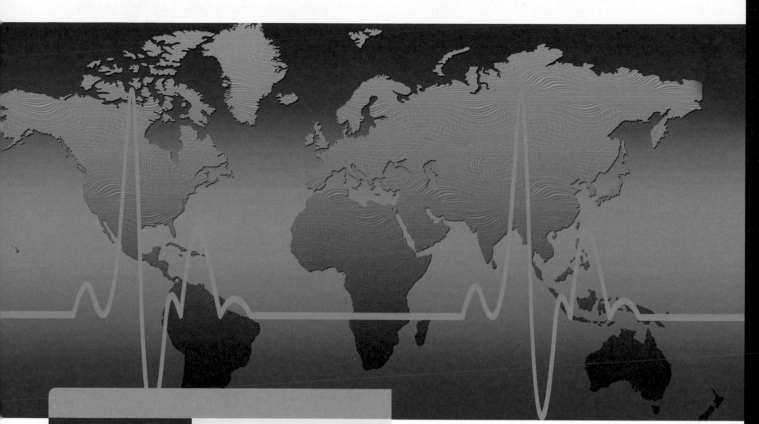

Objectives

1. Assemble a team and prepare to resuscitate an injured patient.

2. Identify the correct sequence of priorities for assessment of a severely injured patient.

3. Apply the principles outlined in the primary and secondary surveys to the assessment of a multiply injured patient.

4. Apply guidelines and techniques to the initial resuscitative and definitive-care phases of the treatment of a multiply injured patient.

5. Explain how a patient's medical history and the mechanism of injury contribute to the identification of injuries.

6. Identify the pitfalls associated with the initial assessment and management of an injured patient and describe steps to minimize their impact.

7. Conduct an initial assessment survey on a simulated multiply injured patient, using the correct sequence of priorities and explaining management techniques for primary treatment and stabilization.

8. Reevaluate a patient who is not responding appropriately to resuscitation and management.

9. Explain the importance of teamwork in the initial assessment of a trauma patient.

10. Recognize patients who will require transfer for definitive management.

The treatment of seriously injured patients requires the rapid assessment of injuries and institution of life-preserving therapy. Because timing is crucial, a systematic approach that can be rapidly and accurately applied is essential. This approach is termed the "initial assessment" and includes the following elements:

- Preparation
- Triage
- Primary survey (ABCDEs)
- Resuscitation
- Adjuncts to primary survey and resuscitation
- Consideration of the need for patient transfer
- Secondary survey (head-to-toe evaluation and patient history)
- Adjuncts to the secondary survey
- Continued postresuscitation monitoring and reevaluation
- Definitive care

The primary and secondary surveys should be repeated frequently to identify any change in the patient's status that indicates the need for additional intervention. The

assessment sequence presented in this chapter reflects a linear, or longitudinal, progression of events. In an actual clinical situation, many of these activities occur in parallel, or simultaneously. The longitudinal progression of the assessment process allows clinicians an opportunity to mentally review the progress of an actual trauma resuscitation.

ATLS® principles guide the assessment and resuscitation of injured patients. Judgment is required to determine which procedures are necessary, because not all patients require all of these procedures.

Preparation

? *How do I prepare for a smooth transition from the prehospital to the hospital environment?*

Preparation for a trauma patient occurs in two different clinical settings. First, during the prehospital phase, all events must be coordinated with the clinicians at the receiving hospital. Second, during the hospital phase, preparations must be made to rapidly facilitate the trauma patient's resuscitation.

PREHOSPITAL PHASE

Coordination with prehospital agencies and personnel can greatly expedite treatment in the field (■ FIGURE 1-1). The prehospital system should be set up to notify the receiving hospital before personnel transport the patient from the scene. This allows for mobilization of the hospital's trauma team members so that all necessary personnel and resources are present in the emergency department (ED) at the time of the patient's arrival.

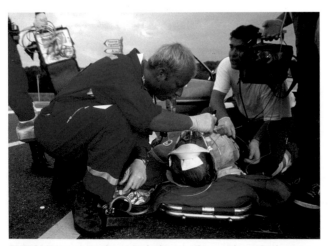

■ **FIGURE 1-1 Prehospital Phase.** The prehospital system should be set up to notify the receiving hospital before personnel transport the patient from the scene.

During the prehospital phase, emphasis should be placed on airway maintenance, control of external bleeding and shock, immobilization of the patient, and immediate transport to the closest appropriate facility, preferably a verified trauma center. Every effort should be made to minimize scene time, a concept that is supported by the Field Triage Decision Scheme, shown in ■ FIGURE 1-2.

Emphasis also should be placed on obtaining and reporting information needed for triage at the hospital, including time of injury, events related to the injury, and patient history. The mechanisms of injury can suggest the degree of injury as well as specific injuries for which the patient must be evaluated.

The National Association of Emergency Medical Technicians' Prehospital Trauma Life Support Committee, in cooperation with the Committee on Trauma (COT) of the American College of Surgeons (ACS), has developed a course with a format similar to the ATLS Course that addresses the prehospital care of injured patients, which is called Prehospital Trauma Life Support (PHTLS).

The use of prehospital care protocols and the ability to access online medical direction (direct medical control) can facilitate and improve care initiated in the field. Periodic multidisciplinary review of the care provided through quality improvement activities is essential.

HOSPITAL PHASE

Advance planning for the trauma patient's arrival is essential. A resuscitation area should be available for trauma patients. Properly functioning airway equipment (e.g., laryngoscopes and tubes) should be organized, tested, and strategically placed where it is immediately accessible. Warmed intravenous crystalloid solutions should be immediately available for infusion, as should appropriate monitoring devices. A protocol to summon additional medical assistance should be in place, as well as a means to ensure prompt responses by laboratory and radiology personnel. Transfer agreements with verified trauma centers should be established and operational. See American College of Surgeons Committee on Trauma (ACS COT), Resources for Optimal Care of the Injured Patient, 2006) (electronic version only). Periodic review of patient care through the quality improvement process is an essential component of each hospital's trauma program.

All personnel who are likely to have contact with the patient must wear standard precaution devices. Due to concerns about communicable diseases, particularly hepatitis and acquired immunodeficiency syndrome (AIDS), the Centers for Disease Control and Prevention (CDC) and other health agencies strongly recommend the use of standard precautions (e.g., face

■ FIGURE 1-2 Field Triage Decision Scheme

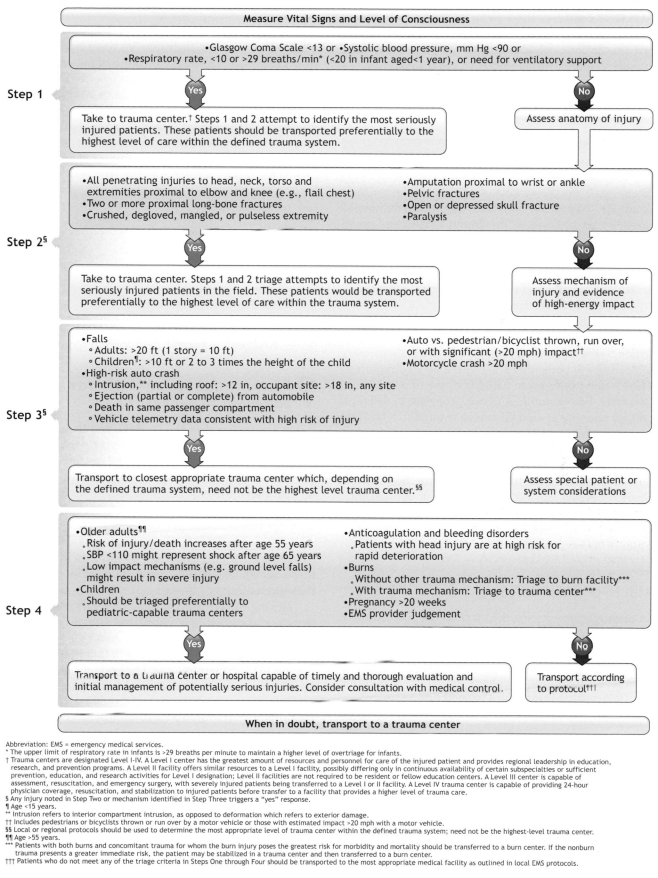

Abbreviation: EMS = emergency medical services.
* The upper limit of respiratory rate in infants is >29 breaths per minute to maintain a higher level of overtriage for infants.
† Trauma centers are designated Level I-IV. A Level I center has the greatest amount of resources and personnel for care of the injured patient and provides regional leadership in education,
  research, and prevention programs. A Level II facility offers similar resources to a Level I facility, possibly differing only in continuous availability of certain subspecialties or sufficient
  prevention, education, and research activities for Level I designation; Level II facilities are not required to be resident or fellow education centers. A Level III center is capable of
  assessment, resuscitation, and emergency surgery, with severely injured patients being transferred to a Level I or II facility. A Level IV trauma center is capable of providing 24-hour
  physician coverage, resuscitation, and stabilization to injured patients before transfer to a facility that provides a higher level of trauma care.
§ Any injury noted in Step Two or mechanism identified in Step Three triggers a "yes" response.
¶ Age <15 years.
** Intrusion refers to interior compartment intrusion, as opposed to deformation which refers to exterior damage.
†† Includes pedestrians or bicyclists thrown or run over by a motor vehicle or those with estimated impact >20 mph with a motor vehicle.
§§ Local or regional protocols should be used to determine the most appropriate level of trauma center within the defined trauma system; need not be the highest-level trauma center.
¶¶ Age >55 years.
*** Patients with both burns and concomitant trauma for whom the burn injury poses the greatest risk for morbidity and mortality should be transferred to a burn center. If the nonburn
    trauma presents a greater immediate risk, the patient may be stabilized in a trauma center and then transferred to a burn center.
††† Patients who do not meet any of the triage criteria in Steps One through Four should be transported to the most appropriate medical facility as outlined in local EMS protocols.

mask, eye protection, water-impervious gown, and gloves) when coming into contact with body fluids. The ACS COT considers these to be minimum precautions and protection for all healthcare providers. Standard precautions are also an Occupational Safety and Health Administration (OSHA) requirement in the United States.

Triage

Triage involves the sorting of patients based on their needs for treatment and the resources available to provide that treatment. Treatment is rendered based on the ABC priorities (Airway with cervical spine protection, Breathing, and Circulation with hemorrhage control). Other factors that may affect triage and treatment priority include injury severity, salvageability, and available resources.

Triage also includes the sorting of patients in the field so that a decision can be made regarding the appropriate receiving medical facility. It is the responsibility of prehospital personnel and their medical directors to ensure that appropriate patients arrive at appropriate hospitals. For example, it is inappropriate to deliver a patient who has sustained severe trauma to a hospital other than a trauma center when such a center is available (see ■ FIGURE 1-2). Prehospital trauma scoring may be helpful in identifying severely injured patients who should be transported to a trauma center. See Trauma Scores: Revised and Pediatric (electronic version only) and Appendix D: Triage Scenarios in this textbook.

Triage situations are categorized as multiple casualties or mass casualties.

MULTIPLE CASUALTIES

In multiple-casualty incidents, although there is more than one patient, the number of patients and the severity of their injuries do not exceed the capability of the facility to render care. In such situations, patients with life-threatening problems and those sustaining multiple-system injuries are treated first.

MASS CASUALTIES

In mass-casualty events, the number of patients and the severity of their injuries exceed the capability of the facility and staff. In such situations, the patients having the greatest chance of survival and requiring the least expenditure of time, equipment, supplies, and personnel, are treated first. (See Appendix C: Disaster Management and Emergency Preparedness.)

Primary Survey

Patients are assessed, and their treatment priorities are established, based on their injuries, vital signs, and the injury mechanisms. In severely injured patients, logical and sequential treatment priorities must be established based on overall patient assessment (■ FIGURE 1-3). The patient's vital functions must be assessed quickly and efficiently. Management consists of a rapid primary survey, resuscitation of vital functions, a more detailed secondary survey, and, finally, the initiation of definitive care. This process constitutes the ABCDEs of trauma care and identifies life-threatening conditions by adhering to the following sequence:

Airway maintenance with cervical spine protection

Breathing and ventilation

Circulation with hemorrhage control

Disability: Neurologic status

Exposure/**E**nvironmental control: Completely undress the patient, but prevent hypothermia

? *What is a quick, simple way to assess a patient in 10 seconds?*

A quick assessment of the A, B, C, and D in a trauma patient can be conducted by identifying oneself, asking the patient for his or her name, and asking what happened. An appropriate response suggests that there is no major airway compromise (ability to speak clearly), breathing is not severely compromised (ability to generate air movement to permit speech), and there is no major decrease in level of consciousness (alert enough to describe what happened). Failure to respond to these questions suggests abnormalities in A, B, or C that warrant urgent assessment and management.

During the primary survey, life-threatening conditions are identified in a prioritized sequence based on the effects of the injuries on the patient's physiology because it is frequently not possible to initially identify the specific anatomic injuries. For example, airway compromise can occur secondary to head trauma, injuries causing shock, or direct physical trauma to the airway. Regardless of the injury causing airway compromise, the first priority is airway management, including clearing the airway, suctioning, administering oxygen, and securing the airway. The prioritized sequence is based on the degree of life threat so that the abnormality that poses the greatest threat to life is addressed first.

The prioritized assessment and management procedures described in this chapter are presented as sequential steps in order of importance and for the purpose of clarity. However, these steps are frequently

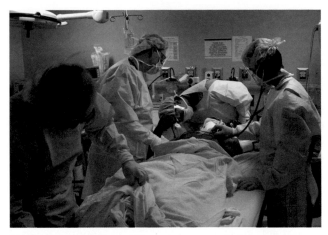

■ **FIGURE 1-3 Primary Survey.** In severely injured patients, logical and sequential treatment priorities must be established based on overall patient assessment.

accomplished simultaneously by a team of health professionals. To perform effectively, the members of such a team must constantly communicate with each other under a team leader (see Teamwork, below).

SPECIAL POPULATIONS

Patient populations that warrant special consideration are children, pregnant females, older adults, athletes, and obese patients.

Priorities for the care of pediatric patients are the same as those for adults. Although the anatomic and physiologic differences from the adult; the quantities of blood, fluids, and medications; size of the child; degree and rapidity of heat loss; and injury patterns may differ, the assessment and management priorities are identical. Specific issues related to pediatric trauma patients are addressed in Chapter 10: Pediatric Trauma.

Priorities for the care of pregnant females are similar to those for nonpregnant females, but the anatomic and physiologic changes of pregnancy can modify the patient's response to injury. Early recognition of pregnancy by palpation of the abdomen for a gravid uterus and laboratory testing (e.g., human chorionic gonadotropin, or hCG) and early fetal assessment are important for maternal and fetal survival. Specific issues related to pregnant patients are addressed in Chapter 12: Trauma in Pregnancy and Intimate Partner Violence.

Trauma is a common cause of death in the elderly, although cardiovascular disease and cancer overtake the incidence of injury as the leading causes of death in this population. Resuscitation of older adults warrants special attention. The aging process diminishes the physiologic reserve of elderly trauma patients, and chronic cardiac, respiratory, and metabolic diseases can impair their ability to respond to injury in the same manner as younger patients. Comorbidities such as diabetes, congestive heart failure, coronary artery disease, restrictive and obstructive pulmonary disease, coagulopathy, liver disease, and peripheral vascular disease are more common in older patients and may adversely affect outcomes following injury. In addition, the long-term use of medications can alter the usual physiologic response to injury and frequently leads to over-resuscitation or under-resuscitation in this patient population. Despite these facts, most elderly trauma patients recover if appropriately treated. Prompt, aggressive resuscitation and the early recognition of preexisting medical conditions and medication use can improve survival in this patient group. Early use of invasive monitoring may be a valuable adjunct to management. See Chapter 11: Geriatric Trauma.

Obese patients pose a particular challenge in the trauma setting, as their anatomy can make procedures such as intubation difficult and hazardous. Diagnostic tests, such as ultrasound, diagnostic peritoneal lavage (DPL), and computed tomography (CT) are also more difficult. In addition, obese patients typically have cardiopulmonary disease, which limits their ability to compensate for injury and stress. Rapid fluid resuscitation may exacerbate their underlying comorbidities.

Because of their excellent conditioning, athletes may not manifest early signs of shock, such as tachycardia and tachypnea. They may also have normally low systolic and diastolic blood pressure.

AIRWAY MAINTENANCE WITH CERVICAL SPINE PROTECTION

Upon initial evaluation of a trauma patient, the airway should be assessed first to ascertain patency. This rapid assessment for signs of airway obstruction should include suctioning and inspection for foreign bodies and facial, mandibular, or tracheal/laryngeal fractures that can result in airway obstruction. Measures to establish a patent airway should be instituted while protecting the cervical spine. Initially, the chin-lift or jaw-thrust maneuver is recommended to achieve airway patency.

If the patient is able to communicate verbally, the airway is not likely to be in immediate jeopardy; however, repeated assessment of airway patency is prudent. In addition, patients with severe head injuries who have an altered level of consciousness or a Glasgow Coma Scale (GCS) score of 8 or less usually require the placement of a definitive airway (i.e., cuffed, secured tube in the trachea). The finding of nonpurposeful motor responses strongly suggests the need for definitive airway management. Management of the airway in pediatric patients requires knowledge of the unique anatomic features of the position and size of the larynx in children, as well as special equipment. See Chapter 10: Pediatric Trauma.

While assessing and managing a patient's airway, great care should be taken to prevent excessive movement of the cervical spine. The patient's head and neck should not be hyperextended, hyperflexed, or rotated to establish and maintain the airway. Based on the history of a traumatic incident, loss of stability of the cervical spine should be assumed. Neurologic examination alone does not exclude a diagnosis of cervical spine injury. Initially, protection of the patient's spinal cord with appropriate immobilization devices should be accomplished and maintained. Evaluation and diagnosis of specific spinal injury, including imaging, should be done later. If immobilization devices must be removed temporarily, one member of the trauma team should manually stabilize the patient's head and neck using inline immobilization techniques (■ FIGURE 1-4).

Cervical spine radiographs may be obtained to confirm or exclude injury once immediate or potentially life-threatening conditions have been addressed, although it is important to remember that a lateral film identifies only 85% of all injuries. **Assume a cervical spine injury in patients with blunt multisystem trauma, especially those with an altered level of consciousness or a blunt injury above the clavicle.** See Chapter 7: Spine and Spinal Cord Trauma.

Every effort should be made to recognize airway compromise promptly and secure a definitive airway. Equally important is the necessity to recognize the potential for progressive airway loss. Frequent reevaluation of airway patency is essential to identify and treat patients who are losing the ability to maintain an adequate airway.

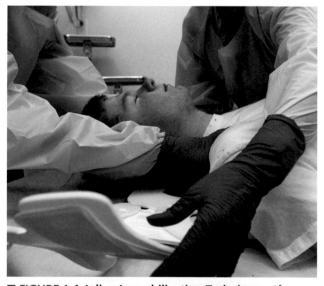

■ FIGURE 1-4 Inline Immobilization Techniques. If immobilization devices must be removed temporarily, one member of the trauma team should manually stabilize the patient's head and neck using inline immobilization techniques.

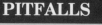

PITFALLS

- Despite the efforts of even the most prudent and attentive clinician, there are circumstances in which airway management is exceptionally difficult and occasionally even impossible to achieve. Equipment failure often cannot be anticipated, for example, the light on the laryngoscope burns out or the cuff on the endotracheal tube that was placed with exceptional difficulty leaks because it was torn on the patient's teeth during intubation.

- These include patients in whom intubation cannot be performed after neuromuscular blockade and patients in whom a surgical airway cannot be established expediently because of their obesity.

- Endotracheal intubation of a patient with an unknown laryngeal fracture or incomplete upper airway transection can precipitate total airway occlusion or complete airway transection. This can occur in the absence of clinical findings that suggest the potential for an airway problem, or when the urgency of the situation dictates the immediate need for a secure airway or ventilation.

These pitfalls cannot always be prevented. However, they should be anticipated, and preparations should be made to minimize their impact.

BREATHING AND VENTILATION

Airway patency alone does not ensure adequate ventilation. Adequate gas exchange is required to maximize oxygenation and carbon dioxide elimination. Ventilation requires adequate function of the lungs, chest wall, and diaphragm. Each component must be rapidly examined and evaluated.

The patient's neck and chest should be exposed to adequately assess jugular venous distention, position of the trachea, and chest wall excursion. Auscultation should be performed to ensure gas flow in the lungs. Visual inspection and palpation can detect injuries to the chest wall that may compromise ventilation. Percussion of the thorax can also identify abnormalities, but during a noisy resuscitation this may be difficult or produce unreliable results.

Injuries that severely impair ventilation in the short term include tension pneumothorax, flail chest with pulmonary contusion, massive hemothorax, and open pneumothorax. These injuries should be identified during the primary survey and may require immediate attention for ventilatory efforts to be effective. Simple pneumothorax or hemothorax, fractured ribs, and pulmonary contusion can compromise ventilation to a lesser degree and are usually identified during the secondary survey.

PITFALLS

Differentiating between ventilation problems and airway compromise can be difficult:

- Patients who have profound dyspnea and tachypnea appear as though their primary problem is related to an inadequate airway. However, if the ventilation problem is caused by a pneumothorax or tension pneumothorax, intubation with vigorous bag-mask ventilation can rapidly lead to further deterioration of the patient.

- When intubation and ventilation are necessary in an unconscious patient, the procedure itself can unmask or aggravate a pneumothorax, and the patient's chest must be reevaluated. Chest x-rays should be obtained as soon after intubation and initiation of ventilation as is practical.

CIRCULATION WITH HEMORRHAGE CONTROL

Circulatory compromise in trauma patients can result from many different injuries. Blood volume, cardiac output, and bleeding are major circulatory issues to consider.

Blood Volume and Cardiac Output

Hemorrhage is the predominant cause of preventable deaths after injury. Identifying and stopping hemorrhage are therefore crucial steps in the assessment and management of such patients. Once tension pneumothorax has been eliminated as a cause of shock, hypotension following injury must be considered to be hypovolemic in origin until proven otherwise. Rapid and accurate assessment of an injured patient's hemodynamic status is essential. The elements of clinical observation that yield important information within seconds are level of consciousness, skin color, and pulse.

Level of Consciousness   When circulating blood volume is reduced, cerebral perfusion may be critically impaired, resulting in altered levels of consciousness. However, a conscious patient also may have lost a significant amount of blood.

Skin Color   Skin color can be a helpful sign in evaluating injured hypovolemic patients. A patient with pink skin, especially in the face and extremities, rarely has critical hypovolemia after injury. Conversely, the patient with hypovolemia may have ashen, gray facial skin and pale extremities.

Pulse   The pulse, typically an easily accessible central pulse (e.g., femoral or carotid artery), should be as-

sessed bilaterally for quality, rate, and regularity. Full, slow, and regular peripheral pulses are usually signs of relative normovolemia in a patient who is not taking ß-adrenergic blocking medications. A rapid, thready pulse is typically a sign of hypovolemia, but the condition may have other causes. A normal pulse rate does not necessarily indicate normovolemia, but an irregular pulse does warn of potential cardiac dysfunction. Absent central pulses that are not attributable to local factors signify the need for immediate resuscitative action to restore depleted blood volume and effective cardiac output.

Bleeding

The source of bleeding should be identified as either external or internal. External hemorrhage is identified and controlled during the primary survey. Rapid, external blood loss is managed by direct manual pressure on the wound. Tourniquets are effective in massive exsanguination from an extremity, but carry a risk of ischemic injury to that extremity and should only be used when direct pressure is not effective. The use of hemostats can result in damage to nerves and veins.

The major areas of internal hemorrhage are the chest, abdomen, retroperitoneum, pelvis, and long bones. The source of the bleeding is usually identified by physical examination and imaging (e.g., chest x-ray, pelvic x-ray, or focused assessment sonography in trauma [FAST]). Management may include chest decompression, pelvic binders, splint application, and surgical intervention.

PITFALLS

Trauma respects no patient population barrier. The elderly, children, athletes, and individuals with chronic medical conditions do not respond to volume loss in a similar or even in a "normal" manner.

- Elderly patients have a limited ability to increase their heart rate in response to blood loss, which obscures one of the earliest signs of volume depletion—tachycardia. Blood pressure has little correlation with cardiac output in older patients. Anticoagulation therapy for medical conditions such as atrial fibrillation, coronary artery disease, and transient ischemic attacks can increase blood loss.

- Children usually have abundant physiologic reserve and often have few signs of hypovolemia, even after severe volume depletion. When deterioration does occur, it is precipitous and catastrophic.

- Well-trained athletes have similar compensatory mechanisms, may have bradycardia, and may not have the usual level of tachycardia with blood loss.

(continued)

■ Often, the AMPLE history, described later in this chapter, is not available, so the healthcare team is not aware of the patient's use of medications for chronic conditions.

Anticipation and an attitude of skepticism regarding the patient's "normal" hemodynamic status are appropriate.

DISABILITY (NEUROLOGIC EVALUATION)

A rapid neurologic evaluation is performed at the end of the primary survey. This neurologic evaluation establishes the patient's level of consciousness, pupillary size and reaction, lateralizing signs, and spinal cord injury level.

The GCS is a quick, simple method for determining the level of consciousness that is predictive of patient outcome, particularly the best motor response. See Chapter 6: Head Trauma in this text and Trauma Scores: Revised and Pediatric (electronic version only).

A decrease in the level of consciousness may indicate decreased cerebral oxygenation and/or perfusion, or it may be caused by direct cerebral injury. An altered level of consciousness indicates the need for immediate reevaluation of the patient's oxygenation, ventilation, and perfusion status. Hypoglycemia and alcohol, narcotics, and other drugs also can alter the patient's level of consciousness. However, if these factors are excluded, changes in the level of consciousness should be considered to be of traumatic central nervous system origin until proven otherwise.

Primary brain injury results from the structural effect of the injury to the brain. Prevention of secondary brain injury by maintaining adequate oxygenation and perfusion are the main goals of initial management.

EXPOSURE AND ENVIRONMENTAL CONTROL

The patient should be completely undressed, usually by cutting off his or her garments to facilitate a thorough examination and assessment. After the patient's clothing has been removed and the assessment is completed, the patient should be covered with warm blankets or an external warming device to prevent hypothermia in the trauma receiving area. Intravenous fluids should be warmed before being infused, and a warm environment (i.e., room temperature) should be maintained. **The patient's body temperature is more important than the comfort of the healthcare providers.**

PITFALLS

Despite proper attention to all aspects of treating a patient with a closed head injury, neurologic deterioration can occur—often rapidly. The lucid interval classically associated with acute epidural hematoma is an example of a situation in which the patient will "talk and die." Frequent neurologic reevaluation can minimize this problem by allowing for early detection of changes. It may be necessary to return to the primary survey and to confirm that the patient has a secure airway, adequate ventilation and oxygenation, and adequate cerebral perfusion. Early consultation with a neurosurgeon also is necessary to guide additional management efforts.

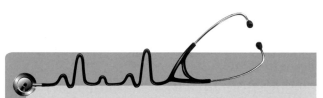

Scenario ■ *continued*   Consider our patient, who was reported unresponsive and required assisted ventilations after a head-on crash. What abnormalities in the primary survey do you suspect? How can you best assess this patient quickly?

Resuscitation

Resuscitation and the management of life-threatening injuries as they are identified are essential to maximize patient survival. Resuscitation also follows the ABC sequence and occurs simultaneously with evaluation.

AIRWAY

The airway should be protected in all patients and secured when there is a potential for airway compromise. The jaw-thrust or chin-lift maneuver may suffice as an initial intervention. If the patient is unconscious and has no gag reflex, the establishment of an oropharyngeal airway can be helpful temporarily. **A definitive airway (i.e., intubation) should be established if there is any doubt about the patient's ability to maintain airway integrity.**

Definitive control of the airway in patients who have compromised airways due to mechanical factors, have ventilatory problems, or are unconscious is achieved by endotracheal intubation. This procedure should be performed with continuous protection of the cervical spine. An airway should be established surgically if intubation is contraindicated or cannot be accomplished.

BREATHING, VENTILATION, AND OXYGENATION

A tension pneumothorax compromises ventilation and circulation dramatically and acutely; if one is suspected, chest decompression should follow immediately. Every injured patient should receive supplemental oxygen. If not intubated, the patient should have oxygen delivered by a mask-reservoir device to achieve optimal oxygenation. The pulse oximeter should be used to monitor adequacy of oxygen hemoglobin saturation. See Chapter 2: Airway and Ventilatory Management.

CIRCULATION AND HEMORRHAGE CONTROL

Definitive bleeding control is essential along with appropriate replacement of intravascular volume. A minimum of two large-caliber intravenous (IV) catheters should be introduced. The maximum rate of fluid administration is determined by the internal diameter of the catheter and inversely by its length—not by the size of the vein in which the catheter is placed. Establishment of upper-extremity peripheral IV access is preferred. Other peripheral lines, cutdowns, and central venous lines should be used as necessary in accordance with the skill level of the clinician who is caring for the patient. See Skill Station IV: Shock Assessment and Management, and Skill Station V: Venous Cutdown, in Chapter 3: Shock. At the time of IV insertion, blood should be drawn for type and crossmatch and baseline hematologic studies, including a pregnancy test for all females of childbearing age. Blood gases and/or lactate level should be obtained to assess the presence and degree of shock.

Aggressive and continued volume resuscitation is not a substitute for definitive control of hemorrhage. Definitive control includes surgery, angioembolization, and pelvic stabilization. IV fluid therapy with crystalloids should be initiated. A bolus of 1 to 2 L of an isotonic solution may be required to achieve an appropriate response in the adult patient. All IV solutions should be warmed either by storage in a warm environment (i.e., 37°C to 40°C, or 98.6°F to 104°F) or fluid-warming devices. Shock associated with injury is most often hypovolemic in origin. If the patient is unresponsive to initial crystalloid therapy, blood transfusion should be given.

Hypothermia may be present when the patient arrives, or it may develop quickly in the ED if the patient is uncovered and undergoes rapid administration of room-temperature fluids or refrigerated blood. Hypothermia is a potentially lethal complication in injured patients, and aggressive measures should be taken to prevent the loss of body heat and restore body temperature to normal. The temperature of the resuscitation area should be increased to minimize the loss of body heat. The use of a high-flow fluid warmer or microwave oven to heat crystalloid fluids to 39°C (102.2°F) is recommended. However blood products should not be warmed in a microwave oven. See Chapter 3: Shock.

Adjuncts to Primary Survey and Resuscitation

Adjuncts that are used during the primary survey include electrocardiographic monitoring; urinary and gastric catheters; other monitoring, such as ventilatory rate, arterial blood gas (ABG) levels, pulse oximetry, blood pressure, and x-ray examinations (e.g., chest and pelvis) (■ FIGURE 1-5).

ELECTROCARDIOGRAPHIC MONITORING

Electrocardiographic (ECG) monitoring of all trauma patients is important. Dysrhythmias—including unexplained tachycardia, atrial fibrillation, premature ventricular contractions, and ST segment changes—can indicate blunt cardiac injury. Pulseless electrical activity (PEA) can indicate cardiac tamponade, tension pneumothorax, and/or profound hypovolemia. When bradycardia, aberrant conduction, and premature beats are present, hypoxia and hypo-perfusion should be suspected immediately. Extreme hypothermia also produces these dysrhythmias. See Chapter 3: Shock.

URINARY AND GASTRIC CATHETERS

The placement of urinary and gastric catheters occurs during the resuscitation phase. A urine specimen should be submitted for routine laboratory analysis.

Urinary Catheters

Urinary output is a sensitive indicator of the patient's volume status and reflects renal perfusion. Monitoring of urinary output is best accomplished by the insertion of

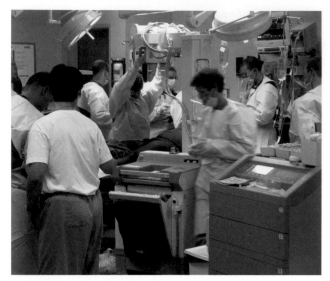

■ **FIGURE 1-5** Radiographic studies are important adjuncts to the primary survey.

an indwelling bladder catheter. Transurethral bladder catheterization is contraindicated in patients in whom urethral injury is suspected. Urethral injury should be suspected in the presence of one of the following:

- Blood at the urethral meatus

- Perineal ecchymosis

- High-riding or nonpalpable prostate

Accordingly, a urinary catheter should not be inserted before the rectum and genitalia have been examined, if urethral injury is suspected. Urethral integrity should be confirmed by a retrograde urethrogram before the catheter is inserted.

PITFALLS

Sometimes anatomic abnormalities (e.g., urethral stricture or prostatic hypertrophy) preclude placement of an indwelling bladder catheter, despite meticulous technique. Nonspecialists should avoid excessive manipulation of the urethra or use of specialized instrumentation. Consult a urologist early.

Gastric Catheters

A gastric tube is indicated to reduce stomach distention, decrease the risk of aspiration, and assess for upper gastrointestinal hemorrhage from trauma. Decompression of the stomach reduces the risk of aspiration, but does not prevent it entirely. Thick or semisolid gastric contents will not return through the tube, and actual passage of the tube can induce vomiting. For the tube to be effective, it must be positioned

properly, be attached to appropriate suction, and be functional. Blood in the gastric aspirate can be indicative of oropharyngeal (swallowed) blood, traumatic insertion, or actual injury to the upper digestive tract. If the cribriform plate is known to be fractured or a fracture is suspected, the gastric tube should be inserted orally to prevent intracranial passage. In this situation, any nasopharyngeal instrumentation is potentially dangerous.

OTHER MONITORING

Adequate resuscitation is best assessed by improvement in physiologic parameters, such as pulse rate, blood pressure, pulse pressure, ventilatory rate, ABG levels, body temperature, and urinary output, rather than the qualitative assessment done during the primary survey. Actual values for these parameters should be obtained as soon as is practical after completing the primary survey, and periodic reevaluation is important.

Ventilatory Rate and Arterial Blood Gases

Ventilatory rate and ABG levels should be used to monitor the adequacy of respirations. Endotracheal tubes can be dislodged whenever the patient is moved. A colorimetric carbon dioxide detector is a device capable of detecting carbon dioxide in exhaled gas. Colorimetry, or capnography, is useful in confirming that the endotracheal tube is properly located in the respiratory tract of the patient on mechanical ventilation and not in the esophagus. However, it does not confirm proper placement of the tube in the trachea. See Chapter 2: Airway and Ventilatory Management.

Pulse Oximetry

Pulse oximetry is a valuable adjunct for monitoring oxygenation in injured patients. The pulse oximeter measures the oxygen saturation of hemoglobin colorimetrically, but it does not measure the partial pressure of oxygen. It also does not measure the partial pressure of carbon dioxide, which reflects the adequacy of ventilation. A small sensor is placed on the finger, toe, earlobe, or another convenient place. Most devices display pulse rate and oxygen saturation continuously.

Hemoglobin saturation from the pulse oximeter should be compared with the value obtained from the ABG analysis. Inconsistency indicates that at least one of the two determinations is in error.

Blood Pressure

The patient's blood pressure should be measured, although it may be a poor measure and late indicator of actual tissue perfusion.

PITFALLS

- Placement of a gastric catheter can induce vomiting or gagging and produce the specific problem that its placement is intended to prevent—aspiration. Functional suction equipment should be immediately available.

- Combative trauma patients can occasionally extubate themselves. They can also occlude their endotracheal tube or deflate the cuff by biting it. Frequent reevaluation of the airway is necessary.

- The pulse oximeter sensor should not be placed distal to the blood pressure cuff. Misleading information regarding hemoglobin saturation and pulse can be generated when the cuff is inflated and occludes blood flow.

- Normalization of hemodynamics in injured patients requires more than simply a normal blood pressure; a return to normal peripheral perfusion must be established. This can be problematic in the elderly, and consideration should be given to early invasive monitoring of cardiac function in these patients.

X-RAY EXAMINATIONS AND DIAGNOSTIC STUDIES

X-ray examination should be used judiciously and should not delay patient resuscitation. Anteroposterior (AP) chest and AP pelvic films often provide information that can guide resuscitation efforts of patients with blunt trauma. Chest x-rays can show potentially life-threatening injuries that require treatment, and pelvic films can show fractures of the pelvis that indicate the need for early blood transfusion. These films can be taken in the resuscitation area with a portable x-ray unit, but should not interrupt the resuscitation process.

Essential diagnostic x-rays should be obtained, even in pregnant patients.

PITFALLS

Technical problems may be encountered when performing any diagnostic procedure, including those necessary to identify intraabdominal hemorrhage. Obesity and intraluminal bowel gas can compromise the images obtained by abdominal ultrasonography. Obesity, previous abdominal operations, and pregnancy also can make DPL difficult. Even in the hands of an experienced surgeon, the effluent volume from the lavage may be minimal or zero. In these circumstances, an alternative diagnostic tool should be chosen. A surgeon should be involved in the evaluation process and guide further diagnostic and therapeutic procedures.

FAST and DPL are useful tools for the quick detection of occult intraabdominal blood. Their use depends on the skill and experience of the clinician. Identification of the source of occult intraabdominal blood loss may indicate the need for operative control of hemorrhage.

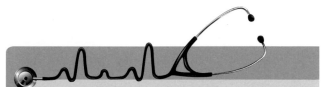

Scenario ▪ *continued* Having completed the primary survey, the patient now has a definitive airway and chest tube in place. Stop to consider whether the abnormalities you have identified indicate the need for transfer to definitive care before proceeding with adjuncts and the secondary survey.

Consider Need for Patient Transfer

During the primary survey and resuscitation phase, the evaluating physician frequently obtains enough information to indicate the need to transfer the patient to another facility. This transfer process may be initiated immediately by administrative personnel at the direction of the examining doctor while additional evaluation and resuscitative measures are being performed. Once the decision to transfer the patient has been made, communication between the referring and receiving doctors is essential. ▪ **FIGURE 1-6** shows a patient monitored during critical care transport by ground ambulance.

Secondary Survey

❓ *What is the secondary survey, and when does it start?*

The secondary survey does not begin until the primary survey (ABCDEs) is completed, resuscitative efforts are underway, and the normalization of vital functions has been demonstrated. When additional personnel are available, part of the secondary survey may be conducted while the other personnel attend to the primary survey. In this setting the conduction of the secondary survey should not interfere with the primary survey, which takes first priority.

The secondary survey is a head-to-toe evaluation of the trauma patient, that is, a complete history

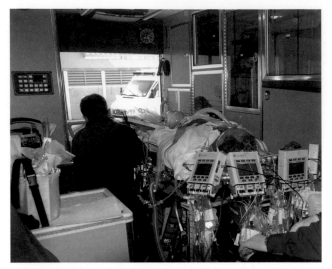

■ **FIGURE 1-6** Careful patient monitoring during critical care transport is essential to prevent and/or manage complications and any deterioration in patient status.

and physical examination, including reassessment of all vital signs. Each region of the body is completely examined. The potential for missing an injury or failure to appreciate the significance of an injury is great, especially in an unresponsive or unstable patient. See Table I-1: Secondary Survey, in Skill Station I: Initial Assessment and Management.

During the secondary survey, a complete neurologic examination is performed, including a repeat GCS score determination. X-rays are also obtained, as indicated by the examination. Such examinations can be interspersed into the secondary survey at appropriate times. Special procedures, such as specific radiographic evaluations and laboratory studies, also are performed at this time. Complete patient evaluation requires repeated physical examinations.

History

Every complete medical assessment includes a history of the mechanism of injury. Often, such a history cannot be obtained from a patient who has sustained trauma; therefore, prehospital personnel and family must be consulted to obtain information that can enhance the understanding of the patient's physiologic state. The AMPLE history is a useful mnemonic for this purpose:

Allergies

Medications currently used

Past illnesses/**P**regnancy

Last meal

Events/**E**nvironment related to the injury

The patient's condition is greatly influenced by the mechanism of injury, and some injuries can be predicted based on the direction and amount of energy behind the mechanism of injury. Injury usually is classified into two broad categories: blunt and penetrating trauma. Prehospital personnel can provide valuable information on such mechanisms and should report pertinent data to the examining doctor. See Biomechanics of Injury (electronic version only). Other types of injuries for which historical information is important include thermal injuries and those caused by hazardous environments.

Blunt Trauma

Blunt trauma often results from automobile collisions, falls, and other injuries related to transportation, recreation, and occupations.

Important information to obtain about automobile collisions includes seat-belt use, steering wheel deformation, direction of impact, damage to the automobile in terms of major deformation or intrusion into the passenger compartment, and whether the patient was ejected from the vehicle. Ejection from the vehicle greatly increases the possibility of major injury.

Injury patterns can often be predicted by the mechanism of injury. Such injury patterns also are influenced by age groups and activities **(Table 1.1: Mechanisms of Injury and Related Suspected Injury Patterns)**.

Penetrating Trauma

The incidence of penetrating trauma (e.g., injuries from firearms, stabbings, and impalement) is increasing. Factors that determine the type and extent of injury and subsequent management include the region of the body that was injured, the organs in the path of the penetrating object, and the velocity of the missile. Therefore, in gunshot victims, the velocity, caliber, presumed path of the bullet, and distance from the weapon to the wound can provide important clues regarding the extent of injury. See Biomechanics of Injury (electronic version only).

Thermal Injury

Burns are a significant type of trauma that can occur alone or be coupled with blunt and penetrating trauma resulting from, for example, a burning automobile, explosion, falling debris, and a patient's attempt to escape a fire. Inhalation injury and carbon monoxide poisoning often complicate burn injuries. Therefore, it is important to know the circumstances of the burn injury, such as the environment in which the burn injury occurred (open or closed space), the substances consumed by the flames (e.g., plastics and chemicals),

TABLE 1.1
Mechanisms of Injury and Suspected Injury Patterns

MECHANISM OF INJURY	SUSPECTED INJURY PATTERNS
Frontal impact automobile collision • Bent steering wheel • Knee imprint, dashboard • Bull's-eye fracture, windscreen	• Cervical spine fracture • Anterior flail chest • Myocardial contusion • Pneumothorax • Traumatic aortic disruption • Fractured spleen or liver • Posterior fracture/dislocation of hip and/or knee
Side impact automobile collision	• Contralateral neck sprain • Cervical spine fracture • Lateral flail chest • Pneumothorax • Traumatic aortic disruption • Diaphragmatic rupture • Fractured spleen/liver and/or kidney, depending on side of impact • Fractured pelvis or acetabulum
Rear impact automobile collision	• Cervical spine injury • Soft tissue injury to neck
Ejection from vehicle	• Ejection from the vehicle precludes meaningful prediction of injury patterns, but places patient at greater risk from virtually all injury mechanisms
Motor vehicle impact with pedestrian	• Head injury • Traumatic aortic disruption • Abdominal visceral injuries • Fractured lower extremities/pelvis

and any possible associated injuries sustained. These factors are critical for patient management.

Acute or chronic hypothermia without adequate protection against heat loss produces either local or generalized cold injuries. Significant heat loss can occur at moderate temperatures (15°C to 20°C or 59°F to 68°F) if wet clothes, decreased activity, and/or vasodilation caused by alcohol or drugs compromise the patient's ability to conserve heat. Such historical information can be obtained from prehospital personnel. Thermal injuries are addressed in more detail in Chapter 9: Thermal Injuries.

Hazardous Environment

A history of exposure to chemicals, toxins, and radiation is important to obtain for two main reasons: first,

these agents can produce a variety of pulmonary, cardiac, and internal organ dysfunctions in injured patients. Second, these same agents may also present a hazard to healthcare providers. Frequently, the clinician's only means of preparation is to understand the general principles of management of such conditions and establish immediate contact with a Regional Poison Control Center.

PHYSICAL EXAMINATION

During the secondary survey, physical examination follows the sequence of head, maxillofacial structures, cervical spine and neck, chest, abdomen, perineum/rectum/vagina, musculoskeletal system, and neurologic system.

Head

The secondary survey begins with evaluating the head and identifying all related neurologic injuries and other significant injuries. The entire scalp and head should be examined for lacerations, contusions, and evidence of fractures. See Chapter 6: Head Trauma.

Because edema around the eyes can later preclude an in-depth examination, the eyes should be reevaluated for:

- Visual acuity
- Pupillary size
- Hemorrhage of the conjunctiva and/or fundi
- Penetrating injury
- Contact lenses (remove before edema occurs)
- Dislocation of the lens
- Ocular entrapment

A quick visual-acuity examination of both eyes can be performed by asking the patient to read printed material such as a hand held Snellen chart, or words on an IV container or dressing package. Ocular mobility should be evaluated to exclude entrapment of extraocular muscles due to orbital fractures. These procedures frequently identify ocular injuries that are not otherwise apparent. See Appendix A: Ocular Trauma.

Maxillofacial Structures

Examination of the face should include palpation of all bony structures, assessment of occlusion, intraoral examination, and assessment of soft tissues.

Maxillofacial trauma that is not associated with airway obstruction or major bleeding should be treated only after the patient is stabilized completely and

PITFALLS

- Facial edema in patients with massive facial injury or in comatose patients can preclude a complete eye examination. Such difficulties should not deter the clinician from performing the components of the ocular examination that are possible.

- Some maxillofacial fractures, such as nasal fracture, nondisplaced zygomatic fractures, and orbital rim fractures, can be difficult to identify early in the evaluation process. Therefore, frequent reassessment is crucial.

life-threatening injuries have been managed. At the discretion of appropriate specialists, definitive management may be safely delayed without compromising care. Patients with fractures of the midface may also have a fracture of the cribriform plate. For these patients, gastric intubation should be performed via the oral route. See Chapter 6: Head Trauma, and Skill Station IX: Head and Neck Trauma: Assessment and Management.

Cervical Spine and Neck

Patients with maxillofacial or head trauma should be presumed to have an unstable cervical spine injury (e.g., fracture and/or ligament injury), and the neck should be immobilized until all aspects of the cervical spine have been adequately studied and an injury has been excluded. The absence of neurologic deficit does not exclude injury to the cervical spine, and such injury should be presumed until a complete cervical spine radiographic series and CT are reviewed by a doctor experienced in detecting cervical spine fractures radiographically.

Examination of the neck includes inspection, palpation, and auscultation. Cervical spine tenderness, subcutaneous emphysema, tracheal deviation, and laryngeal fracture can be discovered on a detailed examination. The carotid arteries should be palpated and auscultated for bruits. Evidence of blunt injury over these vessels should be noted and, if present, should arouse a high index of suspicion for carotid artery injury. A common sign of potential injury is a seatbelt mark. Occlusion or dissection of the carotid artery can occur late in the injury process without antecedent signs or symptoms. Angiography or duplex ultrasonography may be required to exclude the possibility of major cervical vascular injury when the mechanism of injury suggests this possibility. Most major cervical vascular injuries are the result of penetrating injury; however, blunt force to the neck or a traction injury from a shoulder-harness restraint can result in intimal disruption, dissection, and thrombosis. See Chapter 7: Spine and Spinal Cord Trauma.

Protection of a potentially unstable cervical spine injury is imperative for patients who are wearing any type of protective helmet, and extreme care must be taken when removing the helmet. Helmet removal is described in Chapter 2: Airway and Ventilatory Management.

Penetrating injuries to the neck can potentially injure several organ systems. Wounds that extend through the platysma should not be explored manually, probed with instruments, or treated by individuals in the ED who are not trained to manage such injuries. EDs are not typically equipped to deal with the problems that may arise with these injuries; they require evaluation by a surgeon operatively or with specialized diagnostic procedures under the direct supervision of a surgeon. The finding of active arterial bleeding, an expanding hematoma, arterial bruit, or airway compromise usually requires operative evaluation. Unexplained or isolated paralysis of an upper extremity should raise the suspicion of a cervical nerve root injury and should be accurately documented.

PITFALLS

- Blunt injury to the neck can produce injuries in which the clinical signs and symptoms develop late and may not be present during the initial examination. Injury to the intima of the carotid arteries is an example.

- The identification of cervical nerve root or brachial plexus injury may not be possible in a comatose patient. Consideration of the mechanism of injury might be the clinician's only clue.

- In some patients, decubitus ulcers can develop quickly over the sacrum and other areas from immobilization on a rigid spine board and from the cervical collar. Efforts to exclude the possibility of spinal injury should be initiated as soon as is practical, and these devices should be removed. However, resuscitation and efforts to identify life-threatening or potentially life-threatening injuries should not be deferred.

Chest

Visual evaluation of the chest, both anterior and posterior, can identify conditions such as open pneumothorax and large flail segments. A complete evaluation of the chest wall requires palpation of the entire chest cage, including the clavicles, ribs, and sternum. Sternal pressure can be painful if the sternum is fractured or costochondral separations exist. Contusions and hematomas of the chest wall should alert the clinician to the possibility of occult injury.

Significant chest injury can manifest with pain, dyspnea, and hypoxia. Evaluation includes auscultation of the chest and a chest x-ray. Auscultation is conducted high on the anterior chest wall for pneumothorax and at the posterior bases for hemothorax. Although auscultatory findings can be difficult to evaluate in a noisy environment, they may be extremely helpful. Distant heart sounds and decreased pulse pressure can indicate cardiac tamponade. In addition, cardiac tamponade and tension pneumothorax are suggested by the presence of distended neck veins, although associated hypovolemia can minimize or eliminate this finding. Decreased breath sounds, hyperresonance to percussion, and shock may be the only indications of tension pneumothorax and the need for immediate chest decompression.

A chest x-ray may confirm the presence of a hemothorax or simple pneumothorax. Rib fractures may be present, but they may not be visible on the x-ray. A widened mediastinum or other radiographic signs can suggest an aortic rupture. See Chapter 4: Thoracic Trauma.

PITFALLS

- Elderly patients may not tolerate even relatively minor chest injuries. Progression to acute respiratory insufficiency must be anticipated, and support should be instituted before collapse occurs.

- Children often sustain significant injury to the intrathoracic structures without evidence of thoracic skeletal trauma, so a high index of suspicion is essential.

Abdomen

Abdominal injuries must be identified and treated aggressively. The specific diagnosis is not as important as recognizing that an injury exists that requires surgical intervention. A normal initial examination of the abdomen does not exclude a significant intraabdominal injury. Close observation and frequent reevaluation of the abdomen, preferably by the same observer, is important in managing blunt abdominal trauma, because over time, the patient's abdominal findings can change. Early involvement of a surgeon is essential.

Patients with unexplained hypotension, neurologic injury, impaired sensorium secondary to alcohol and/or other drugs, and equivocal abdominal findings should be considered candidates for peritoneal lavage, abdominal ultrasonography, or, if hemodynamic findings are normal, CT of the abdomen. Fractures of the pelvis or lower rib cage also can hinder accurate diagnostic examination of the abdomen, because palpating the abdomen can elicit pain from these areas. See Chapter 5: Abdominal and Pelvic Trauma.

PITFALLS

- Excessive manipulation of the pelvis should be avoided, because it can precipitate additional hemorrhage. The AP pelvic x-ray examination, performed as an adjunct to the primary survey and resuscitation, can provide valuable information regarding the presence of pelvic fractures, which are potentially associated with significant blood loss.

- Injury to the retroperitoneal organs may be difficult to identify, even with the use of CT. Classic examples include duodenal and pancreatic injuries.

- Knowledge of injury mechanism, identification of associated injuries, and a high index of suspicion are required.

- Female urethral injury, although uncommon, does occur in association with pelvic fractures and straddle injuries. When present, such injuries are difficult to detect.

Perineum, Rectum, and Vagina

The perineum should be examined for contusions, hematomas, lacerations, and urethral bleeding. See Chapter 5: Abdominal and Pelvic Trauma.

A rectal examination may be performed before placing a urinary catheter. If a rectal examination is required, the clinician should assess for the presence of blood within the bowel lumen, a high-riding prostate, the presence of pelvic fractures, the integrity of the rectal wall, and the quality of sphincter tone.

Vaginal examination should be performed in patients who are at risk of vaginal injury, including all women with a pelvic fracture. The clinician should assess for the presence of blood in the vaginal vault and vaginal lacerations. In addition, pregnancy tests should be performed on all females of childbearing age.

Musculoskeletal System

The extremities should be inspected for contusions and deformities. Palpation of the bones and examination for tenderness and abnormal movement aids in the identification of occult fractures.

Pelvic fractures can be suspected by the identification of ecchymosis over the iliac wings, pubis, labia, or scrotum. Pain on palpation of the pelvic ring is an important finding in alert patients. Mobility of the pelvis in response to gentle anterior-to-posterior pressure with the heels of the hands on both anterior iliac spines and the symphysis pubis can suggest pelvic ring disruption in unconscious patients. Because such manipulation can initiate unwanted bleeding, it should be done only once (if at all), and preferably by the orthopedic surgeon responsible for the patient's care. In addition, assessment of peripheral pulses can identify vascular injuries.

Significant extremity injuries can exist without fractures being evident on examination or x-rays. Ligament ruptures produce joint instability. Muscle-tendon unit injuries interfere with active motion of the affected structures. Impaired sensation and/or loss of voluntary muscle contraction strength can be caused by nerve injury or ischemia, including that due to compartment syndrome.

Thoracic and lumbar spinal fractures and/or neurologic injuries must be considered based on physical findings and mechanism of injury. Other injuries can mask the physical findings of spinal injuries, and they can remain undetected unless the clinician obtains the appropriate x-rays.

The musculoskeletal examination is not complete without an examination of the patient's back. Unless the patient's back is examined, significant injuries can be missed. See Chapter 7: Spine and Spinal Cord Trauma, and Chapter 8: Musculoskeletal Trauma.

PITFALLS

■ Blood loss from pelvic fractures that increase pelvic volume can be difficult to control, and fatal hemorrhage can result. A sense of urgency should accompany the management of these injuries.

■ Fractures involving the bones of the hands, wrists, and feet are often not diagnosed in the secondary survey performed in the ED. Sometimes, it is only after the patient has regained consciousness and/or other major injuries are resolved that pain in the area of an occult injury is noted.

■ Injuries to the soft tissues around joints are frequently diagnosed after the patient begins to recover. Therefore, frequent reevaluation is essential.

■ A high level of suspicion must be maintained to prevent the development of compartment syndrome.

Neurological System

A comprehensive neurologic examination includes not only motor and sensory evaluation of the extremities, but reevaluation of the patient's level of consciousness and pupillary size and response. The GCS score facilitates detection of early changes and trends in the neurologic status. See Trauma Scores: Revised and Pediatric (electronic version only).

Early consultation with a neurosurgeon is required for patients with head injury. Patients should be monitored frequently for deterioration in level of consciousness and changes in the neurologic examination, as these findings can reflect worsening of the intracranial injury. If a patient with a head injury deteriorates neurologically, oxygenation and perfusion of the

brain and adequacy of ventilation (i.e., the ABCDEs) must be reassessed. Intracranial surgical intervention or measures for reducing intracranial pressure may be necessary. The neurosurgeon will decide whether conditions such as epidural and subdural hematomas require evacuation, and whether depressed skull fractures need operative intervention. See Chapter 6: Head Trauma, and Chapter 7: Spine and Spinal Cord Trauma.

Any evidence of loss of sensation, paralysis, or weakness suggests major injury to the spinal column or peripheral nervous system. Neurologic deficits should be documented when identified, even when transfer to another facility or doctor for specialty care is necessary. **Protection of the spinal cord is required at all times until a spine injury is excluded. Early consultation with a neurosurgeon or orthopedic surgeon is necessary if a spinal injury is detected.**

PITFALLS

■ Any increase in intracranial pressure (ICP) can reduce cerebral perfusion pressure and lead to secondary brain injury. Most of the diagnostic and therapeutic maneuvers necessary for the evaluation and care of patients with brain injury will increase ICP. Tracheal intubation is a classic example; in patients with brain injury, it should be performed expeditiously and as smoothly as possible. Rapid neurologic deterioration of patients with brain injury can occur despite the application of all measures to control ICP and maintain appropriate support of the central nervous system.

■ Immobilization of the entire patient, using a long spine board, semirigid cervical collar, and/or other cervical immobilization devices, must be maintained until spinal injury can be excluded. The common mistake of immobilizing the head but freeing the torso allows the cervical spine to flex with the body as a fulcrum.

Adjuncts to the Secondary Survey

❓ How can I minimize missed injuries?

Missed injuries can be minimized by maintaining a high index of suspicion and providing continuous monitoring of the patient's status. Specialized diagnostic tests may be performed during the secondary survey to identify specific injuries. These include additional x-ray examinations of the spine and extremities; CT scans of the head, chest, abdomen, and spine; contrast urography and angiography; transesophageal ultrasound; bronchoscopy; esophagoscopy; and other diagnostic procedures (■ FIGURE 1-7).

During the secondary survey, complete cervical and thoracolumbar spine imaging may be obtained with a portable x-ray unit if the patient's care is not compromised and the mechanism of injury suggests the possibility of spinal injury. In a patient with obtundation who requires CT of the brain, CT of the spine may be used as the method of radiographic assessment. Many trauma centers forego plain films and use CT instead for detecting spine injury. Spinal cord protection that was established during the primary survey should be maintained. An AP chest film and additional films pertinent to the site(s) of suspected injury should be obtained.

Often these procedures require transportation of the patient to other areas of the hospital, where equipment and personnel to manage life-threatening contingencies may not be immediately available. Therefore, these specialized tests should not be performed until the patient has been carefully examined and his or her hemodynamic status has been normalized.

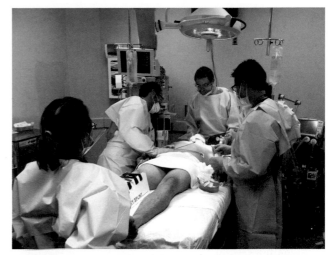

■ **FIGURE 1-7** Specialized diagnostic tests may be performed during the secondary survey to identify specific injuries.

The relief of severe pain is an important part of the treatment of trauma patients. Many injuries, especially musculoskeletal injuries, produce pain and anxiety in conscious patients. Effective analgesia usually requires the administration of opiates or anxiolytics intravenously (intramuscular injections should be avoided). These agents should be used judiciously and in small doses to achieve the desired level of patient comfort and relief of anxiety, while avoiding respiratory depression, the masking of subtle injuries, and changes in the patient's status.

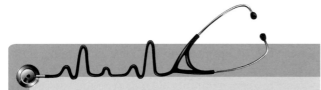

Scenario ■ *continued* The patient becomes tachycardic and hypotensive, with a pulse of 120 and a systolic blood pressure of 90 mm Hg. What do you do?

Reevaluation

Trauma patients must be reevaluated constantly to ensure that new findings are not overlooked and to discover deterioration in previously noted findings. As initial life-threatening injuries are managed, other equally life-threatening problems and less severe injuries may become apparent. Underlying medical problems that can significantly affect the ultimate prognosis of the patient may become evident. A high index of suspicion facilitates early diagnosis and management.

Continuous monitoring of vital signs and urinary output is essential. For adult patients, maintenance of urinary output at 0.5 mL/kg/h is desirable. In pediatric patients who are older than 1 year, an output of 1 mL/kg/h is typically adequate. ABG analyses and cardiac monitoring devices should be used. Pulse oximetry on critically injured patients and end-tidal carbon dioxide monitoring on intubated patients should be initiated.

Definitive Care

❓ *Which patients do I transfer to a higher level of care? When should the transfer occur?*

Transfer should be considered whenever the patient's treatment needs exceed the capability of the receiving institution. This decision requires a detailed assessment of the patient's injuries and the capabilities of the institution, including equipment, resources, and personnel.

Interhospital triage criteria will help determine the level, pace, and intensity of initial treatment of the multiply injured patient. See ACS COT, Resources for Optimal Care of the Injured Patient, 2006 (electronic version only). These criteria take into account the patient's physiologic status, obvious anatomic injury, mechanisms of injury, concurrent diseases, and other factors that can alter the patient's prognosis. ED and surgical personnel should use these criteria to determine whether the patient requires transfer to a trauma center or the closest appropriate hospital capable of providing more specialized care. The closest appropriate local facility should be chosen based on its overall capabilities to care for the injured patient. See Chapter 13: Transfer to Definitive Care and Figure 1-2.

Disaster

Disasters frequently overwhelm local and regional resources. Plans for management of such conditions must be developed, reevaluated, and rehearsed frequently to enhance the possibility of saving the maximum number of injured patients. ATLS providers should understand their role in disaster management within their healthcare institutions and remember the principles of ATLS relevant to patient care. See Appendix C: Disaster Management and Emergency Preparedness.

Records and Legal Considerations

Specific legal considerations, including records, consent for treatment, and forensic evidence, are relevant to ATLS providers.

RECORDS

Meticulous record keeping during patient assessment and management, including documenting the time for all events, is very important. Often more than one clinician cares for an individual patient, and precise records are essential for subsequent practitioners to evaluate the patient's needs and clinical status. Accurate record keeping during resuscitation can be facilitated by a member of the nursing staff whose primary responsibility is to record and collate all patient care information.

Medicolegal problems arise frequently, and precise records are helpful for all individuals concerned. Chronologic reporting with flow sheets helps both the attending doctor and the consulting doctor to assess changes in the patient's condition quickly. See Sample Trauma Flow Sheet (electronic version only), and Chapter 13: Transfer to Definitive Care, in this textbook.

CONSENT FOR TREATMENT

Consent is sought before treatment, if possible. In life-threatening emergencies, it is often not possible to obtain such consent. In these cases, treatment should be provided first, with formal consent obtained later.

FORENSIC EVIDENCE

If criminal activity is suspected in conjunction with a patient's injury, the personnel caring for the patient must preserve the evidence. All items, such as clothing and bullets, must be saved for law enforcement personnel. Laboratory determinations of blood alcohol concentrations and other drugs may be particularly pertinent and have substantial legal implications.

Teamwork

In many centers, trauma patients are assessed by a team, the size and composition of which varies from institution to institution. **In order to perform effectively, one team member should assume the role of team leader.** The team leader supervises, checks, and directs the assessment; ideally he/she is not involved hands-on in the assessment itself. The team leader is not necessarily the most senior person present. He/she should be trained in ATLS and what is involved in leading a medical team.

The team leader supervises and checks the preparation stage to ensure a smooth transition from the prehospital to hospital environment, assigning tasks to the other members of the team. Team function is related to team training; during training, duties are assigned to a particular role, which is reviewed with individual team members by the team leader as the team prepares for a specific patient. Depending on the size and composition of the team, it is helpful to have team members assigned to the following roles: patient assessment; undressing/exposing the patient and applying monitoring equipment; and recording the resuscitation activity.

On arrival of the patient, the team leader supervises the hand-over by EMS personnel, making certain that no team member begins working on the patient unless immediate life-threatening conditions are obvious ("hands-off hand-over"). A useful format is the MIST acronym:

Mechanism (and time) of injury

Injuries found and suspected

Symptoms and Signs

Treatment initiated

As assessment of "A," "B," and "C" proceed, it is extremely important that each member knows what the other members have found and/or are doing. This is facilitated by verbalizing each action and each finding out loud without more than one member speaking at the same time. Requests and orders should not be stated in general terms, but instead should be directed to an individual, by name. That individual then repeats the request/order, and later confirms its completion and, if applicable, its outcome.

The team leader checks the progression of the assessment, at intervals summarizes the findings and the condition of the patient, calls for consultants as required, orders additional examinations, and suggests/directs transfer of the patient.

During the entire process, all team members are expected to make remarks, ask questions and make suggestions, when appropriate. In that case, all other team members should pay attention and then act as directed by the team leader.

When the patient has left the ED, it is optimal for the team leader to conduct an "After Action" session, during which the technical and emotional aspects of the resuscitation are addressed.

Scenario ■ conclusion The 44-year-old patient, who was involved in a head-on MVC, was initially unresponsive at the scene. He was intubated on arrival at the hospital and a chest tube placed for a left pneumothorax. Correct position of the tube was confirmed with chest x-ray, and a pelvic fracture was identified on pelvic x-ray. The patient received 2 units of blood for tachycardia and hypotension, and is now normotensive. His GCS is 6T. A cervical collar remains in place. He will need further evaluation for possible head injury and abdominal injury.

Chapter Summary

1 The correct sequence of priorities for assessment of a multiply injured patient is preparation; triage; primary survey; resuscitation; adjuncts to primary survey and resuscitation; consider need for patient transfer; secondary survey, adjuncts to secondary survey; reevaluation; and definitive care.

2 The principles of the primary and secondary surveys are appropriate for the assessment of all multiply injured patients.

3 The guidelines and techniques included in the initial resuscitative and definitive-care phases of treatment should be applied to all multiply injured patients.

4 A patient's medical history and the mechanism of injury are critical to identifying injuries.

5 Pitfalls associated with the initial assessment and management of injured patients must be anticipated and managed to minimize their impact.

6 The primary survey should be repeated frequently, and any abnormalities should prompt a thorough reassessment.

7 Early identification of patients requiring transfer to a higher level of care improves outcomes.

▶ BIBLIOGRAPHY

1. American College of Surgeons Committee on Trauma. *Resources for Optimal Care of the Injured Patient.* Chicago, IL: American College of Surgeons Committee on Trauma; 2006.

2. Battistella FD. Emergency department evaluation of the patient with multiple injuries. In: Wilmore DW, Cheung LY, Harken AH, et al., eds. *Scientific American Surgery.* New York, NY: Scientific American; 1988–2000.

3. Lubbert PH, Kaasschieter EG, Hoorntje LE, et al. Video registration of trauma team performance in the emergency department: the results of a 2-year analysis in a level 1 trauma center. *J Trauma.* 2009; 67:1412–1420.

4. Enderson BL, Reath DB, Meadors J, et al. The tertiary trauma survey: a prospective study of missed injury. *J Trauma* 1990;30:666–670.

5. Esposito TJ, Ingraham A, Luchette FA, et al. Reasons to omit digital rectal exam in trauma patients: no fingers, no rectum, no useful additional information. *J Trauma* 2005;59(6):1314–1319.

6. Esposito TJ, Kuby A, Unfred C, et al. General surgeons and the Advanced Trauma Life Support course. Chicago, IL: American College of Surgeons, 2008.

7. McSwain NE Jr., Salomone J, et al., eds. *PHTLS: Prehospital Trauma Life Support.* 7th ed. St. Louis, MO: Mosby/Jems; 2011.: Is it time to refocus? *J Trauma* 1995;39:929–934.

8. Morris JA, MacKinzie EJ, Daminso AM, et al. Mortality in trauma patients: interaction between host factors and severity. *J Trauma* 1990;30:1476–1482.

9. Nahum AM, Melvin J, eds. *The Biomechanics of Trauma.* Norwalk, CT: Appleton-Century-Crofts; 1985.

10. Rhodes M, Brader A, Lucke J, et al: Direct transport to the operating room for resuscitation of trauma patients. *J Trauma* 1989;29:907-915.

11. Holcomb JB, Dumire RD, Crommett JW, et al. Evaluation of trauma team performance using an advanced human patient simulator for resuscitation training. *J Trauma* 2002;52:1078–1086.

12. Manser T. Teamwork and patient safety in dynamic domains of healthcare: a review of the literature. *Acta Anaesthesiol Scand* 2009;53:143–151.

13. Kappel D, Rossi D, Polack E, Avtgis T, Martin M. Time to decision to transfer in the rural system. Paper presented at: 39th Annual WTA Meeting; 2009; Crested Butte.

Initial Assessment and Management

▶▶ INTERACTIVE SKILL PROCEDURES

THE FOLLOWING PROCEDURES ARE INCLUDED IN THIS SKILL STATION:

▶▶ **Skill I-A:** Primary Survey and Resuscitation

▶▶ **Skill I-B:** Secondary Survey and Management

▶▶ **Skill I-C:** Patient Reevaluation

▶▶ **Skill I-D:** Transfer to Definitive Care

▶▶ **Skill I-E:** After-Action Review

Objectives

Performance at this station will allow the participant to practice and demonstrate the following activities in a simulated clinical situation:

1 Communicate and demonstrate to the instructor the systematic initial assessment and treatment of each patient.

2 Using the primary survey assessment techniques, determine and demonstrate
- Airway patency and cervical spine control
- Breathing and ventilation
- Circulatory status with hemorrhage control
- Disability: Neurologic status
- Exposure/environment: Undress the patient, but prevent hypothermia

3 Establish resuscitation (management) priorities in a multiply injured patient based on findings from the primary survey.

4 Integrate appropriate history taking as an invaluable aid in patient assessment.

5 Identify the injury-producing mechanism and describe the injuries that may exist and/or may be anticipated as a result of the mechanism of injury.

6 Using secondary survey techniques, assess the patient from head to toe.

7 Using the primary and secondary survey techniques, reevaluate the patient's status and response to therapy instituted.

8 Given a series of x-rays:
- Diagnose fractures
- Differentiate associated injuries

9 Outline the definitive care necessary to stabilize each patient in preparation for possible transport to a trauma center or to the closest appropriate facility.

10 In the role of referring doctor, communicate with the receiving doctor (instructor) in a logical, sequential manner:
- Patient's history, including mechanism of injury
- Physical findings
- Treatment instituted
- Patient's response to therapy
- Diagnostic tests performed and results
- Need for transport
- Method of transportation
- Anticipated time of arrival

▶ Skill I-A: Primary Survey and Resuscitation

The student should: (1) outline preparations that must be made to facilitate the rapid progression of assessment and resuscitation of the patient; (2) indicate the need to wear appropriate clothing to protect both the caregivers and the patient from communicable diseases; and (3) indicate that the patient is to be completely undressed, but that hypothermia should be prevented. *Note: Standard precautions are required whenever caring for trauma patients.*

▶▶ AIRWAY MAINTENANCE WITH CERVICAL SPINE PROTECTION

STEP 1.   Assessment
  A. Ascertain patency.
  B. Rapidly assess for airway obstruction.

STEP 2.   Management—Establish a patent airway
  A. Perform a chin-lift or jaw-thrust maneuver.
  B. Clear the airway of foreign bodies.
  C. Insert an oropharyngeal airway.
  D. Establish a definitive airway.
    1) Intubation
    2) Surgical cricothyroidotomy
  E. Describe jet insufflation of the airway, noting that it is only a temporary procedure.

STEP 3.   Maintain the cervical spine in a neutral position with manual immobilization as necessary when establishing an airway.

STEP 4.   Reinstate immobilization of the c-spine with appropriate devices after establishing an airway.

▶▶ BREATHING: VENTILATION AND OXYGENATION

STEP 1.   Assessment
  A. Expose the neck and chest, and ensure immobilization of the head and neck.
  B. Determine the rate and depth of respirations.
  C. Inspect and palpate the neck and chest for tracheal deviation, unilateral and bilateral chest movement, use of accessory muscles, and any signs of injury.
  D. Percuss the chest for presence of dullness or hyperresonance.
  E. Auscultate the chest bilaterally.

STEP 2.   Management
  A. Administer high-concentration oxygen.
  B. Ventilate with a bag-mask device.
  C. Alleviate tension pneumothorax.
  D. Seal open pneumothorax.
  E. Attach a CO_2 monitoring device to the endotracheal tube.
  F. Attach a pulse oximeter to the patient.

▶▶ CIRCULATION WITH HEMORRHAGE CONTROL

STEP 1.   Assessment
  A. Identify source of external, exsanguinating hemorrhage.
  B. Identify potential source(s) of internal hemorrhage.
  C. Assess pulse: Quality, rate, regularity, and paradox.
  D. Evaluate skin color.
  E. Measure blood pressure, if time permits.

STEP 2.   Management
  A. Apply direct pressure to external bleeding site(s).
  B. Consider presence of internal hemorrhage and potential need for operative intervention, and obtain surgical consult.
  C. Insert two large-caliber IV catheters.
  D. Simultaneously obtain blood for hematologic and chemical analyses; pregnancy test, when appropriate; type and crossmatch; and ABCs.
  E. Initiate IV fluid therapy with warmed crystalloid solution and blood replacement.
  F. Prevent hypothermia.

▶▶ DISABILITY: BRIEF NEUROLOGIC EXAMINATION

STEP 1.   Determine the level of consciousness using the GCS.

STEP 2.   Check pupils for size and reaction.

STEP 3.   Assess for lateralizing signs and spinal cord injury.   ↳ pupil size, symmetry and rxn to light, movement in all 04 limbs, deep tendon reflexes, plantar response

▶▶ EXPOSURE/ENVIRONMENTAL CONTROL

STEP 1.   Completely undress the patient, but prevent hypothermia.

▶▶ ADJUNCTS TO PRIMARY SURVEY AND RESUSCITATION

STEP 1. Obtain ABG analysis and ventilatory rate.

STEP 2. Monitor the patient's exhaled CO_2 with an appropriate monitoring device.

STEP 3. Attach an ECG monitor to the patient.

STEP 4. Insert urinary and gastric catheters unless contraindicated, and monitor the patient's hourly output of urine.

STEP 5. Consider the need for and obtain AP chest and AP pelvic x-rays.

STEP 6. Consider the need for and perform FAST or DPL.

▶▶ REASSESS PATIENT'S ABCDEs AND CONSIDER NEED FOR PATIENT TRANSFER

▶ Skill I-B: Secondary Survey and Management
(Also See Table I.1: Secondary Survey)

▶▶ SAMPLE HISTORY AND MECHANISM OF INJURY

STEP 1. Obtain AMPLE history from patient, family, or prehospital personnel.

STEP 2. Obtain history of injury-producing event and identify injury mechanisms.

▶▶ HEAD AND MAXILLOFACIAL

STEP 3. Assessment
  A. Inspect and palpate entire head and face for lacerations, contusions, fractures, and thermal injury.
  B. Reevaluate pupils.
  C. Reevaluate level of consciousness and GCS score.
  D. Assess eyes for hemorrhage, penetrating injury, visual acuity, dislocation of lens, and presence of contact lenses.
  E. Evaluate cranial-nerve function.
  F. Inspect ears and nose for cerebrospinal fluid leakage.
  G. Inspect mouth for evidence of bleeding and cerebrospinal fluid, soft-tissue lacerations, and loose teeth.

STEP 4. Management
  A. Maintain airway, and continue ventilation and oxygenation as indicated.
  B. Control hemorrhage.
  C. Prevent secondary brain injury.
  D. Remove contact lenses.

▶▶ CERVICAL SPINE AND NECK

STEP 5. Assessment
  A. Inspect for signs of blunt and penetrating injury, tracheal deviation, and use of accessory respiratory muscles.
  B. Palpate for tenderness, deformity, swelling, subcutaneous emphysema, tracheal deviation, and symmetry of pulses.
  C. Auscultate the carotid arteries for bruits.
  D. Obtain a CT of the cervical spine or a lateral, cross-table cervical spine x-ray.

STEP 6. Management: Maintain adequate in-line immobilization and protection of the cervical spine.

▶▶ CHEST

STEP 7. Assessment
  A. Inspect the anterior, lateral, and posterior chest wall for signs of blunt and penetrating injury, use of accessory breathing muscles, and bilateral respiratory excursions.
  B. Auscultate the anterior chest wall and posterior bases for bilateral breath sounds and heart sounds.
  C. Palpate the entire chest wall for evidence of blunt and penetrating injury, subcutaneous emphysema, tenderness, and crepitation.
  D. Percuss for evidence of hyperresonance or dullness.

STEP 8.   Management

    A. Perform needle decompression of pleural space or tube thoracostomy, as indicated.

    B. Attach the chest tube to an underwater seal-drainage device.

    C. Correctly dress an open chest wound.

    D. Perform pericardiocentesis, as indicated.

    E. Transfer the patient to the operating room, if indicated.

▶▶ ABDOMEN

STEP 9.   Assessment

    A. Inspect the anterior and posterior abdomen for signs of blunt and penetrating injury and internal bleeding.

    B. Auscultate for the presence of bowel sounds.

    C. Percuss the abdomen to elicit subtle rebound tenderness.

    D. Palpate the abdomen for tenderness, involuntary muscle guarding, unequivocal rebound tenderness, and a gravid uterus.

    E. Obtain a pelvic x-ray film.

    F. Perform DPL/abdominal ultrasound, if warranted.

    G. Obtain CT of the abdomen if the patient is hemodynamically normal.

STEP 10.   Management

    A. Transfer the patient to the operating room, if indicated.

    B. Wrap a sheet around the pelvis or apply a pelvic compression binder as indicated to reduce pelvic volume and control hemorrhage from a pelvic fracture.

▶▶ PERINEUM/RECTUM/VAGINA

STEP 11.   Perineal assessment.
Assess for:

    A. Contusions and hematomas

    B. Lacerations

    C. Urethral bleeding

STEP 12.   Rectal assessment in selected patients.
Assess for:

    A. Rectal blood

    B. Anal sphincter tone

    C. Bowel wall integrity

    D. Bony fragments

    E. Prostate position

STEP 13.   Vaginal assessment in selected patients.
Assess for:

    A. Presence of blood in vaginal vault

    B. Vaginal lacerations

▶▶ MUSCULOSKELETAL

STEP 14.   Assessment

    A. Inspect the upper and lower extremities for evidence of blunt and penetrating injury, including contusions, lacerations, and deformity.

    B. Palpate the upper and lower extremities for tenderness, crepitation, abnormal movement, and sensation.

    C. Palpate all peripheral pulses for presence, absence, and equality.

    D. Assess the pelvis for evidence of fracture and associated hemorrhage.

    E. Inspect and palpate the thoracic and lumbar spines for evidence of blunt and penetrating injury, including contusions, lacerations, tenderness, deformity, and sensation.

    F. Evaluate the pelvic x-ray film for evidence of a fracture.

    G. Obtain x-ray films of suspected fracture sites as indicated.

STEP 15.   Management

    A. Apply and/or readjust appropriate splinting devices for extremity fractures as indicated.

    B. Maintain immobilization of the patient's thoracic and lumbar spines.

    C. Wrap a sheet around the pelvis or apply a pelvic compression binder as indicated to reduce pelvic volume and control hemorrhage associated with a pelvic fracture.

    D. Apply a splint to immobilize an extremity injury.

    E. Administer tetanus immunization.

    F. Administer medications as indicated or as directed by specialist.

    G. Consider the possibility of compartment syndrome.

    H. Perform a complete neurovascular examination of the extremities.

▶▶ NEUROLOGIC

STEP 16.   Assessment

    A. Reevaluate the pupils and level of consciousness.

    B. Determine the GCS score.

    C. Evaluate the upper and lower extremities for motor and sensory functions.

    D. Observe for lateralizing signs.

STEP 17.   Management

    A. Continue ventilation and oxygenation.

    B. Maintain adequate immobilization of the entire patient.

▶▶ ADJUNCTS TO SECONDARY SURVEY

STEP 18. Consider the need for and obtain these diagnostic tests as the patient's condition permits and warrants:

- Spinal x-rays
- CT of the head, chest, abdomen, and/or spine

- Contrast urography
- Angiography
- Extremity x-rays
- Transesophageal ultrasound
- Bronchoscopy
- Esophagoscopy

■ TABLE I.1 SECONDARY SURVEY

ITEM TO ASSESS	ESTABLISHES/IDENTIFIES	ASSESS	FINDING	CONFIRM BY
Level of Consciousness	• Severity of head injury	• GCS score	• 8, Severe head injury • 9–12, Moderate head injury • 13–15, Minor head injury	• CT scan • Repeat without paralyzing agents
Pupils	• Type of head injury • Presence of eye injury	• Size • Shape • Reactivity	• Mass effect • Diffuse brain injury • Ophthalmic injury	• CT scan
Head	• Scalp injury • Skull injury	• Inspect for lacerations and skull fractures • Palpable defects	• Scalp laceration • Depressed skull fracture • Basilar skull fracture	• CT scan
Maxillofacial	• Soft-tissue injury • Bone injury • Nerve injury • Teeth/mouth injury	• Visual deformity • Malocclusion • Palpation for crepitation	• Facial fracture • Soft-tissue injury	• Facial-bone x-ray • CT scan of facial bones
Neck	• Laryngeal injury • C-spine injury • Vascular injury • Esophageal injury • Neurologic deficit	• Visual inspection • Palpation • Auscultation	• Laryngeal deformity • Subcutaneous emphysema • Hematoma • Bruit • Platysmal penetration • Pain, tenderness of c-spine	• C-spine x-ray or CT • Angiography/duplex exam • Esophagoscopy • Laryngoscopy
Thorax	• Thoracic-wall injury • Subcutaneous emphysema • Pneumothorax/hemothorax • Bronchial injury • Pulmonary contusion • Thoracic aortic disruption	• Visual inspection • Palpation • Auscultation	• Bruising, deformity, or paradoxical motion • Chest-wall tenderness, crepitation • Diminished breath sounds • Muffled heart tones • Mediastinal crepitation • Severe back pain	• Chest x-ray • CT scan • Angiography • Bronchoscopy • Tube thoracostomy • Pericardiocentesis • TE ultrasound
Abdomen/Flank	• Abdominal-wall injury • Intraperitoneal injury • Retroperitoneal injury	• Visual inspection • Palpation • Auscultation • Determine path of penetration	• Abdominal-wall pain/tenderness • Peritoneal irritation • Visceral injury • Retroperitoneal organ injury	• DPL/ultrasound • CT scan • Laparotomy • Contrast GI x-ray studies • Angiography
Pelvis	• Genitourinary (GU) tract injuries • Pelvic fracture(s)	• Palpate symphysis pubis for widening • Palpate bony pelvis for tenderness • Determine pelvic stability only once • Inspect perineum • Rectal/vaginal exam	• GU tract injury (hematuria) • Pelvic fracture • Rectal, vaginal, and/or perineal injury	• Pelvic x-ray • GU contrast studies • Urethrogram • Cystogram • IVP • Contrast-enhanced CT

■ TABLE I.1 (continued)

ITEM TO ASSESS	ESTABLISHES/IDENTIFIES	ASSESS	FINDING	CONFIRM BY
Spinal Cord	• Cranial injury • Cord injury • Peripheral nerve(s) injury	• Motor response • Pain response	• Unilateral cranial mass effect • Quadriplegia • Paraplegia • Nerve root injury	• Plain spine x-rays • CT scan • MRI
Vertebral Column	• Column injury • Vertebral instability • Nerve injury	• Verbal response to pain, lateralizing signs • Palpate for tenderness • Deformity	• Fracture versus dislocation	• Plain x-rays • CT scan • MRI
Extremities	• Soft-tissue injury • Bony deformities • Joint abnormalities • Neurovascular defects	• Visual inspection • Palpation	• Swelling, bruising, pallor • Malalignment • Pain, tenderness, crepitation • Absent/diminished pulses • Tense muscular compartments • Neurologic deficits	• Specific x-rays • Doppler examination • Compartment pressures • Angiography

▶ Skill I-C: Patient Reevaluation

Reevaluate the patient, noting, reporting, and documenting any changes in the patient's condition and responses to resuscitative efforts. Judicious use of analgesics may be instituted. Continuous monitoring of vital signs, urinary output, and the patient's response to treatment is essential.

▶ Skill I-D: Transfer to Definitive Care

Outline rationale for patient transfer, transfer procedures, and patient's needs during transfer, and state the need for direct doctor-to-doctor communication.

▶ Skill I-E: After-Action Review

Outline the rationale for conducting an after-action review, and identify what went well and what could have been improved upon **medically**. Attention should be paid to breakdowns in **intra-team communication and interactions** that may have occurred.

2 Airway and Ventilatory Management

Prevention of hypoxemia requires a protected, unobstructed airway and adequate ventilation, which take priority over management of all other conditions.

Scenario A 34-year-old motorcyclist lost control and crashed into a fence at a high rate of speed. He was not wearing a helmet and has obvious facial trauma. The patient smells of alcohol. He was combative and belligerent at the scene, although he is now lethargic and not communicating. His breath sounds are sonorous. Pulse oximeter reading is 85%.

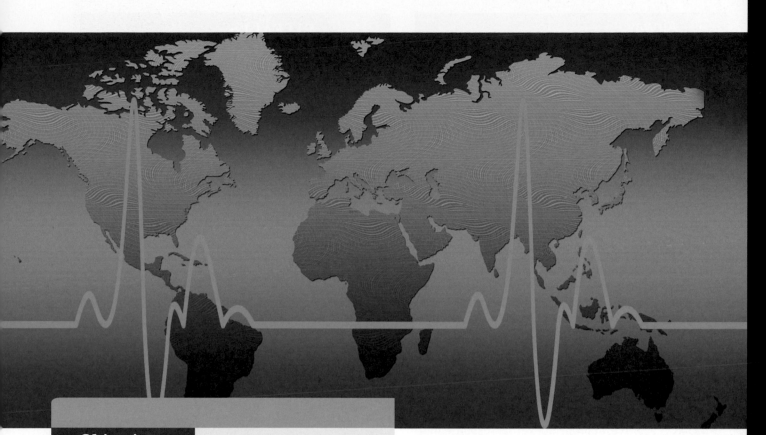

Objectives

1 Identify the clinical situations in which airway compromise is likely to occur.

2 Recognize the signs and symptoms of acute airway obstruction.

3 Recognize ventilatory compromise and signs of inadequate ventilation.

4 Describe the techniques for establishing and maintaining a patent airway.

5 Describe the techniques for confirming the adequacy of ventilation and oxygenation, including pulse oximetry and end-tidal CO_2 monitoring.

6 Define the term definitive airway.

7 List the indications for rapid sequence intubation.

8 Outline the steps necessary for maintaining oxygenation before, during, and after establishing a definitive airway.

The inadequate delivery of oxygenated blood to the brain and other vital structures is the quickest killer of injured patients. Prevention of hypoxemia requires a protected, unobstructed airway and adequate ventilation, which take priority over management of all other conditions. An airway must be secured, oxygen delivered, and ventilatory support provided. **Supplemental oxygen must be administered to all trauma patients.**

Early preventable deaths from airway problems after trauma often result from:

- Failure to recognize the need for an airway intervention

- Inability to establish an airway

- Inability to recognize the need for an alternative airway plan in the setting of repeated failed intubation attempts

- Failure to recognize an incorrectly placed airway

- Displacement of a previously established airway

- Failure to recognize the need for ventilation

- Aspiration of gastric contents

Airway and ventilation are the first priorities.

Airway

? How do I know the airway is adequate?

The first steps toward identifying and managing potentially life-threatening airway compromise are to recognize the problems involving maxillofacial, neck, and laryngeal trauma, and to identify objective signs of airway obstruction.

PROBLEM RECOGNITION

Airway compromise can be sudden and complete, insidious and partial, and/or progressive and recurrent. Although it is often related to pain or anxiety, or both, tachypnea can be a subtle but early sign of airway or ventilatory compromise. Therefore, assessment and frequent reassessment of airway patency and adequacy of ventilation are critical.

During initial assessment of the airway, the "talking patient" provides reassurance (at least for the moment) that the airway is patent and not compromised. Therefore, the most important early measure is to talk to the patient and stimulate a verbal response. A positive, appropriate verbal response indicates that the airway is patent, ventilation is intact, and brain perfusion is adequate. Failure to respond or an inappropriate response suggests an altered level of consciousness, airway and ventilatory compromise, or both.

Patients with an altered level of consciousness are at particular risk for airway compromise and often require a definitive airway. A definitive airway is defined as a tube placed in the trachea with the cuff inflated below the vocal cords, the tube connected to some form of oxygen-enriched assisted ventilation, and the airway secured in place with tape. Unconscious patients with head injuries, patients who are obtunded because of the use of alcohol and/or other drugs, and patients with thoracic injuries all can have a compromised ventilatory effort. In these patients, the purpose of endotracheal intubation is to provide an airway, deliver supplementary oxygen, support ventilation, and prevent aspiration. **Maintaining oxygenation and preventing hypercarbia are critical in managing trauma patients, especially those who have sustained head injuries.**

It is important to anticipate vomiting in all injured patients and be prepared to manage the situation. The presence of gastric contents in the oropharynx represents a significant risk of aspiration with the patient's next breath. Therefore, immediate suctioning and rotation of the entire patient to the lateral position are indicated.

PITFALLS

Aspiration is a danger for trauma patients. Functional suction equipment must be immediately available to aid clinicians in ensuring a secure, patent airway in all trauma patients.

Maxillofacial Trauma

Trauma to the face demands aggressive but careful airway management (■ FIGURE 2-1). The mechanism for this injury is exemplified by an unbelted automobile passenger who is thrown into the windshield and dashboard. Trauma to the midface can produce fractures and dislocations that compromise the nasopharynx and oropharynx. Facial fractures can be associated with hemorrhage, increased secretions, and dislodged teeth, which cause additional difficulties in maintaining a patent airway. Fractures of the mandible, especially bilateral body fractures, can cause loss of normal airway *structural* support. Airway obstruction can result if the patient is in a supine position. Patients who refuse to lie down may be experiencing difficulty in maintaining their airway or handling secretions. Furthermore, providing general anesthesia, sedation, or muscle relaxation can lead to the total loss of airway due to diminished or absent muscle tone. See Chapter 6: Head Trauma.

Neck Trauma

Penetrating injury to the neck can cause vascular injury with significant hematoma, which can result in

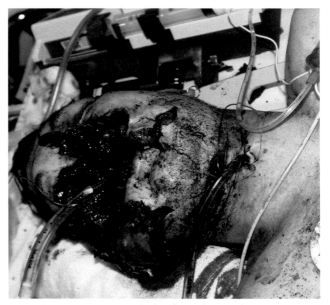

■ FIGURE 2-1 Trauma to the face demands aggressive but careful airway management.

displacement and obstruction of the airway. Emergency placement of a surgical airway may be necessary if this displacement and obstruction make endotracheal intubation impossible. Hemorrhage from adjacent vascular injury can be massive, and operative control may be required.

Blunt or penetrating injury to the neck can cause disruption of the larynx or trachea, resulting in airway obstruction and/or severe bleeding into the tracheobronchial tree. A definitive airway is urgently required in this situation.

Neck injuries involving disruption of the larynx and trachea or compression of the airway from hemorrhage into the soft tissues of the neck can cause partial airway obstruction. Initially, a patient with this type of serious airway injury may be able to maintain airway patency and ventilation. However, if airway compromise is suspected, a definitive airway is required. To prevent exacerbating an existing airway injury, an endotracheal tube must be inserted cautiously and preferably under direct visualization. Loss of airway patency can be precipitous, and an early surgical airway usually is indicated. See Skill Station IX: Head and Neck Trauma: Assessment and Management.

Laryngeal Trauma

Although fracture of the larynx is a rare injury, it can present with acute airway obstruction. It is indicated by the following triad of clinical signs:

1. Hoarseness
2. Subcutaneous emphysema
3. Palpable fracture

# of LARYNX

Complete obstruction of the airway or severe respiratory distress warrants an attempt at intubation. Flexible endoscopic intubation may be helpful in this situation, but only if it can be performed promptly. If intubation is unsuccessful, an emergency tracheostomy is indicated, followed by operative repair. However, a tracheostomy is difficult to perform under emergency conditions, can be associated with profuse bleeding, and can be time-consuming. Surgical cricothyroidotomy, although not preferred for this situation, can be a lifesaving option.

Penetrating trauma to the larynx or trachea is overt and requires immediate management. Complete tracheal transection or occlusion of the airway with blood or soft tissue can cause acute airway compromise that requires immediate correction. These injuries are often associated with trauma to the esophagus, carotid artery, or jugular vein, as well as extensive tissue destruction. Noisy breathing indicates partial airway obstruction that can suddenly become complete, whereas the absence of breathing suggests that complete obstruction already exists. When the patient's level of consciousness is depressed, detection of significant airway obstruction is more subtle. Labored respiratory effort may be the only clue to airway obstruction and tracheobronchial injury.

If a fracture of the larynx is suspected, based on the mechanism of injury and subtle physical findings, computed tomography (CT) can help to identify this injury.

OBJECTIVE SIGNS OF AIRWAY OBSTRUCTION

Several objective signs of airway obstruction can be identified by taking the following steps:

1. Observe the patient to determine whether he or she is agitated or obtunded. Agitation suggests hypoxia, and obtundation suggests hypercarbia. Cyanosis indicates hypoxemia due to inadequate oxygenation; it is identified by inspection of the nail beds and circumoral skin. However, cyanosis is a late finding of hypoxia. Pulse oximetry is used early in the airway assessment to detect inadequate oxygenation prior to the development of cyanosis. Look for retractions and the use of accessory muscles of ventilation that, when present, provide additional evidence of airway compromise.

2. Listen for abnormal sounds. Noisy breathing is obstructed breathing. Snoring, gurgling, and crowing sounds (stridor) can be associated with partial occlusion of the pharynx or larynx. Hoarseness (dysphonia) implies functional, laryngeal obstruction.

3. Feel for the location of the trachea and quickly determine whether it is in the midline position.

4. Evaluate patient behavior. **Abusive and belligerent patients may in fact have hypoxia and should not be presumed to be intoxicated.**

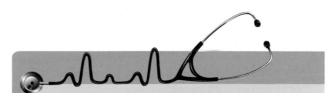

Scenario ▪ *continued* The patient's breath sounds become more labored, and he remains unresponsive. Using inline cervical immobilization, you perform the chin-lift maneuver and bag-mask ventilation, increasing his oxygenation saturation from 85% to 92%.

Ventilation

Ensuring a patent airway is an important step in providing oxygen to the patient, but it is only the first step. An unobstructed airway is not likely to benefit the patient unless there is also adequate ventilation. The clinician must look for any objective signs of inadequate ventilation.

PROBLEM RECOGNITION

Ventilation can be compromised by airway obstruction, altered ventilatory mechanics, and/or central nervous system (CNS) depression. If a patient's breathing is not improved by clearing the airway, other causes of the problem must be found and managed. Direct trauma to the chest, especially with rib fractures, causes pain with breathing and leads to rapid, shallow ventilation and hypoxemia. Elderly patients and individuals with preexisting pulmonary dysfunction are at significant risk for ventilatory failure under these circumstances. Intracranial injury can cause abnormal breathing patterns and compromise adequacy of ventilation. Cervical spinal cord injury can result in diaphragmatic breathing and interfere with the ability to meet increased oxygen demands. Complete cervical cord transection, which spares the phrenic nerves (C3 and C4), results in abdominal breathing and paralysis of the intercostal muscles; assisted ventilation may be required.

OBJECTIVE SIGNS OF INADEQUATE VENTILATION

? *How do I know ventilation is adequate?*

Several objective signs of inadequate ventilation can be identified by taking the following steps:

1. Look for symmetrical rise and fall of the chest and adequate chest wall excursion. Asymmetry suggests splinting of the rib cage or a flail chest. Labored breathing may indicate an imminent threat to the patient's ventilation.

2. Listen for movement of air on both sides of the chest. Decreased or absent breath sounds over one or both hemithoraces should alert the examiner to the presence of thoracic injury. See Chapter 4: Thoracic Trauma. Beware of a rapid respiratory rate—tachypnea can indicate respiratory distress.

3. Use a pulse oximeter. This device provides information regarding the patient's oxygen saturation and peripheral perfusion, but does not measure the adequacy of ventilation.

PITFALLS

Patients who are breathing high concentrations of oxygen can maintain their oxygen saturation although breathing inadequately. Measure arterial or end-tidal carbon dioxide.

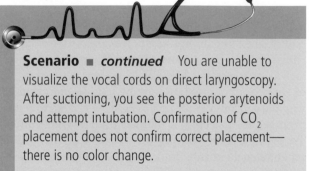

Scenario ■ *continued* You are unable to visualize the vocal cords on direct laryngoscopy. After suctioning, you see the posterior arytenoids and attempt intubation. Confirmation of CO_2 placement does not confirm correct placement—there is no color change.

Airway Management

? *How do I manage the airway of a trauma patient?*

Airway patency and adequacy of ventilation must be assessed quickly and accurately. Pulse oximetry and end-tidal CO_2 measurement are essential. If problems are identified or suspected, measures should be instituted immediately to improve oxygenation and reduce the risk of further ventilatory compromise. These measures include airway maintenance techniques, definitive airway measures (including surgical airway), and methods of providing supplemental ventilation. **Because all of these actions can require some neck motion, it is important to maintain cervical spine (c-spine) protection in all patients, especially patients who are known to have an unstable c-spine injury and those who have been incompletely evaluated and are at risk.** The spinal cord must be protected until the possibility of a spinal injury has been excluded by clinical assessment and appropriate radiographic studies.

High-flow oxygen is required both before and immediately after airway management measures are instituted. A rigid suction device is essential and should be readily available. Patients with facial injuries can have associated cribriform plate fractures, and the insertion of any tube through the nose can result in passage into the cranial vault.

Patients who are wearing a helmet and require airway management need their head and neck held in a neutral position while the helmet is removed. This is

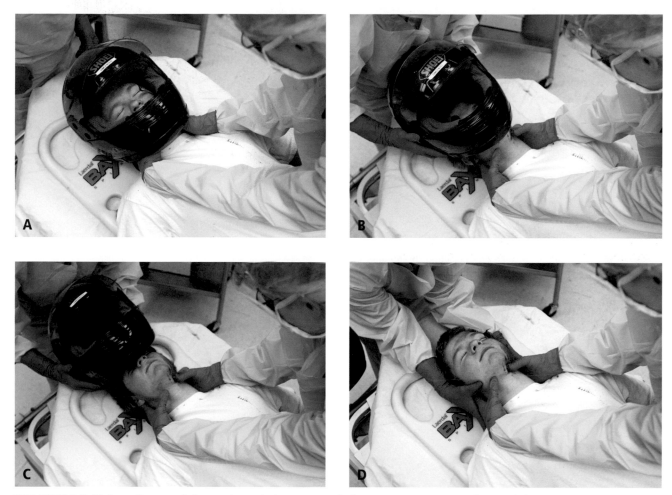

■ **FIGURE 2-2 Helmet Removal.** Removing a helmet properly is a two-person procedure. While one person provides manual, inline stabilization of the head and neck (**A**), the second person expands the helmet laterally. The second person then removes the helmet (**B**), with attention paid to the helmet clearing the nose and occiput. Once removed, the first person supports the weight of the patient's head (**C**), and the second person takes over inline stabilization (**D**).

a two-person procedure: One person provides manual inline stabilization from below, while the second person expands the helmet laterally and removes it from above (■ **FIGURE 2-2**). Then, inline stabilization is reestablished from above, and the patient's head and neck are secured during airway management. Removal of the helmet using a cast cutter while stabilizing the head and neck can minimize c-spine motion in patients with known c-spine injury.

PREDICTING DIFFICULT AIRWAYS

❓ *How do I predict a potentially difficult airway?*

It is important to assess the patient's airway prior to attempting intubation in order to predict the likely difficulty of the maneuver. Factors that may predict dif-

ficulties with airway maneuvers include c-spine injury, severe arthritis of the c-spine, significant maxillofacial or mandibular trauma, limited mouth opening, obesity, and anatomical variations (e.g., receding chin, overbite, and a short, muscular neck). In such cases, skilled clinicians should assist in the event of difficulty.

The mnemonic LEMON is helpful as a prompt when assessing the potential for a difficult intubation (Box 2-1). Several components of LEMON are particularly useful in trauma. Look for evidence of a difficult airway (small mouth or jaw, large overbite, or facial trauma). Any obvious airway obstruction presents an immediate challenge. All blunt trauma patients necessitate c-spine immobilization, which increases the difficulty of establishing an airway. Clinical judgment and experience will determine whether to proceed immediately with drug-assisted intubation or to exercise caution.

Box 2-1 LEMON Assessment for Difficult Intubation

L = Look Externally: Look for characteristics that are known to cause difficult intubation or ventilation.

E = Evaluate the 3-3-2 Rule: To allow for alignment of the pharyngeal, laryngeal, and oral axes and therefore simple intubation, the following relationships should be observed.

- The distance between the patient's incisor teeth should be at least 3 finger breadths (3)

- The distance between the hyoid bone and the chin should be at least 3 finger breadths (3)

- The distance between the thyroid notch and floor of the mouth should be at least 2 finger breadths (2)

M = Mallampati: The hypopharynx should be visualized adequately. This has been done traditionally by assessing the Mallampati classification. When possible, the patient is asked to sit upright, open the mouth fully, and protrude the tongue as far as possible. The examiner then looks into the mouth with a light torch to assess the degree of hypopharynx visible. In supine patients, the Mallampati score can be estimated by asking the patient to open the mouth fully and protrude the tongue; a laryngoscopy light is then shone into the hypopharynx from above.

O = Obstruction: Any condition that can cause obstruction of the airway will make laryngoscopy and ventilation difficult. Such conditions include epiglottitis, peritonsillar abscess, and trauma.

N = Neck Mobility: This is a vital requirement for successful intubation. It can be assessed easily by asking the patient to place his or her chin onto the chest and then extending the neck so that he or she is looking toward the ceiling. **Patients in hard collar neck immobilization obviously have no neck movement and are therefore more difficult to intubate.**

Modified with permission from: MJ Reed, MJG Dunn and DW McKeown. Can an airway assessment score predict difficulty at intubation in the emergency department? *Emerg Med J* 2005;22;99-102

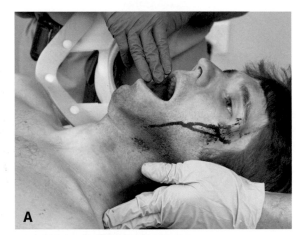

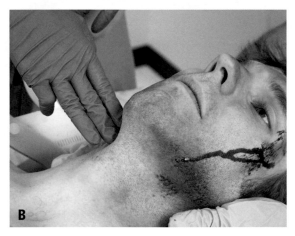

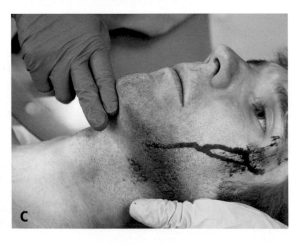

The 3-3-2 Rule. To allow for alignment of the pharyngeal, laryngeal, and oral axes, and therefore simple intubation, the following relationships should be observed: The distance between the patient's incisor teeth should be at least 3 finger breadths (**A**); The distance between the hyoid bone and the chin should be at least 3 finger breadths (**B**); and the distance between the thyroid notch and floor of the mouth should be at least 2 finger breadths (**C**).

(continued)

Box 2-1 *(continued)*

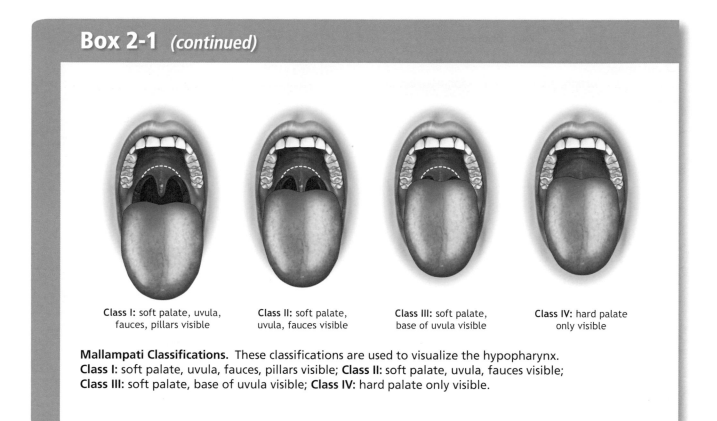

Class I: soft palate, uvula, fauces, pillars visible

Class II: soft palate, uvula, fauces visible

Class III: soft palate, base of uvula visible

Class IV: hard palate only visible

Mallampati Classifications. These classifications are used to visualize the hypopharynx. **Class I:** soft palate, uvula, fauces, pillars visible; **Class II:** soft palate, uvula, fauces visible; **Class III:** soft palate, base of uvula visible; **Class IV:** hard palate only visible.

AIRWAY DECISION SCHEME

■ **FIGURE 2-3** provides a scheme for deciding the appropriate route of airway management. This algorithm applies only to patients who are in acute respiratory distress or who have apnea, are in need of an immediate airway, and in whom a c-spine injury is suspected because of the mechanism of injury or suggested by the physical examination. The first priority is to ensure continued oxygenation with maintenance of c-spine immobilization. This is accomplished initially by position (i.e., chin-lift or jaw-thrust maneuver) and the preliminary airway techniques (i.e., oropharyngeal airway or nasopharyngeal airway). An endotracheal tube is then passed while a second person provides inline immobilization. If an endotracheal tube cannot be inserted and the patient's respiratory status is in jeopardy, ventilation via a laryngeal mask airway or other extraglottic airway device may be attempted as a bridge to a definitive airway. If this fails, a cricothyroidotomy should be performed. All of these methods are described below.

Oxygenation and ventilation must be maintained before, during, and immediately upon completion of insertion of the definitive airway. Prolonged periods of inadequate or absent ventilation and oxygenation should be avoided.

AIRWAY MAINTENANCE TECHNIQUES

In patients who have a decreased level of consciousness, the tongue can fall backward and obstruct the hypopharynx. This form of obstruction can be corrected readily by the chin-lift or jaw-thrust maneuvers. The airway can then be maintained with an oropharyngeal or nasopharyngeal airway. **Maneuvers used to establish an airway can produce or aggravate c-spine injury, so inline immobilization of the c-spine is essential during these procedures.**

Chin-Lift Maneuver

In the chin-lift maneuver, the fingers of one hand are placed under the mandible, which is then gently lifted upward to bring the chin anterior. The thumb of the same hand lightly depresses the lower lip to open the mouth (■ **FIGURE 2-4**). The thumb also may be placed behind the lower incisors and, simultaneously, the chin is gently lifted. The chin-lift maneuver should not hyperextend the neck. This maneuver is useful for trauma victims because it can prevent converting a cervical fracture without cord injury into one with cord injury.

Jaw-Thrust Maneuver

The jaw-thrust maneuver is performed by grasping the angles of the lower jaw, one hand on each side, and

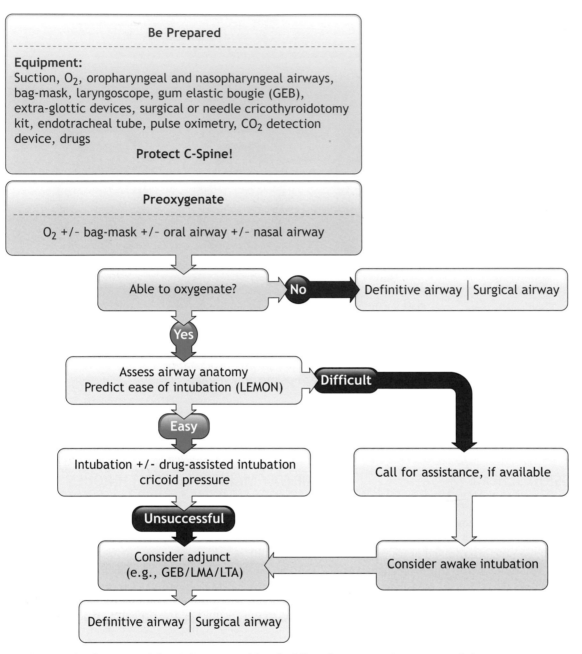

■ **FIGURE 2-3 Airway Decision Scheme** Used for deciding the appropriate route of airway management. *Note: The ATLS Airway Decision Scheme provides a general approach to airway management in trauma. Many centers have developed detailed airway management algorithms. It is important to review and learn the standard used by teams in your trauma system.*

displacing the mandible forward (■ **FIGURE 2-5**). When this method is used with the face mask of a bag-mask device, a good seal and adequate ventilation can be achieved. Care must be taken to prevent neck extension.

Oropharyngeal Airway

Oral airways are inserted into the mouth behind the tongue. The preferred technique is to use a tongue blade to depress the tongue and then insert the air-

way posteriorly, taking care not to push the tongue backward, which would block—rather than clear—the airway. This device must not be used in conscious patients because it can induce gagging, vomiting, and aspiration. Patients who tolerate an oropharyngeal airway are highly likely to require intubation.

An alternative technique is to insert the oral airway upside down, so its concavity is directed upward, until the soft palate is encountered. At this point,

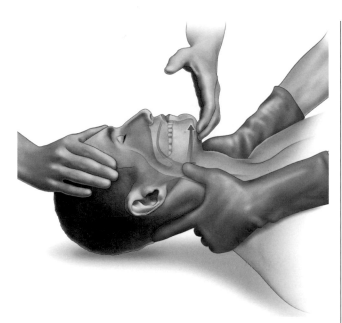

■ **FIGURE 2-4 The Chin-Lift Maneuver to Establish an Airway.** This maneuver is useful for trauma victims because it can prevent converting a cervical fracture without cord injury into one with cord injury.

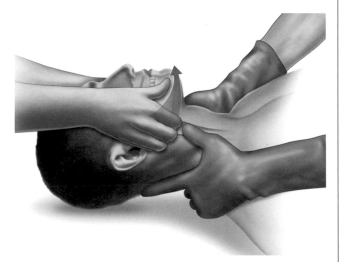

■ **FIGURE 2-5 The Jaw-Thrust Maneuver to Establish an Airway.** Care must be taken to prevent neck extension.

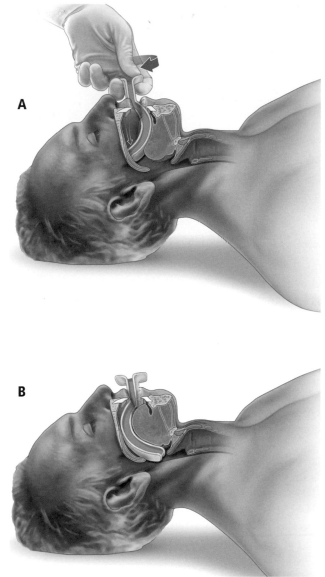

■ **FIGURE 2-6 Alternative Technique for Inserting Oral Airway.** In this technique, the oral airway is inserted upside down (**A**) until the soft palate is encountered, at which point the device is rotated 180 degrees and slipped into place over the tongue (**B**). This method should not be used in children.

with the device rotated 180 degrees, the concavity is directed inferiorly, and the device is slipped into place over the tongue (■ **FIGURE 2-6**). This alternative method should not be used in children, because the rotation of the device can damage the mouth and pharynx. See Skill Station II: Airway and Ventilatory Management, <u>Skill II-A: Oropharyngeal Airway Insertion</u>.

Nasopharyngeal Airway

Nasopharyngeal airways are inserted in one nostril and passed gently into the posterior oropharynx. They should

be well lubricated and inserted into the nostril that appears to be unobstructed. If obstruction is encountered during introduction of the airway, stop and try the other nostril. **This procedure should not be attempted in patients with suspected or potential cribriform plate fracture.** See Skill Station II: Airway and Ventilatory Management, <u>Skill II-B: Nasopharyngeal Airway Insertion</u>.

Extraglottic and Supraglottic Devices

The following extraglottic, or supraglottic, devices have a role in managing patients who require an advanced

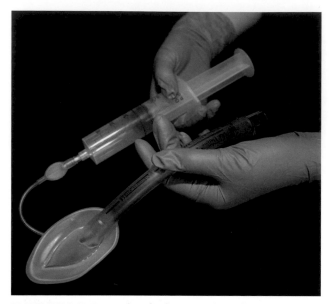

■ **FIGURE 2-7** Example of a laryngeal mask airway.

airway adjunct, but in whom intubation has failed or is unlikely to succeed: laryngeal mask airway, multilumen esophageal airway, and laryngeal tube airway. Other supraglottic devices used in trauma patient are currently being investigated.

Laryngeal Mask Airway and Intubating LMA There is an established role for the laryngeal mask airway (LMA) and the intubating laryngeal mask airway (ILMA), in the treatment of patients with difficult airways, particularly if attempts at endotracheal intubation or bag-mask ventilation have failed (■ **FIGURE 2-7**). The LMA does not provide a definitive airway, and proper placement of this device is difficult without appropriate training. The ILMA is an evolution of the device that allows for intubation through the LMA. When a patient has an LMA or an ILMA in place on arrival in the emergency department (ED), clinicians must plan for a definitive airway. See Skill Station II: Airway and Ventilatory Management, <u>Skill II-E: Laryngeal Mask Airway (LMA) and Intubating LMA (ILMA) Insertion</u>.

Laryngeal Tube Airway The laryngeal tube airway (LTA) is an extraglottic airway device with capabilities similar to those of the LMA in providing successful patient ventilation (■ **FIGURE 2-8**). The LTA is not a definitive airway device, and plans to provide a definitive airway are necessary. As with the LMA, the LTA is placed without direct visualization of the glottis and does not require significant manipulation of the head and neck for placement. See Skill Station II: Airway and Ventilatory Management, <u>Skill II-F: Laryngeal Tube Airway (LTA) Insertion</u>.

Multilumen Esophageal Airway Multilumen esophageal airway devices are used by some prehospital personnel to achieve an airway when a definitive airway is not feasible (■ **FIGURE 2-9**). One of the ports communicates with the esophagus and the other with the airway. The personnel who use this device are trained to observe which port occludes the esophagus and which provides air to the trachea. The esophageal port is then occluded with a balloon, and the other port is ventilated. A CO_2 detector improves the accuracy of this apparatus. The multilumen esophageal airway device must be removed and/or a definitive airway provided after appropriate assessment.

AIRWAYS

A definitive airway requires a tube placed in the trachea with the cuff inflated below the vocal cords, the tube connected to some form of oxygen-enriched assisted ventilation, and the airway secured in place with tape. There are three types of definitive airways: orotracheal tubes, nasotracheal tubes, and surgical airways (cricothyroidotomy or tracheostomy). The criteria for establishing a definitive airway are based on clinical findings and include (see Table 2.1):

- Airway problems—Inability to maintain a patent airway by other means, with impending or potential compromise of the airway (e.g., following inhalation injury, facial fractures, or retropharyngeal hematoma)

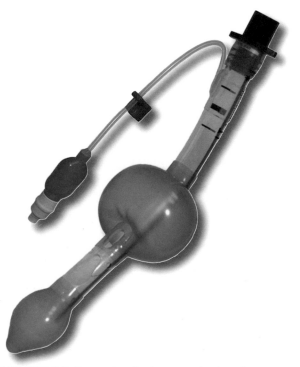

■ **FIGURE 2-8** Example of a laryngeal tube airway.

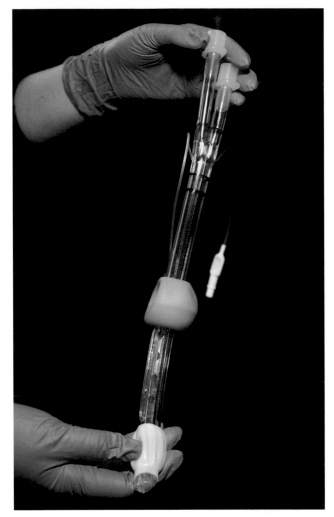

■ **FIGURE 2-8** Example of a multilumen esophageal airway.

■ **TABLE 2.1**
Indications for Definitive Airway

NEED FOR AIRWAY PROTECTION	NEED FOR VENTILATION OR OXYGENATION
Severe maxillofacial fractures	Inadequate respiratory efforts • Tachypnea • Hypoxia • Hypercarbia • Cyanosis
Risk for obstruction • Neck hematoma • Laryngeal or tracheal injury • Stridor	Massive blood loss and need for volume resuscitation
Risk for aspiration • Bleeding • Vomiting	Severe closed head injury with need for brief hyperventilation if acute neurologic deterioration occurs
Unconscious	Apnea • Neuromuscular paralysis • Unconscious

- Breathing problems— Inability to maintain adequate oxygenation by face-mask oxygen supplementation, and presence of apnea

- Disability problems—Presence of a closed head injury requiring assisted ventilation (Glasgow Coma Scale [GCS] score of 8 or less), need to protect the lower airway from aspiration of blood or vomitus, or sustained seizure activity

The urgency of the situation and the circumstances indicating the need for airway intervention dictate the specific route and method to be used. Continued assisted ventilation is aided by supplemental sedation, analgesics, or muscle relaxants, as indicated. Assessment of the patient's clinical status and the use of a pulse oximeter can be helpful in determining the need for a definitive airway, the urgency of the need, and, by inference, the effectiveness of airway placement. The potential for concomitant c-spine injury is of major concern in the patient requiring an airway.

Endotracheal Intubation

Although it is important to establish the presence or absence of a c-spine fracture, obtaining radiological studies (CT scan or c-spine x-rays) should not impede or delay placement of a definitive airway when one is clearly indicated. **Patients with GCS scores of 8 or less require prompt intubation. If there is no immediate need for intubation, radiological clearance of the c-spine may be obtained.** However, a normal lateral c-spine film does not exclude the possibility of a c-spine injury.

The most important determinants of whether to proceed with orotracheal or nasotracheal intubation are the experience of the clinician and the presence of a spontaneously breathing patient. Both techniques are safe and effective when performed properly, although the orotracheal route is more commonly used and has fewer intensive care unit (ICU)-related complications (e.g., sinusitis and pressure necrosis). **If the patient has apnea, orotracheal intubation is indicated.**

Blind nasotracheal intubation requires a patient who is spontaneously breathing and is contraindicated in patients with apnea. The deeper the patient breathes, the easier it is to follow the airflow through the larynx. Facial, frontal sinus, basilar skull, and cribriform plate fractures are relative contraindications to nasotracheal intubation. Evidence of nasal fracture, raccoon eyes (bilateral ecchymosis in the periorbital region), Battle's sign (postauricular ecchymosis), and possible cerebrospinal fluid (CSF) leaks (rhinorrhea or otorrhea) are all signs of these injuries. Precautions regarding c-spine immobilization should be followed, as with orotracheal intubation.

If the decision to perform orotracheal intubation is made, the two-person technique with manual inline stabilization is necessary (■ FIGURE 2-10).

Laryngeal manipulation by backward, upward, and rightward pressure (BURP) on the thyroid cartilage can aid in visualizing the vocal cords. Additional hands are required for drug administration and the BURP maneuver.

Alternative intubation devices have been developed over the years with the integration of video and optic imaging techniques. Their use in trauma patients may be beneficial in specific cases by experienced providers. Careful assessment of the situation, equipment, and personnel available is mandatory, and rescue plans must be available. See Skill Station II: Airway and Ventilatory Management, Skill II-D: Adult Orotracheal Intubation (with and without Gum Elastic Bougie Device, and Skill II-G: Infant Endotracheal Intubation.

An excellent tool when faced with a difficult airway is the Eschmann Tracheal Tube Introducer (ETTI), also known as the gum elastic bougie (GEB) (■ FIGURE 2-11). The GEB is used when vocal cords cannot be visualized on direct laryngoscopy. With the laryngoscope in place, the GEB is passed blindly beyond the epiglottis, with the angled tip positioned anteriorly (■ FIGURE 2-12 and ■ FIGURE 2-13). Tracheal position is confirmed by feeling clicks as the distal tip rubs along the cartilaginous tracheal rings (present in 65%–90% of GEB placements [■ FIGURE 2-14]), when the tube rotates to the right or left when entering the bronchus, or when the tube is held up at the bronchial tree (10%–13%), which is usually at about the 50-cm mark. None of these indications occur if the GEB has entered the esophagus.

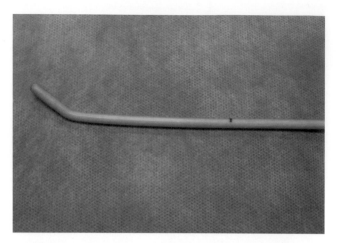

■ **FIGURE 2-11 Eschmann Tracheal Tube Introducer (ETTI).** This is also known as the gum elastic bougie.

? How do I know the tube is in the right place?

Following direct laryngoscopy and insertion of the orotracheal tube, the cuff is inflated, and assisted ventilation is instituted. Proper placement of the tube is suggested—but not confirmed—by hearing equal breath sounds bilaterally and detecting no borborygmi (i.e., rumbling or gurgling noises) in the epigastrium. The presence of borborygmi in the epigastrium with inspiration suggests esophageal intubation and warrants repositioning of the tube. A carbon dioxide detector (ideally a capnograph, but, if that is not available, a colorimetric CO_2 monitoring device) is indicated to help confirm proper intubation of the airway. The presence of CO_2 in exhaled air indicates that the airway has been successfully intubated, but does not ensure the correct position of the endotracheal tube. If CO_2 is not detected, esophageal intubation has occurred. Proper position of the tube is best confirmed by chest x-ray, once the possibility of esophageal intubation is excluded. Colorimetric CO_2 indicators are not useful for physiologic monitoring or assessing the adequacy of ventilation, which requires arterial blood gas analysis or continual end-tidal carbon dioxide analysis. See Skill Station II: Airway and Ventilatory Management, Skill II-H: Pulse Oximetry Monitoring, and Skill II-I: Carbon Dioxide Detection.

When the proper position of the tube is determined, it is secured in place. If the patient is moved, tube placement is reassessed by auscultation of both lateral lung fields for equality of breath sounds and by reassessment for exhaled CO_2.

If orotracheal intubation is unsuccessful on the first attempt or if the cords are difficult to visualize, a gum elastic bougie should be used, and further preparations for difficult airway should be undertaken.

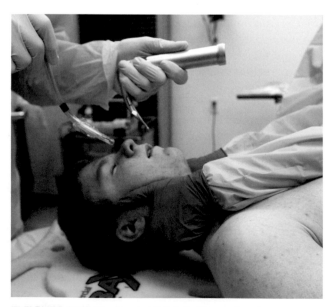

■ **FIGURE 2-10** Orotracheal intubation using two-person technique with inline cervical spine immobilization.

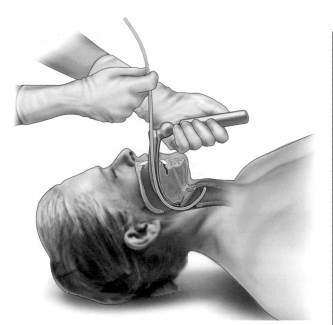

■ **FIGURE 2-12** Cervical spine immobilization needs to happen but has been eliminated from the image for clarity.

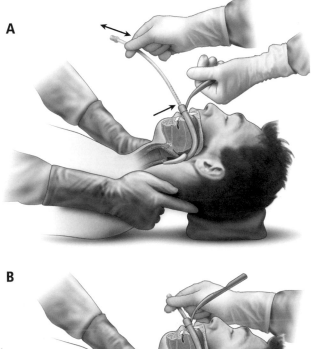

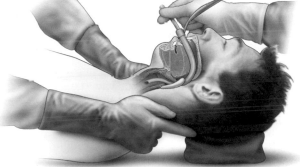

■ **FIGURE 2-13 Intubation through an "Intubating Laryngeal Mask."** Once the laryngeal mask is introduced, a dedicated endotracheal tube is inserted into it, allowing therefore a "blind" intubation technique.

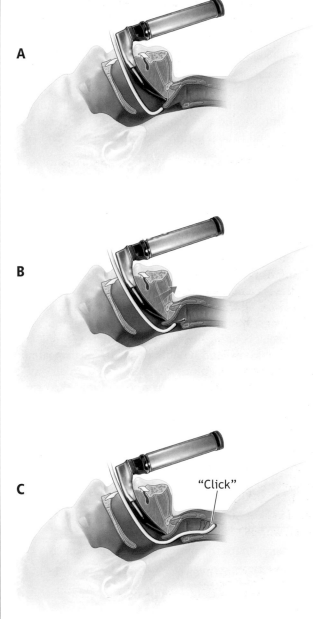

■ **FIGURE 2-14 Insertion of the GEB designed to aid in difficult intubations. (A)** The GEB is lubricated and directed posterior to the epiglottis with the tip angled anteriorly. **(B)** It slides under the epiglottis and is maneuvered in a semiblind or blind fashion anteriorly into the trachea. **(C)** Placement of the GEB into the trachea may be detected by the palpable "clicks" as the tip passes over the cartilaginous rings of the trachea.

Gum Elastic Bougie

Once the position is confirmed, the proximal end is lubricated, and a 6.0-cm internal diameter or larger endotracheal tube is passed over the GEB beyond the vocal cords. If the endotracheal tube is held up at the arytenoids or aryepiglottic folds, the tube is withdrawn slightly and turned 90 degrees to facilitate advancement beyond the obstruction. The GEB is then removed, and tube position is confirmed with the auscultation of breath sounds and capnography.

Use of the GEB has allowed for the rapid intubation of nearly 80 percent of prehospital patients in whom direct laryngoscopy is difficult.

Rapid Sequence Intubation

The use of anesthetic, sedative, and neuromuscular blocking drugs for endotracheal intubation in trauma patients, is potentially dangerous. In certain cases, the need for an airway justifies the risk of administering these drugs, but it is important to understand their pharmacology, be skilled in the techniques of endotracheal intubation, and be able to secure a surgical airway if necessary. In many cases in which an airway is acutely needed during the primary survey, the use of paralyzing or sedating drugs is not necessary.

The technique for rapid sequence intubation (RSI) is as follows:

1. Have a plan in the event of failure that includes the possibility of performing a surgical airway. Know where your rescue airway equipment is located.

2. Ensure that suction and the ability to deliver positive pressure ventilation are ready.

3. Preoxygenate the patient with 100% oxygen.

4. Apply pressure over the cricoid cartilage.

5. Administer an induction drug (e.g., etomidate, 0.3 mg/kg) or sedate, according to local practice.

6. Administer 1 to 2 mg/kg succinylcholine intravenously (usual dose is 100 mg).

7. After the patient relaxes, intubate the patient orotracheally.

8. Inflate the cuff and confirm tube placement by auscultating the patient's chest and determining the presence of CO_2 in exhaled air.

9. Release cricoid pressure.

10. Ventilate the patient.

The drug etomidate (Amidate) does not have a significant effect on blood pressure or intracranial pressure, but it can depress adrenal function and is not universally available. This drug does provide adequate sedation, which is advantageous in these patients. Etomidate and other sedatives must be used with great care to avoid loss of the airway as the patient becomes sedated. Then, succinylcholine, which is a short-acting drug, is administered. It has a rapid onset of paralysis (<1 minute) and a duration of 5 minutes or less.

The most dangerous complication of using sedation and neuromuscular blocking agents is the inability to establish an airway. If endotracheal intubation is unsuccessful, the patient must be ventilated with a bag-mask device until the paralysis resolves; long-acting drugs are not routinely used for RSI for this reason. Because of the potential for severe hyperkalemia, succinylcholine must be used carefully in patients with severe crush injuries, major burns, and electrical injuries. Particular attention must be paid in cases of preexisting chronic renal failure, chronic paralysis, and chronic neuromuscular disease.

Induction agents, such as thiopental and sedatives, are potentially dangerous in trauma patients with hypovolemia. Small doses of diazepam or midazolam are appropriate to reduce anxiety in paralyzed patients. Flumazenil must be available to reverse the sedative effects after benzodiazepines have been administered. Practice patterns, drug preferences, and specific procedures for airway management vary among institutions. The critical principle is that the individual using these techniques needs to be skilled in their use, knowledgeable of the inherent pitfalls associated with rapid sequence intubation, and capable of managing the potential complications.

PITFALLS

Equipment failure can occur at the most inopportune times and cannot always be anticipated. For example, the light on the laryngoscope burns out, the laryngoscope batteries are weak, the endotracheal tube cuff leaks, or the pulse oximeter does not function properly. Have spares available.

Surgical Airway

The inability to intubate the trachea is a clear indication for an alternate airway plan, including laryngeal mask airway, intubating laryngeal mask airway, or a surgical airway. A surgical airway (i.e., cricothyroidotomy or tracheostomy) is established when edema of the glottis, fracture of the larynx, or severe oropharyngeal hemorrhage obstructs the airway or an endotracheal tube cannot be placed through the vocal cords. A surgical cricothyroidotomy is preferable to a tracheostomy for most patients who require establishment of an emergency surgical airway, because it is easier to perform, associated with less bleeding, and requires less time to perform than an emergency tracheostomy.

Needle Cricothyroidotomy Needle cricothyroidotomy involves insertion of a needle through the cricothyroid membrane or into the trachea in an emergency situation to provide oxygen on a short-term basis until a definitive airway can be placed. Needle cricothyroidotomy can provide temporary, supplemental oxygenation so that intubation can be accomplished on an urgent rather than an emergent basis.

The jet insufflation technique is performed by placing a large-caliber plastic cannula, 12- to 14-gauge for adults, and 16- to 18-gauge in children, through the cricothyroid membrane into the trachea below the level of the obstruction (■ FIGURE 2-15). The cannula is then connected to oxygen at 15 L/min (40 to 50 psi) with a Y-connector or a side hole cut in the tubing between the oxygen source and the plastic cannula. Intermittent insufflation, 1 second on and 4 seconds off, can then be achieved by placing the thumb over the open end of the Y-connector or the side hole.

The patient can be adequately oxygenated for 30 to 45 minutes using this technique, and only patients with normal pulmonary function who do not have a significant chest injury may be oxygenated in this manner. During the 4 seconds that the oxygen is not being delivered under pressure, some exhalation occurs. Because of the inadequate exhalation, CO_2 slowly accumulates, limiting the use of this technique, especially in patients with head injuries. See Skill Station III: Cricothyroidotomy, Skill III-A: Needle Cricothyroidotomy.

Jet insufflation must be used with caution when complete foreign-body obstruction of the glottic area is suspected. Although high pressure can expel the impacted material into the hypopharynx, where it can be removed readily, significant barotrauma can occur, including pulmonary rupture with tension pneumothorax. Therefore, particular attention must be paid to effective airflow, and low flow rates (5 to 7 L/min) should be used when persistent glottic obstruction is present.

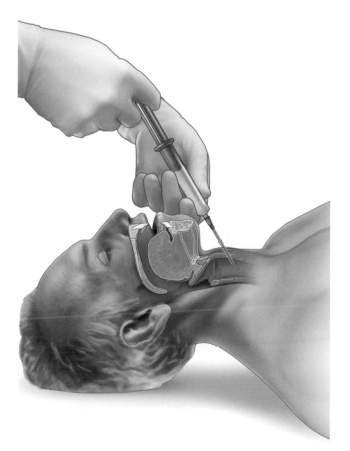

■ FIGURE 2-15 **Needle Cricothyroidotomy.** This procedure is performed by placing a large-caliber plastic cannula through the cricothyroid membrane into the trachea below the level of the obstruction.

> ## PITFALLS
>
> The inability to intubate a patient expediently, provide a temporary airway with a supraglottic device, or establish a surgical airway results in hypoxia and patient deterioration. Remember that performing a needle cricothyroidotomy with jet insufflation can provide the time necessary to establish a definitive airway.

Surgical Cricothyroidotomy Surgical cricothyroidotomy is performed by making a skin incision that extends through the cricothyroid membrane. A curved hemostat may be inserted to dilate the opening, and a small endotracheal tube or tracheostomy tube (preferably 5 to 7 mm OD) can be inserted. See Skill Station III: Cricothyroidotomy, Skill III-B: Surgical Cricothyroidotomy.

When an endotracheal tube is used, the cervical collar can be reapplied. It is possible for the endotracheal tube to become malpositioned and therefore easily advanced into a bronchus. Care must be taken, especially with children, to avoid damage to the cricoid cartilage, which is the only circumferential support for the upper trachea. Therefore, surgical cricothyroidotomy is not recommended for children under 12 years of age. See Chapter 10: Pediatric Trauma.

In recent years, percutaneous tracheostomy has been reported as an alternative to open tracheostomy. This is not a safe procedure in the acute trauma situation, because the patient's neck must be hyperextended to properly position the head to perform the procedure safely. Percutaneous tracheostomy requires the use of a heavy guidewire and sharp dilator, or a guidewire and multiple or single large-bore dilators. This procedure can be dangerous and time-consuming, depending on the type of equipment used.

> **Scenario ■ *continued***   You are able to increase oxygenation saturation to 92% again using bag-mask ventilation. Which advanced airway techniques will you use?

Management of Oxygenation

❓ *How do I know oxygenation is adequate?*

Oxygenated inspired air is best provided via a tight-fitting oxygen reservoir face mask with a flow rate of at least 11 L/min. Other methods (e.g., nasal catheter, nasal cannula, and nonrebreather mask) can improve inspired oxygen concentration.

Because changes in oxygenation occur rapidly and are impossible to detect clinically, pulse oximetry must be used at all times. It is invaluable when difficulties are anticipated in intubation or ventilation, including during transport of critically injured patients. Pulse oximetry is a noninvasive method of continuously measuring the oxygen saturation (O_2 sat) of arterial blood. It does not measure the partial pressure of oxygen (PaO_2) and, depending on the position of the oxyhemoglobin dissociation curve, the PaO_2 can vary widely (see Table 2.2). However, a measured saturation of 95% or greater by pulse oximetry is strong corroborating evidence of adequate peripheral arterial oxygenation (PaO_2 >70 mm Hg, or 9.3 kPa).

Pulse oximetry requires intact peripheral perfusion and cannot distinguish oxyhemoglobin from carboxyhemoglobin or methemoglobin, which limits its usefulness in patients with severe vasoconstriction and those with carbon monoxide poisoning. Profound anemia (hemoglobin <5 g/dL) and hypothermia (<30°C, or <86°F) decrease the reliability of the technique. However, in most trauma patients, pulse oximetry is useful, as the continuous monitoring of oxygen saturation provides an immediate assessment of therapeutic interventions.

Management of Ventilation

❓ *How do I know ventilation is adequate?*

Effective ventilation can be achieved by bag-mask techniques. However, one-person ventilation techniques using a bag-mask are less effective than two-person techniques in which both hands can be used to ensure a good seal. Bag-mask ventilation should be performed by two people whenever possible. See Skill Station II: Airway and Ventilatory Management, <u>Skill II-C: Bag-Mask Ventilation: Two-Person Technique</u>.

Intubation of patients with hypoventilation and/or apnea may not be successful initially and may require multiple attempts. The patient must be ventilated periodically during prolonged efforts to intubate. The clinician should practice taking a deep breath and holding it when intubation is first attempted. When the individual performing the intubation must breathe, the attempted intubation should be aborted and the patient ventilated.

With intubation of the trachea accomplished, assisted ventilation follows, using positive-pressure breathing techniques. A volume- or pressure-regulated respirator can be used, depending on availability of the equipment. The clinician should be alert to the complications of changes in intrathoracic pressure, which can convert a simple pneumothorax to a tension pneumothorax, or even create a pneumothorax secondary to barotrauma.

▶ PITFALLS

Gastric distention can occur when ventilating the patient with a bag-mask device, which can result in the patient vomiting and aspirating. It also can cause distention of the stomach against the vena cava, resulting in hypotension and bradycardia.

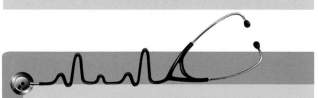

> **Scenario ■ conclusion**   You successfully intubated the patient using a GEB, confirmed correct placement with a colorimetric CO_2 exchanger and bilateral breath sounds, and ordered a chest radiograph.

■ TABLE 2.2
Approximate PaO_2 Versus O_2 Hemoglobin Saturation Levels

PaO_2 LEVELS	O_2 HEMOGLOBIN SATURATION LEVELS
90 mm Hg	100%
60 mm Hg	90%
30 mm Hg	60%
27 mm Hg	50%

Chapter Summary

1 Clinical situations in which airway compromise is likely to occur include maxillofacial trauma, neck trauma, laryngeal trauma, and airway obstruction.

2 Actual or impending airway obstruction should be suspected in all injured patients. Objective signs of airway obstruction include agitation, presentation with obtundation, cyanosis, abnormal sounds, and a displaced trachea.

3 Recognition of ventilatory compromise and ensuring accuracy of ventilations is of primary importance.

4 Techniques for establishing and maintaining a patent airway include the chin-lift and jaw-thrust maneuvers, oropharyngeal and nasopharyngeal airways, laryngeal mask airway, multilumen esophageal airway, and laryngeal tube airway. The selection of orotracheal or nasotracheal routes for intubation is based on the experience and skill level of the clinician. A surgical airway is indicated whenever an airway is needed and intubation is unsuccessful.

5 With all airway maneuvers, the cervical spine must be protected by inline immobilization.

6 The assessment of airway patency and adequacy of ventilation must be performed quickly and accurately. Pulse oximetry and end-tidal CO_2 measurement are essential.

7 A definitive airway requires a tube placed in the trachea with the cuff inflated below the vocal cords, the tube connected to some form of oxygen-enriched assisted ventilation, and the airway secured in place with tape. Examples of definitive airways include endotracheal intubation and surgical airways (e.g., needle cricothyroidotomy and surgical cricothyroidotomy). A definitive airway should be established if there is any doubt about the integrity of the patient's airway. A definitive airway should be placed early after the patient has been ventilated with oxygen-enriched air, to prevent prolonged periods of apnea.

8 Rapid sequence intubation or other pharmacologic assistance may be necessary in patients with active gag reflex.

9 To maintain a patient's oxygenation, oxygenated inspired air is best provided via a tight-fitting oxygen reservoir face mask with a flow rate of greater than 11 L/min. Other methods (e.g., nasal catheter, nasal cannula, and nonrebreather mask) can improve inspired oxygen concentration.

▶ BIBLIOGRAPHY

1. Alexander R, Hodgson P, Lomax D, Bullen C. A comparison of the laryngeal mask airway and Guedel airway, bag and facemask for manual ventilation following formal training. *Anaesthesia* 1993;48(3):231-234.

2. Aoi Y, Inagawa G, Hashimoto K, Tashima H, Tsuboi S, Takahata T, Nakamura K, Goto T. Airway scope laryngoscopy under manual inline stabilization and cervical collar immobilization: a crossover in vivo cinefluoroscopic study. *J Trauma* 2010;Aug 27.

3. Aprahamian C, Thompson BM, Finger WA, et al. Experimental cervical spine injury model: evaluation of airway management and splinting techniques. *Ann Emerg Med* 1984;13(8):584-587.

4. Arslan ZI, Yildiz T, Baykara ZN, Solak M, Toker K. Tracheal intubation in patients with rigid collar immobilisation of the cervical spine: a comparison of Airtraq and LMA CTrach devices. *Anaesthesia* 2009Dec;64(12):1332-6. Epub 2009;Oct 22.

5. Asai T, Shingu K. The laryngeal tube. *Br J Anaesth* 2005;95(6):729-736.

6. Bathory I, Frascarolo P, Kern C, Schoettker P. Evaluation of the GlideScope for tracheal intubation in patients with cervical spine immobilisation by a semi-rigid collar. *Anaesthesia* 2009Dec;64(12):1337-41.

7. Bergen JM, Smith DC. A review of etomidate for rapid sequence intubation in the emergency department. *J Emerg Med* 1997;15(2):221-230.

8. Brantigan CO, Grow JB Sr. Cricothyroidotomy: elective use in respiratory problems requiring tracheotomy. *J Thorac Cardiovasc Surg* 1976;71:72-81.

9. Combes X, Dumerat M, Dhonneur G. Emergency gum elastic bougie-assisted tracheal intubation in four patients with upper airway distortion. *Can J Anaesth* 2004;51(10):1022-1024.

10. Crosby ET, Cooper RM, Douglas MJ, et al. The unanticipated difficult airway with recommendations for management. *Can J Anaesth* 1998;45(8):757-776.

11. Danzl DF, Thomas DM. Nasotracheal intubation in the emergency department. *Crit Care Med* 1980;8(11):667-682.

12. Davies PR, Tighe SQ, Greenslade GL, Evans GH. Laryngeal mask airway and tracheal tube insertion by unskilled personnel. *Lancet* 1990;336(8721):977-979.

13. Dogra S, Falconer R, Latto IP. Successful difficult intubation. Tracheal tube placement over a gum-elastic bougie. *Anaesthesia* 1990;45(9):774-776.

14. Dorges V, Ocker H, Wenzel V, Sauer C, Schmucker P. Emergency airway management by non-anaesthesia house officers—a comparison of three strategies. *Emerg Med J* 2001;18(2):90-94.

15. El-Orbany MI, Salem MR, Joseph NJ. The Eschmann tracheal tube introducer is not gum, elastic, or a bougie. *Anesthesiology* 2004;101(5);1240; author reply 1242-1240; author reply 1244.

16. Frame SB, Simon JM, Kerstein MD, et al. Percutaneous transtracheal catheter ventilation (PTCV) in complete airway obstructions canine model. *J Trauma* 1989;29(6):774-781.

17. Fremstad JD, Martin SH. Lethal complication from insertion of nasogastric tube after severe basilar skull fracture. *J Trauma* 1978;18:820-822.

18. Gataure PS, Vaughan RS, Latto IP. Simulated difficult intubation: comparison of the gum elastic bougie and the stylet. *Anaesthesia* 1996;1:935-938.

19. Greenberg RS, Brimacombe J, Berry A, Gouze V, Piantadosi S, Dake EM. A randomized controlled trial comparing the cuffed oropharyngeal airway and the laryngeal mask airway in spontaneously breathing anesthetized adults. *Anesthesiology* 1998;88(4):970-977.

20. Grein AJ, Weiner GM. Laryngeal mask airway versus bag-mask ventilation or endotracheal intubation for neonatal resuscitation. *Cochrane Database Syst Rev* 2005;(2):CD003314.

21. Grmec S, Mally S. Prehospital determination of tracheal tube placement in severe head injury. *Emerg Med J* 2004;21(4):518-520.

22. Guildner CV. Resuscitation—opening the airway: a comparative study of techniques for opening an airway obstructed by the tongue. *J Am Coll Emerg Physicians* 1976;5:588-590.

23. Hagberg C, Bogomolny Y, Gilmore C, Gibson V, Kaitner M, Khurana S. An evaluation of the insertion and function of a new supraglottic airway device, the King LT, during spontaneous ventilation. *Anesth Analg* 2006;102(2):621-625.

24. Iserson KV. Blind nasotracheal intubation. *Ann Emerg Med* 1981;10:468.

25. Jabre P, Combes X, Leroux B, Aaron E, Auger H, Margenet A, Dhonneur G. Use of the gum elastic bougie for prehospital difficult intubation. *Am J Emerg Med* 2005;23(4):552-555.

26. Jorden RC, Moore EE, Marx JA, et al. A comparison of PTV and endotracheal ventilation in an acute trauma model. *J Trauma* 1985;25(10):978-983.

27. Kidd JF, Dyson A, Latto IP. Successful difficult intubation. Use of the gum elastic bougie. *Anaesthesia* 1988;43:437-438.

28. Kress TD, et al. Cricothyroidotomy. *Ann Emerg Med* 1982;11:197.

29. Latto IP, Stacey M, Mecklenburgh J, Vaughan RS. Survey of the use of the gum elastic bougie in clinical practice. *Anaesthesia* 2002;57(4):379-384.

30. Levinson MM, Scuderi PE, Gibson RL, et al. Emergency percutaneous and transtracheal ventilation. *J Am Coll Emerg Physicians* 1979;8(10):396-400.

31. Levitan R, Ochroch EA. Airway management and direct laryngoscopy. A review and update. *Crit Care Clin* 2000;16(3):373-88, v.

32. Liu EH, Goy RW, Tan BH, Asai T. Tracheal intubation with videolaryngoscopes in patients with cervical spine

immobilization: a randomized trial of the Airway Scope and the GlideScope. *Br J Anaesth* 2009 Sep;103(3):446-51.

33. Macintosh RR. An aid to oral intubation. *BMJ* 1949;1:28.

34. Majernick TG, Bieniek R, Houston JB, et al: Cervical spine movement during orotracheal intubation. *Ann Emerg Med* 1986;15(4):417-420.

35. Morton T, Brady S, Clancy M. Difficult airway equipment in English emergency departments. *Anaesthesia* 2000;55(5):485-488.

36. Nocera A. A flexible solution for emergency intubation difficulties. *Ann Emerg Med* 1996;27(5):665-667.

37. Noguchi T, Koga K, Shiga Y, Shigematsu A. The gum elastic bougie eases tracheal intubation while applying cricoid pressure compared to a stylet. *Can J Anaesth* 2003;50(7):712-717.

38. Nolan JP, Wilson ME. An evaluation of the gum elastic bougie. Intubation times and incidence of sore throat. *Anaesthesia* 1992;47(10):878-881.

39. Nolan JP, Wilson ME. Orotracheal intubation in patients with potential cervical spine injuries. An indication for the gum elastic bougie. *Anaesthesia* 1993;48(7):630-633.

40. Oczenski W, Krenn H, Dahaba AA, et al. Complications following the use of the Combitube, tracheal tube and laryngeal mask airway. *Anaesthesia* 1999;54(12):1161-1165.

41. Pennant JH, Pace NA, Gajraj NM. Role of the laryngeal mask airway in the immobile cervical spine. *J Clin Anesth* 1993;5(3):226-230.

42. Phelan MP. Use of the endotracheal bougie introducer for difficult intubations. *Am J Emerg Med* 2004;22(6):479-482.

43. Reed MJ, Dunn MJ, McKeown DW. Can an airway assessment score predict difficulty at intubation in the emergency department? *Emerg Med J* 2005;22(2):99-102.

44. Reed MJ, Rennie LM, Dunn MJ, Gray AJ, Robertson CE, McKeown DW. Is the "LEMON" method an easily applied emergency airway assessment tool? *Eur J Emerg Med* 2004;11(3);154-157.

45. Russi C, Miller L. An out-of-hospital comparison of the King LT to endotracheal intubation and the Esophageal-Tracheal Combitube in a simulated difficult airway patient encounter [in process citation]. *Acad Emerg Med* 2007;14(5 Suppl 1):S22.

46. Seshul MB Sr, Sinn DP, Gerlock AJ Jr. The Andy Gump fracture of the mandible: a cause of respiratory obstruction or distress. *J Trauma* 1978;18:611-612.

47. Silvestri S, Ralls GA, Krauss B, et al. The effectiveness of out-of-hospital use of continuous end-tidal carbon dioxide monitoring on the rate of unrecognized misplaced intubation within a regional emergency medical services system. *Ann Emerg Med* 2005;45(5):497-503.

48. Smith CE, Dejoy SJ. New equipment and techniques for airway management in trauma [In Process Citation]. *Curr Opin Anaesthesiol* 2001;14(2):197-209.

49. Walter J, Doris PE, Shaffer MA. Clinical presentation of patients with acute cervical spine injury. *Ann Emerg Med* 1984;13(7):512-515.

50. Yeston NS. Noninvasive measurement of blood gases. *Infect Surg* 1990;90:18-24.

Airway and Ventilatory Management

Objectives

Performance at this skill station will allow participants to evaluate a series of clinical situations and acquire the cognitive skills for decision making in airway and ventilatory management. Students will practice and demonstrate the following skills on adult and infant intubation manikins:

1 Insert oropharyngeal and nasopharyngeal airways.

2 Using both oral and nasal routes, intubate the trachea of an adult intubation manikin (within the guidelines listed), provide effective ventilation, and use capnography to determine proper placement of the endotracheal tube.

3 Describe and demonstrate methods for managing difficult or failed airways, including laryngeal mask airway (LMA), intubating laryngeal mask airway (ILMA), laryngeal tube airway (LTA), and gum elastic bougie (GEB).

4 Intubate the trachea of an infant intubation manikin with an endotracheal tube (within the guidelines listed) and provide effective ventilation.

5 Describe how trauma affects airway management when performing oral endotracheal intubation and nasotracheal intubation.

6 Using a pulse oximeter:

- State the purpose of pulse oximetry monitoring.
- Demonstrate the proper use of the device.
- Describe the indications for its use, its functional limits of accuracy, and possible reasons for malfunction or inaccuracy.
- Accurately interpret the pulse oximeter monitor readings and relate their significance to the care of trauma patients.

7 Describe the indications for and use of end-tidal CO_2 detector devices.

▶ SCENARIOS

SCENARIO II-1

A 22-year-old male is an unrestrained passenger in a motor vehicle that collides head-on into a retaining wall. He has a strong odor of alcohol on his breath. At the time of the collision, he hits the windshield and sustains a scalp laceration. At the injury scene, he is combative, and his GCS score is 11. His blood pressure is 120/70 mm Hg, his heart rate is 100 beats/min, and his respirations are 20 breaths/min. A semirigid cervical collar is applied, and he is immobilized on a long backboard. He is receiving oxygen via a high-flow oxygen mask. Shortly after his arrival in the ED, he begins to vomit.

SCENARIO II-2

The patient described in Scenario II-1 is now unresponsive and has undergone endotracheal intubation. Ventilation with 100% oxygen is being applied. Part of his evaluation includes a CT scan of his brain. After he is transported to radiology for the scan, the pulse oximeter reveals 82% SaO2.

SCENARIO II-3

A 3-year-old, unrestrained, front-seat passenger is injured when her car crashes into a stone wall. The child is unconscious at the injury scene. In the ED, bruises to her forehead, face, and chest wall are noted, and there is blood around her mouth. The patient's blood pressure is 105/70 mm Hg, heart rate is 120 beats/minute, and respirations are rapid and shallow. Her GCS score is 8.

SCENARIO II-4

A 35-year-old male sustains blunt chest trauma during a single-motor-vehicle collision. In the ED, he is alert with evidence of a right chest-wall contusion. He has point tenderness and fracture crepitation of several right ribs. His GCS score is 14. He is immobilized with a semirigid cervical spine collar and secured to a long backboard. High-flow oxygen is being administered via a face mask.

▶ Skill II-A: Oropharyngeal Airway Insertion

Note: This procedure is used for temporary ventilation while preparing to intubate an unconscious patient.

STEP 1. Select the proper-size airway. A correctly sized airway extends from the corner of the patient's mouth to the ear lobe.

STEP 2. Open the patient's mouth with the chin-lift maneuver or crossed-finger technique (scissors technique).

STEP 3. Insert a tongue blade on top of the patient's tongue far enough back to depress the tongue adequately. Be careful not to cause the patient to gag.

STEP 4. Insert the airway posteriorly, gently sliding the airway over the curvature of the tongue until the device's flange rests on top of the patient's lips. The airway must not push the tongue backward and block the airway. An alternate technique for airway insertion, termed the rotation method, involves inserting the oropharyngeal airway upside down so its tip is facing the roof of the patient's mouth. As the airway is inserted, it is rotated 180 degrees until the flange comes to rest on the patient's lips and/or teeth. This maneuver should not be used in children.

STEP 5. Remove the tongue blade.

STEP 6. Ventilate the patient with a bag-mask device.

▶ Skill II-B: Nasopharyngeal Airway Insertion

Note: This procedure is used when the patient would gag on an oropharyngeal airway.

STEP 1. Assess the nasal passages for any apparent obstruction (e.g., polyps, fractures, or hemorrhage).

STEP 2. Select the proper-size airway, which will easily pass the selected nostril.

STEP 3. Lubricate the nasopharyngeal airway with a water-soluble lubricant or tap water.

STEP 4. Insert the tip of the airway into the nostril and direct it posteriorly and toward the ear.

STEP 5. Gently insert the nasopharyngeal airway through the nostril into the hypopharynx with a slight rotating motion until the flange rests against the nostril.

STEP 6. Ventilate the patient with a bag-mask device.

▶ Skill II-C: Bag-Mask Ventilation: Two-Person Technique

STEP 1. Select the proper-size mask to fit the patient's face.

STEP 2. Connect the oxygen tubing to the bag-mask device and adjust the flow of oxygen to 15 L/min.

STEP 3. Ensure that the patient's airway is patent and secured according to previously described techniques.

STEP 4. The first person applies the mask to the patient's face, performing a jaw-thrust maneuver and ascertaining a tight seal with both hands.

STEP 5. The second person applies ventilation by squeezing the bag with both hands.

STEP 6. Assess the adequacy of ventilation by observing the patient's chest movement.

STEP 7. Ventilate the patient in this manner every 5 seconds.

▶ Skill II-D: Adult Orotracheal Intubation

(With and without Gum Elastic Bougie device)

STEP 1. Ensure proper sterilization.

STEP 2. Inspect all components for visible damage.

STEP 3. Examine the interior of the airway tube to ensure that it is free from blockage and loose particles.

STEP 4. Ensure that adequate ventilation and oxygenation are in progress and that suctioning equipment is immediately available in case the patient vomits.

STEP 5. Inflate the cuff of the endotracheal tube to ascertain that the balloon does not leak, and then deflate the cuff.

STEP 6. Connect the laryngoscope blade to the handle and check the light bulb for brightness.

STEP 7. Assess the patient's airway for ease of intubation, using the LEMON mnemonic. (Box 2-1, page 36.)

STEP 8. Direct an assistant to manually immobilize the head and neck. The patient's neck must not be hyperextended or hyperflexed during the procedure.

STEP 9. Hold the laryngoscope in the left hand.

STEP 10. Insert the laryngoscope into the right side of the patient's mouth, displacing the tongue to the left.

STEP 11. Visually identify the epiglottis and then the vocal cords. External laryngeal manipulation with backward, upward, and rightward pressure (BURP) may be helpful for better visualization.

STEP 12. Gently insert the endotracheal tube into the trachea without applying pressure on the teeth or oral tissues.

STEP 13. Inflate the cuff with enough air to provide an adequate seal. **Do not overinflate the cuff.**

STEP 14. Check the placement of the endotracheal tube by applying bag-to-tube ventilation.

STEP 15. Visually observe chest-valve (bag-valve) excursions with ventilation.

STEP 16. Auscultate the chest and abdomen with a stethoscope to ascertain tube position.

Placement of the tube must be checked carefully. A chest x-ray exam is helpful to assess the position of the tube, but it cannot exclude esophageal intubation.

STEP 17. If endotracheal intubation is not accomplished within seconds or in the same time required to hold your breath before exhaling, discontinue attempts, apply ventilation with a bag-mask device, and try again using a GEB.

STEP 18. Secure the tube. If the patient is moved, the tube placement should be reassessed.

STEP 19. Attach a CO_2 detector to the endotracheal tube between the adapter and the ventilating device to confirm the position of the endotracheal tube in the airway.

STEP 20. Attach a pulse oximeter to one of the patient's fingers (intact peripheral perfusion must exist) to measure and monitor the patient's oxygen saturation levels and provide an immediate assessment of therapeutic interventions.

▶ Skill II-E: Laryngeal Mask Airway (LMA) and Intubating LMA (ILMA) Insertion

STEP 1. Ensure proper sterilization.

STEP 2. Inspect all components for visible damage.

STEP 3. Examine the interior of the airway tube to ensure that it is free from blockage and loose particles.

STEP 4. Ensure that adequate ventilation and oxygenation are in progress and that suctioning equipment is immediately available in case the patient vomits.

STEP 5. Inflate the cuff of the LMA/ILMA to ascertain that the balloon does not leak.

STEP 6. Direct an assistant to manually immobilize the head and neck. The patient's neck must not be hyperextended or hyperflexed during the procedure.

STEP 7. Before attempting insertion, completely deflate the LMA/ILMA cuff by pressing it firmly onto a flat surface, and then lubricate it.

STEP 8. Choose the correct size LMA/ILMA: 3 for a small female, 4 for a large female or small male, and 5 for a large male.

STEP 9. Hold the LMA/ILMA with the dominant hand as you would a pen, with the index finger placed at the junction of the cuff and the shaft and the LMA/ILMA opening oriented over the tongue.

STEP 10. Pass the LMA/ILMA behind the upper incisors, with the shaft parallel to the patient's chest and the index finger pointing toward the intubator.

STEP 11. Push the lubricated LMA/ILMA into position along the palatopharyngeal curve, with the index finger maintaining pressure on the tube and guiding the LMA/ILMA into the final position.

STEP 12. Inflate the cuff with the correct volume of air (indicated on the shaft of the LMA/ILMA).

STEP 13. Check the placement of the LMA/ILMA by applying bag-mask-to-tube ventilation.

STEP 14. Visually observe chest excursions with ventilation.

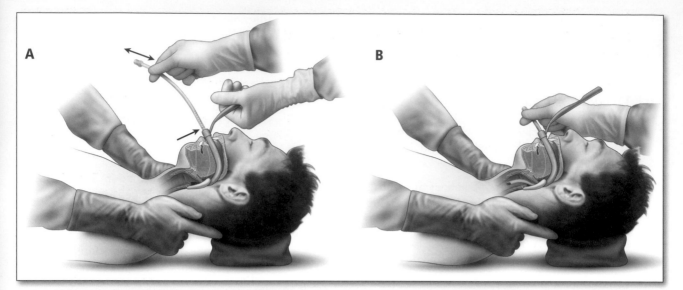

■ **FIGURE II-1 Intubation through an "Intubating Laryngeal Mask."** Once the laryngeal mask is introduced, a dedicated endotracheal tube is inserted into it, allowing therefore a "blind" intubation technique.

STEP 15. If ILMA is available, careful intubation through the ILMA may be attempted (■ **FIGURE II-1**). Inflate the cuff of the endotracheal tube to ascertain that the balloon does not leak, and then deflate the cuff.

STEP 16. Lubricate the endotracheal tube with a water-soluble lubricant.

STEP 17. Carefully insert the lubricated tube into the ILMA.

STEP 18. Inflate the cuff with enough air to provide an adequate seal. **Do not overinflate the cuff.**

STEP 19. Check the placement of the endotracheal tube by applying bag-mask-to-tube ventilation.

STEP 20. Visually observe chest excursions with ventilation.

STEP 21. Auscultate the chest and abdomen with a stethoscope to ascertain tube position.

STEP 22. If endotracheal intubation is not accomplished within seconds or in the same time required to hold your breath before exhaling, discontinue attempts and apply ventilation with a bag-mask device connected to the ILMA.

STEP 23. Secure the tube. If the patient is moved, tube placement should be reassessed.

Note: Removal of the ILMA ideally should be performed in a hospital, due to the risk of accidentally extubating the patient during the maneuver.

▶ Skill II-F: Laryngeal Tube Airway (LTA) Insertion

STEP 1. Ensure proper sterilization.

STEP 2. Inspect all components for visible damage.

STEP 3. Examine the interior of the airway tube to ensure that it is free from blockage and loose particles.

STEP 4. Inflate the cuffs by injecting the maximum recommended volume of air into the cuffs.

STEP 5. Select the correct laryngeal tube size.

STEP 6. Apply a water-soluble lubricant to the beveled distal tip and posterior aspect of the tube, taking care to avoid introduction of lubricant into or near the ventilatory openings.

STEP 7. Preoxygenate the patient.

STEP 8. Achieve the appropriate depth of anesthesia.

STEP 9. Direct an assistant to manually immobilize the head and neck. The patient's neck must not be hyper-extended or hyperflexed during the procedure.

STEP 10. Hold the LTA at the connector with the dominant hand. With the nondominant hand, hold the mouth open and apply the chin-lift maneuver.

STEP 11. With the LTA rotated laterally 45 to 90 degrees, introduce the tip into the mouth and advance it behind the base of the tongue.

STEP 12. Rotate the tube back to the midline as the tip reaches the posterior wall of the pharynx.

STEP 13. Without exerting excessive force, advance the LTA until the base of the connector is aligned with the patient's teeth or gums.

STEP 14. Inflate the LTA cuffs to the minimum volume necessary to seal the airway at the peak ventilatory pressure used (just seal volume).

STEP 15. While gently bagging the patient to assess ventilation, simultaneously withdraw the airway until ventilation is easy and free flowing (large tidal volume with minimal airway pressure).

STEP 16. Reference marks are provided at the proximal end of the LTA; when aligned with the upper teeth, these marks indicate the depth of insertion.

STEP 17. Confirm proper position by auscultation, chest movement, and verification of CO_2 by capnography.

STEP 18. Readjust cuff inflation to seal volume.

STEP 19. Secure LTA to patient using tape or other accepted means. A bite block can also be used, if desired.

▶ Skill II-G: Infant Endotracheal Intubation

STEP 1. Ensure proper sterilization.

STEP 2. Inspect all components for visible damage.

STEP 3. Examine the interior of the airway tube to ensure that it is free from blockage and loose particles.

STEP 4. Ensure that adequate ventilation and oxygenation are in progress and that suctioning equipment is immediately available in case the patient vomits.

STEP 5. Select the proper-size tube, which should be the same size as the infant's nostril or little finger.

STEP 6. Connect the laryngoscope blade and handle; check the light bulb for brightness.

STEP 7. Direct an assistant to manually immobilize the head and neck. The patient's neck must not be hyper-extended or hyperflexed during the procedure.

STEP 8. Hold the laryngoscope in the left hand.

STEP 9. Insert the laryngoscope blade into the right side of the mouth, moving the tongue to the left.

STEP 10. Observe the epiglottis and then the vocal cords. External laryngeal manipulation with

BURP may be helpful for better visualization.

STEP 11. Insert the endotracheal tube not more than 2 cm past the cords.

STEP 12. Check the placement of the tube by applying bag-mask-to-tube ventilation, observing lung inflations, and auscultating the chest and abdomen with a stethoscope. Placement of the tube must be checked carefully. Chest x-ray examination may be helpful to assess the position of the tube, but it cannot exclude esophageal intubation.

STEP 13. If endotracheal intubation is not accomplished within 30 seconds or in the same time required to hold your breath before exhaling,

discontinue attempts, ventilate the patient with a bag-mask device, and try again.

STEP 14. Secure the tube. If the patient is moved, tube placement should be reassessed.

STEP 15. Attach a CO_2 detector to the secured endotracheal tube between the adapter and the ventilating device to confirm the position of the endotracheal tube in the trachea.

STEP 16. Attach a pulse oximeter to one of the patient's fingers (intact peripheral perfusion must exist) to measure and monitor the patient's oxygen saturation levels and provide an immediate assessment of therapeutic interventions.

▶ Skill II-H: Pulse Oximetry Monitoring

The pulse oximeter is designed to measure oxygen saturation and pulse rate in peripheral circulation. This device is a microprocessor that calculates the percentage saturation of oxygen in each pulse of arterial blood that flows past a sensor. It simultaneously calculates the heart rate.

The pulse oximeter works by a low-intensity light beamed from a light-emitting diode (LED) to a light-receiving photodiode. Two thin beams of light, one red and the other infrared, are transmitted through blood and body tissue, and a portion is absorbed by the blood and body tissue. The photodiode measures the portion of the light that passes through the blood and body tissue. The relative amount of light absorbed by oxygenated hemoglobin differs from that absorbed by nonoxygenated hemoglobin. The microprocessor evaluates these differences in the arterial pulse and reports the values as calculated oxyhemoglobin saturation ($\%SaO_2$). Measurements are reliable and correlate well when compared with a cooximeter that directly measures SaO_2.

However, pulse oximetry is unreliable when the patient has poor peripheral perfusion, a condition that can be caused by vasoconstriction, hypotension, a blood pressure cuff that is inflated above the sensor, hypothermia, and other causes of poor blood flow. Severe anemia can likewise influence the reading. Significantly high levels of carboxyhemoglobin or methemoglobin can cause abnormalities, and circulating dye (e.g., indocyanine green and methylene blue) can interfere with the measurement. Excessive patient movement, other electrical devices, and intense ambient light can cause pulse oximeters to malfunction.

Using a pulse oximeter requires knowledge of the particular device being used. Different sensors are appropriate for different patients. The fingertip and earlobe are common sites for sensor application; however, both of these areas can be subject to vasoconstriction. The fingertip or toe tip of an injured extremity or below a blood pressure cuff should not be used.

When analyzing pulse oximetry results, evaluate the initial readings. Does the pulse rate correspond to the electrocardiographic monitor? Is the oxygen saturation appropriate? If the pulse oximeter is giving low readings or very poor readings, look for a physiologic cause, not a mechanical one.

The relationship between partial pressure of oxygen in arterial blood (PaO_2) and $\%SaO_2$ is shown in ■ **FIGURE II-2**. The sigmoid shape of this curve indicates that the relationship between $\%SaO_2$ and PaO_2 is nonlinear. This is particularly important in the middle range of this curve, where small changes in PaO_2 will effect large changes in saturation. Remember, the pulse oximeter measures arterial oxygen saturation, not arterial oxygen partial pressure. Also see Table 2.2: Approximate PaO2 versus O2 Hemoglobin Saturation Levels in Chapter 2: Airway and Ventilatory Management.

Standard blood gas measurements report both PaO_2 and $\%SaO_2$. When oxygen saturation is calculated from blood gas PaO_2, the calculated value can differ from the oxygen saturation measured by the pulse oximeter. This difference can occur because an oxygen saturation value that has been calculated from the blood gas PaO_2 has not necessarily been correctly adjusted for the effects of variables that shift the relationship between PaO_2 and saturation. These variables include temperature, pH, $PaCO_2$ (partial pressure of carbon dioxide), 2,3-DPG (diphosphoglycerates), and the concentration of fetal hemoglobin.

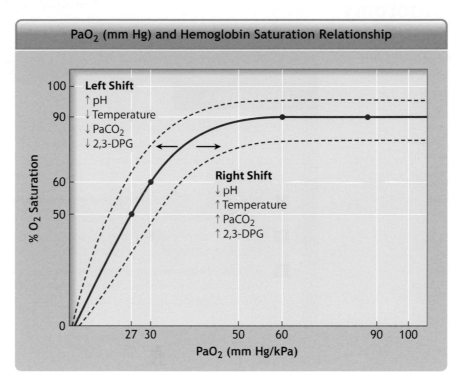

■ **FIGURE II-2** Relationship between partial pressure of oxygen in arterial blood (PaO_2) and $\%SaO_2$.

▶ Skill II-I: Carbon Dioxide Detection

When a patient is intubated, it is essential to check the position of the endotracheal tube. If carbon dioxide is detected in the exhaled air, the tube is in the airway. Methods of determining end-tidal CO_2 should be readily available in all emergency departments and any other locations where patients require intubation. The preferred method is quantitative, such as capnography, capnometry, or mass spectroscopy.

Colorimetric devices use a chemically treated indicator strip that generally reflects the CO_2 level. At very low levels of CO_2, such as atmospheric air, the indicator turns purple. At higher CO_2 levels (e.g., 2%–5%), the indicator turns yellow. A tan color indicates detection of CO_2 levels that are generally lower than those found in the exhaled tracheal gases.

It is important to note that, on rare occasion, patients with gastric distention can have elevated CO_2 levels in the esophagus. These elevated levels clear rapidly after several breaths, and the results of the colorimetric test should not be used until after at least six breaths. If the colorimetric device still shows an intermediate range, six additional breaths should be taken or given. If the patient sustains a cardiac arrest and has no cardiac output, CO_2 is not delivered to the lungs. In fact, with cardiac asystole, this can be a method of determining whether cardiopulmonary resuscitation is adequate.

The colorimetric device is not used for the detection of elevated CO_2 levels. Similarly, it is not used to detect a mainstem bronchial intubation. Physical and chest x-ray examinations are required to determine that the endotracheal tube is properly positioned in the airway. In a noisy ED or when the patient is transported several times, this device is extremely reliable in differentiating between tracheal and esophageal intubation.

Cricothyroidotomy

Objectives

Performance at this skill station will allow students to practice and demonstrate the techniques of needle cricothyroidotomy and surgical cricothyroidotomy on a live, anesthetized animal, fresh human cadaver, or anatomic human body manikin.

1 Identify the surface markings and structures relevant to performing needle and surgical cricothyroidotomies.

2 State the indications and complications of needle and surgical cricothyroidotomies.

3 Perform needle and surgical cricothyroidotomies on a live, anesthetized animal, fresh human cadaver, or anatomic human body manikin, as outlined in this skill station.

▶ Skill III-A: Needle Cricothyroidotomy

STEP 1. Assemble and prepare oxygen tubing by cutting a hole toward one end of the tubing. Connect the other end of the oxygen tubing to an oxygen source capable of delivering 50 psi or greater at the nipple, and ensure the free flow of oxygen through the tubing.

STEP 2. Place the patient in a supine position.

STEP 3. Assemble a 12- or 14-gauge, 8.5-cm, over-the-needle catheter to a 6- to 12-mL syringe.

STEP 4. Surgically prepare the neck, using antiseptic swabs.

STEP 5. Palpate the cricothyroid membrane anteriorly between the thyroid cartilage and the cricoid cartilage. Stabilize the trachea with the thumb and forefinger of one hand to prevent lateral movement of the trachea during the procedure.

STEP 6. Puncture the skin in the midline with a 12- or 14-gauge needle attached to a syringe, directly over the cricothyroid membrane (i.e., midsagittally) (■ FIGURE III-1).

STEP 7. Direct the needle at a 45-degree angle caudally, while applying negative pressure to the syringe.

STEP 8. Carefully insert the needle through the lower half of the cricothyroid membrane, aspirating as the needle is advanced.

STEP 9. Note the aspiration of air, which signifies entry into the tracheal lumen.

STEP 10. Remove the syringe and withdraw the stylet, while gently advancing the catheter downward into position, taking care not to perforate the posterior wall of the trachea (■ FIGURE III-2).

STEP 11. Attach the oxygen tubing over the catheter needle hub, and secure the catheter to the patient's neck.

STEP 12. Apply intermittent ventilation by occluding the open hole cut into the oxygen tubing with your thumb for 1 second and releasing it for 4 seconds. After releasing your thumb from the hole in the tubing, passive

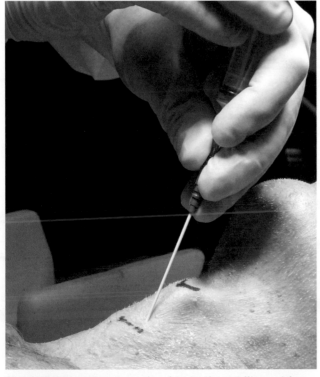

■ **FIGURE III-1** Puncture the skin in the midline with a 12- or 14-gauge needle attached to a syringe, directly over the cricothyroid membrane.

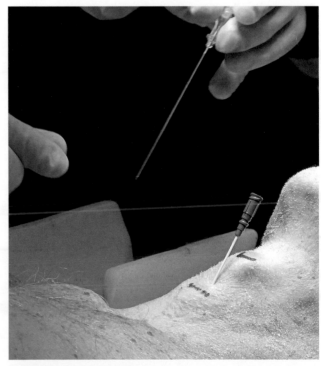

■ **FIGURE III-2** Remove the syringe and withdraw the stylet, while gently advancing the catheter downward into position, taking care not to perforate the posterior wall of the trachea.

exhalation occurs. Note: Adequate PaO_2 can be maintained for only 30 to 45 minutes, and CO_2 accumulation can occur more rapidly.

STEP 13. Continue to observe lung inflation and auscultate the chest for adequate ventilation. Pay special attention to lung deflation in order to avoid barotrauma, which can lead to pneumothorax. If lung deflation is not observed, gentle manual rib cage compression to aid exhalation may be necessary.

▶▶ COMPLICATIONS OF NEEDLE CRICOTHYROIDOTOMY

- Inadequate ventilation, leading to hypoxia and death
- Aspiration (blood)
- Esophageal laceration
- Hematoma
- Perforation of the posterior tracheal wall
- Subcutaneous and/or mediastinal emphysema
- Thyroid perforation
- Pneumothorax

▶ Skill III-B: Surgical Cricothyroidotomy

STEP 1. Place the patient in a supine position with the neck in a neutral position.

STEP 2. Palpate the thyroid notch, cricothyroid interval, and sternal notch for orientation (■ FIGURE III-3A).

STEP 3. Assemble the necessary equipment.

STEP 4. Surgically prepare and anesthetize the area locally, if the patient is conscious.

STEP 5. Stabilize the thyroid cartilage with the left hand and maintain stabilization until the trachea is intubated.

STEP 6. Make a transverse skin incision over the cricothyroid membrane and carefully incise through the membrane transversely (■ FIGURE III-3B). **Caution:** Do not cut or remove the cricoid and/or thyroid cartilages.

STEP 7. Insert hemostat or tracheal spreader into the incision and rotate it 90 degrees to open the airway (■ FIGURE III-3C).

STEP 8. Insert a proper-size, cuffed endotracheal tube or tracheostomy tube (usually a

number 5 or 6) into the cricothyroid membrane incision, directing the tube distally into the trachea (■ FIGURE III-3D).

STEP 9. Inflate the cuff and apply ventilation.

STEP 10. Observe lung inflation and auscultate the chest for adequate ventilation.

STEP 11. Secure the endotracheal or tracheostomy tube to the patient to prevent dislodging.

▶▶ COMPLICATIONS OF SURGICAL CRICOTHYROIDOTOMY

- Aspiration (blood)
- Creation of a false passage into the tissues
- Subglottic stenosis/edema
- Laryngeal stenosis
- Hemorrhage or hematoma formation
- Laceration of the esophagus
- Laceration of the trachea
- Mediastinal emphysema
- Vocal cord paralysis, hoarseness

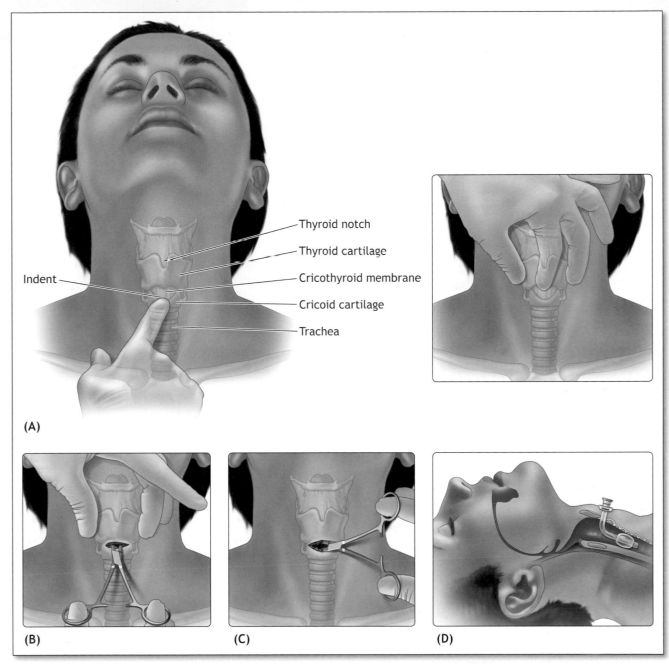

Indent

Thyroid notch
Thyroid cartilage
Cricothyroid membrane
Cricoid cartilage
Trachea

(A)

(B)

(C)

(D)

■ **FIGURE III.3 Surgical Cricothyroidotomy. (A)** Palpate the thyroid notch, cricothyroid interval, and the sternal notch for orientation. **(B)** Make a transverse skin incision over the cricothyroid membrane and carefully incise through the membrane transversely. **(C)** Insert hemostat or tracheal spreader into the incision and rotate it 90 degrees to open the airway. **(D)** Insert a proper-size, cuffed endotracheal tube or tracheostomy tube into the cricothyroid membrane incision, directing the tube distally into the trachea.

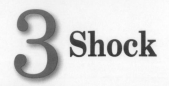

3 Shock

The diagnosis of shock is based on clinical recognition of the presence of inadequate tissue perfusion and oxygenation; the first step in the initial management of shock is to recognize its presence.

Scenario A 28-year-old unrestrained driver is involved in a motor vehicle collision. She is confused and anxious, but is able to tell you her name. Her respiratory rate is 28, pulse 126, and blood pressure 96/70 mm Hg.

Outline

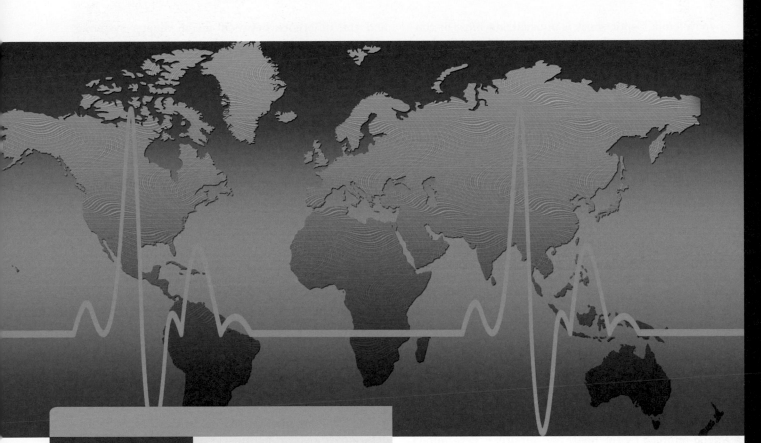

Objectives

1. Define shock and apply this definition to clinical practice.

2. Recognize shock and correlate a patient's acute clinical signs with the degree of volume deficit.

3. Explain the importance of early identification and control of the source of hemorrhage in trauma patients.

4. Compare and contrast the clinical presentation of patients with various classifications of hemorrhage.

5. Describe the initial management of hemorrhagic shock and the ongoing evaluation of fluid resuscitation and organ perfusion.

6. Recognize the physiologic responses to resuscitation in order to continually reassess the patient's response and avoid complications.

7. Explain the role of blood replacement in the management of shock.

8. Describe the special considerations in the diagnosis and treatment of shock, including equating blood pressure with cardiac output, advanced age, athletes, pregnancy, medications, hypothermia, and pacemakers.

The first step in the initial management of shock in trauma patients is to recognize its presence. No vital sign and no laboratory test can diagnose shock; rather, the initial diagnosis is based on clinical recognition of the presence of inadequate tissue perfusion and oxygenation. The definition of shock—an abnormality of the circulatory system that results in inadequate organ perfusion and tissue oxygenation—also becomes an operative tool for diagnosis and treatment.

The second step in the initial management of shock is to identify the probable cause of the shock state. In trauma patients, this process is directly related to the mechanism of injury. Most injured patients in shock have hypovolemia, but they may suffer from cardiogenic, obstructive, neurogenic, and, rarely, septic shock. Tension pneumothorax can reduce venous return and produce obstructive shock, and cardiac tamponade also produces obstructive shock, as blood in the pericardial sac inhibits cardiac contractility and cardiac output. These diagnoses should be considered in patients who may have injuries above the diaphragm. Neurogenic shock results from extensive injury to the cervical or upper thoracic spinal cord. For all practical purposes, shock does not result from isolated brain injuries. Patients with spinal cord injury may initially present in shock resulting from both vasodilation and relative hypovolemia. Septic shock is unusual, but must be considered in patients whose arrival at the emergency facility has been delayed for many hours.

Patient management responsibilities begin with recognizing the presence of shock, and treatment should be initiated simultaneously with the identification of a probable cause. The response to initial treatment, coupled with the findings during the primary and secondary patient surveys, usually provides sufficient information to determine the cause of shock. **Hemorrhage is the most common cause of shock in the injured patient.**

Shock Pathophysiology

? *What is shock?*

An overview of basic cardiac physiology and blood loss pathophysiology is essential to understanding the shock state.

BASIC CARDIAC PHYSIOLOGY

Cardiac output, which is defined as the volume of blood pumped by the heart per minute, is determined by multiplying the heart rate by the stroke volume. Stroke volume, the amount of blood pumped with each cardiac contraction, is classically determined by preload, myocardial contractility, and afterload.

Preload, the volume of venous return to the heart, is determined by venous capacitance, volume status, and the difference between mean venous systemic pressure and right atrial pressure (■ FIGURE 3-1). This pressure differential determines venous flow. The venous system can be considered a reservoir or capacitance system in which the volume of blood is divided into two components:

1. The first component does not contribute to the mean systemic venous pressure and represents the volume of blood that would remain in this capacitance circuit if the pressure in the system was zero.

2. The second and more important component represents the venous volume that contributes to the mean systemic venous pressure. Nearly 70% of the body's total blood volume is estimated to be located in the venous circuit. The relationship between venous volume and venous pressure describes the compliance of the system. It is this pressure gradient that drives venous flow and therefore the volume of venous return to the heart. Blood loss depletes this component of venous volume and reduces the pressure gradient; as a consequence, venous return is reduced.

The volume of venous blood returned to the heart determines myocardial muscle fiber length after ventricular filling at the end of diastole. Muscle fiber length is related to the contractile properties of myocardial muscle according to Starling's law. Myocardial contractility is the pump that drives the system. Afterload is systemic (peripheral) vascular resistance or, simply stated, resistance to the forward flow of blood.

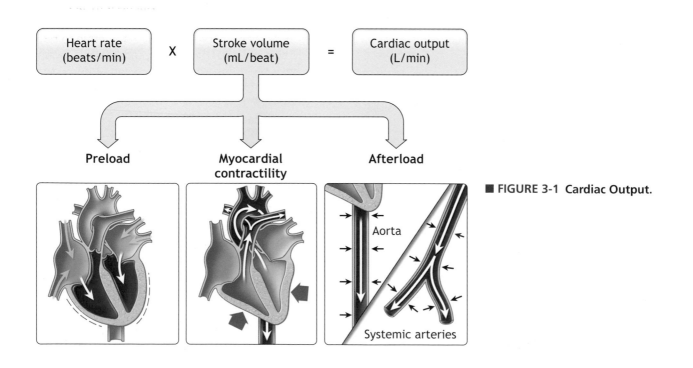

■ FIGURE 3-1 Cardiac Output.

BLOOD LOSS PATHOPHYSIOLOGY

Early circulatory responses to blood loss are compensatory and include progressive vasoconstriction of cutaneous, muscle, and visceral circulation to preserve blood flow to the kidneys, heart, and brain. The usual response to acute circulating volume depletion associated with injury is an increase in heart rate in an attempt to preserve cardiac output. In most cases, tachycardia is the earliest measurable circulatory sign of shock. The release of endogenous catecholamines increases peripheral vascular resistance, which in turn increases diastolic blood pressure and reduces pulse pressure, but does little to increase organ perfusion. Other hormones with vasoactive properties are released into the circulation during shock, including histamine, bradykinin, ß-endorphins, and a cascade of prostanoids and other cytokines. These substances have profound effects on the microcirculation and vascular permeability.

Venous return in early hemorrhagic shock is preserved to some degree by the compensatory mechanism of contraction of the volume of blood in the venous system, which does not contribute to mean systemic venous pressure. However, this compensatory mechanism is limited. **The most effective method of restoring adequate cardiac output and end-organ perfusion is to restore venous return to normal by locating and stopping the source of bleeding, along with appropriate volume repletion.**

At the cellular level, inadequately perfused and oxygenated cells are deprived of essential substrates for normal aerobic metabolism and energy production. Initially, compensation occurs by shifting to anaerobic metabolism, which results in the formation of lactic acid and the development of metabolic acidosis. If shock is prolonged and substrate delivery for the generation of adenosine triphosphate (ATP) is inadequate, the cellular membrane loses the ability to maintain its integrity, and the normal electrical gradient is lost. Proinflammatory mediators, such as inducible nitric oxide synthase (iNOS), tumor necrosis factor (TNF), and other cytokines are released, setting the stage for subsequent end-organ damage and multiple organ dysfunction.

If the process is not reversed, progressive cellular damage, alterations in endothelial permeability, additional tissue swelling, and cellular death can occur. This process compounds the impact of blood loss and hypoperfusion, potentially increasing the volume of fluid required for resuscitation.

The administration of an appropriate quantity of isotonic electrolyte solutions and blood helps combat this process. Patient treatment is directed toward reversing the shock state by providing adequate oxygenation, ventilation, and appropriate fluid resuscitation, as well as stopping the bleeding.

The initial treatment of shock is directed toward restoring cellular and organ perfusion with adequately oxygenated blood. **Definitive control of hemorrhage and restoration of adequate circulating volume are the goals of treatment of hemorrhagic shock.** Vasopressors are contraindicated for the treatment of hemorrhagic shock because they worsen tissue perfusion. Frequent monitoring of the patient's indices of perfusion is necessary to evaluate the response to therapy and detect any deterioration in the patient's condition as early as possible. Reassessment will help to identify patients in compensated shock or those who are unable to mount a compensatory response prior to cardiovascular collapse.

Most injured patients who are in hypovolemic shock require early surgical intervention or angioembolization to reverse the shock state. **The presence of shock in an injured patient warrants the immediate involvement of a surgeon.**

Initial Patient Assessment

Optimally, clinicians will recognize the shock state during the initial patient assessment. To do so, it is important to be familiar with the clinical differentiation of the causes of shock—chiefly, hemorrhagic and nonhemorrhagic.

RECOGNITION OF SHOCK

? *Is the patient in shock?*

Profound circulatory shock—as evidenced by hemodynamic collapse with inadequate perfusion of the skin, kidneys, and central nervous system—is simple to recognize. However, after the airway and adequate ventilation have been ensured, careful evaluation of the patient's circulatory status is necessary to identify the early manifestations of shock, including tachycardia and cutaneous vasoconstriction.

Reliance solely on systolic blood pressure as an indicator of shock can result in delayed recognition of the shock state. Compensatory mechanisms can preclude a measurable fall in systolic pressure until up to 30% of the patient's blood volume is lost. Specific attention should be directed to pulse rate, pulse character, respiratory rate, skin circulation, and pulse pressure (i.e., the difference between systolic and diastolic pressure). Tachycardia and cutaneous vasoconstriction are the typical early physiologic responses to volume loss in most adults. **Any injured patient who is cool and has tachycardia is considered to be in shock until proven otherwise.** Occasionally, a normal heart rate or even bradycardia is associated with an acute reduction of blood volume; other indices of perfusion must be monitored in these situations.

The normal heart rate varies with age. Tachycardia is diagnosed when the heart rate is greater than 160 beats per minutes (BPM) in an infant, 140 BPM in a preschool-aged child, 120 BPM in children from school age to puberty, and 100 BPM in adults. Elderly patients may not exhibit tachycardia because of their limited cardiac response to catecholamine stimulation or the concurrent use of medications, such as ß-adrenergic blocking agents. The ability of the body to increase the heart rate also may be limited by the presence of a pacemaker. A narrowed pulse pressure suggests significant blood loss and involvement of compensatory mechanisms.

Laboratory values for hematocrit or hemoglobin concentration may be unreliable for estimating acute blood loss and should not be used to exclude the presence of shock. **Massive blood loss may produce only a minimal acute decrease in the hematocrit or hemoglobin concentration.** Thus, a very low hematocrit value obtained shortly after injury suggests either massive blood loss or a preexisting anemia, whereas a normal hematocrit does not exclude significant blood loss. Base deficit and/or lactate levels can be useful in determining the presence and severity of shock. Serial measurement of these parameters may be used to monitor a patient's response to therapy.

CLINICAL DIFFERENTIATION OF CAUSE OF SHOCK

❓ *What is the cause of shock?*

Shock in a trauma patient is classified as hemorrhagic or nonhemorrhagic. A patient with injuries above the diaphragm may have evidence of inadequate organ perfusion due to poor cardiac performance from blunt myocardial injury, cardiac tamponade, or a tension pneumothorax that produces inadequate venous return (preload). A high index of suspicion and careful observation of the patient's response to initial treatment will enable clinicians to recognize and manage all forms of shock.

Initial determination of the cause of shock depends on taking an appropriate patient history and performing an expeditious, careful physical examination. Selected additional tests, such as monitoring central venous pressure (CVP), chest and/or pelvic x-ray examinations, and ultrasonography, can provide confirmatory evidence for the cause of the shock state, but should not delay appropriate resuscitation.

Hemorrhagic Shock

Hemorrhage is the most common cause of shock after injury, and virtually all patients with multiple in-

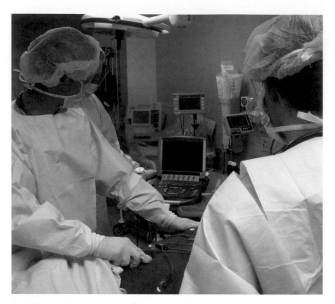

■ **FIGURE 3-2** Using ultrasound in the search for the cause of shock.

juries have an element of hypovolemia. In addition, most nonhemorrhagic shock states respond partially or briefly to volume resuscitation. Therefore, if signs of shock are present, treatment usually is instituted as if the patient is hypovolemic (■ **FIGURE 3-2**). However, as treatment is instituted, it is important to identify the small number of patients whose shock has a different cause (e.g., a secondary condition such as cardiac tamponade, tension pneumothorax, spinal cord injury, or blunt cardiac injury, which complicates hypovolemic/hemorrhagic shock). Specific information about the treatment of hemorrhagic shock is provided in the next section of this chapter. The primary focus in hemorrhagic shock is to promptly identify and stop hemorrhage. Sources of potential blood loss—chest, abdomen, pelvis, retroperitoneum, extremities, and external bleeding—must be quickly assessed by physical examination and appropriate adjunctive studies. Chest x-ray, pelvic x-ray, abdominal assessment with either focused assessment sonography in trauma (FAST) or diagnostic peritoneal lavage (DPL), and bladder catheterization may all be necessary to determine the source of blood loss (■ **FIGURE 3-3**).

Nonhemorrhagic Shock

Nonhemorrhagic shock includes cardiogenic shock, cardiac tamponade, tension pneumothorax, neurogenic shock, and septic shock.

Cardiogenic Shock Myocardial dysfunction can be caused by blunt cardiac injury, cardiac tamponade, an

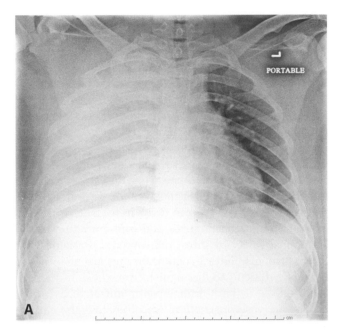

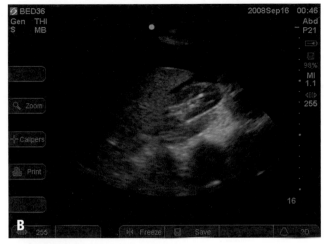

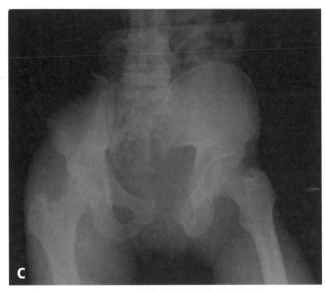

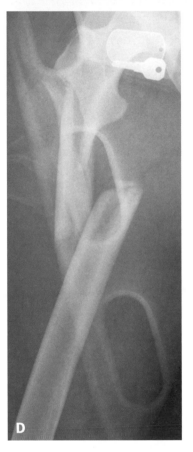

■ **FIGURE 3-3** Assessment of circulation includes a rapid determination of the site of blood loss. In addition to the floor, there are four potential places for blood to be ("on the floor plus four more"): **(A)** the chest; **(B)** the abdomen; **(C)** the pelvis; and **(D)** the femur.

air embolus, or, rarely, a myocardial infarction associated with the patient's injury. Blunt cardiac injury should be suspected when the mechanism of injury to the thorax is rapid deceleration. All patients with blunt thoracic trauma need constant electrocardiographic (ECG) monitoring to detect injury patterns and dysrhythmias. Blood creatine kinase (CK; formerly, creatine phosphokinase [CPK]) isoenzymes, and specific isotope studies of the myocardium rarely assist in diagnosing or treating injured patients in the emergency department

(ED). Echocardiography may be useful in the diagnosis of tamponade and valvular rupture, but it is often not practical or immediately available in the ED. FAST in the ED can identify pericardial fluid and the likelihood of cardiac tamponade as the cause of shock. Blunt cardiac injury may be an indication for early CVP monitoring to guide fluid resuscitation in this situation.

Cardiac Tamponade Cardiac tamponade is most commonly identified in penetrating thoracic trauma, but it can occur as the result of blunt injury to the thorax. Tachycardia, muffled heart sounds, and dilated, engorged neck veins with hypotension resistant to fluid therapy suggest cardiac tamponade. However, the absence of these classic findings does not exclude the presence of this condition. Tension pneumothorax can mimic cardiac tamponade, but it is differentiated from the latter condition by the findings of absent breath sounds, tracheal deviation, and a hyperresonant percussion note over the affected hemithorax. Cardiac tamponade is best managed by thoracotomy. Pericardiocentesis may be used as a temporizing maneuver when thoracotomy is not an available option. See Skill Station VII: Chest Trauma Management, Skill VII-C: Pericardiocentesis.

Tension Pneumothorax Tension pneumothorax is a true surgical emergency that requires immediate diagnosis and treatment. It develops when air enters the pleural space, but a flap-valve mechanism prevents its escape. Intrapleural pressure rises, causing total lung collapse and a shift of the mediastinum to the opposite side with the subsequent impairment of venous return and fall in cardiac output. The presence of acute respiratory distress, subcutaneous emphysema, absent breath sounds, hyperresonance to percussion, and tracheal shift supports the diagnosis and warrants immediate thoracic decompression without waiting for x-ray confirmation of the diagnosis. Appropriate placement of a needle into the pleural space in a case of tension pneumothorax temporarily relieves this life-threatening condition. See Skill Station VII: Chest Trauma Management, Skill VII-A: Needle Thoracentesis.

Neurogenic Shock Isolated intracranial injuries do not cause shock. The presence of shock in a patient with a head injury necessitates the search for a cause other than an intracranial injury. Cervical or upper thoracic spinal cord injury can produce hypotension due to loss of sympathetic tone. Loss of sympathetic tone compounds the physiologic effects of hypovolemia, and hypovolemia compounds the physiologic effects of sympathetic denervation. The classic picture of neurogenic shock is hypotension without tachycardia or cutaneous vasoconstriction. A narrowed pulse pressure is not seen in neurogenic shock. Patients who have

PITFALLS

- Missing tension pneumothorax.
- Assuming there is only one cause for shock.
- Young, healthy patients may have compensation for an extended period and then crash quickly.

sustained a spinal injury often have concurrent torso trauma; therefore, patients with known or suspected neurogenic shock should be treated initially for hypovolemia. The failure of fluid resuscitation to restore organ perfusion suggests either continuing hemorrhage or neurogenic shock. CVP monitoring may be helpful in managing this complex problem. See Chapter 7: Spine and Spinal Cord Trauma.

Septic Shock Shock due to infection immediately after injury is uncommon; however, if a patient's arrival at an emergency facility is delayed for several hours, it can occur. Septic shock can occur in patients with penetrating abdominal injuries and contamination of the peritoneal cavity by intestinal contents. Patients with sepsis who also have hypotension and are afebrile are clinically difficult to distinguish from those in hypovolemic shock, as both groups can manifest tachycardia, cutaneous vasoconstriction, impaired urinary output, decreased systolic pressure, and narrow pulse pressure. Patients with early septic shock can have a normal circulating volume, modest tachycardia, warm skin, systolic pressure near normal, and a wide pulse pressure.

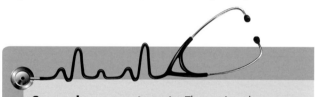

Scenario ■ *continued* The patient has two large-bore peripheral intervenous (IV) catheters placed and has received 1 liter of crystalloid. Her respiratory rate remains 28, pulse is 136, and blood pressure is 90/70 mm Hg.

Hemorrhagic Shock

Hemorrhage is the most common cause of shock in trauma patients. The trauma patient's response to blood loss is made more complex by shifts of fluids among the fluid compartments in the body—particularly in the extracellular fluid compartment. The classic response to blood loss must be considered in the context of fluid shifts associated with soft tissue injury. In addition, the changes associated with severe, prolonged shock and the pathophysiologic results of resuscitation and reperfusion must also be considered, as previously discussed.

DEFINITION OF HEMORRHAGE

Hemorrhage is defined as an acute loss of circulating blood volume. Although there is considerable variability, the normal adult blood volume is approximately 7% of body weight. For example, a 70-kg male has a circulating blood volume of approximately 5 L. The blood volume of obese adults is estimated based on their ideal body weight, because calculation based on actual weight can result in significant overestimation. The blood volume for a child is calculated as 8% to 9% of body weight (80–90 mL/kg). See Chapter 10: Pediatric Trauma.

DIRECT EFFECTS OF HEMORRHAGE

The classification of hemorrhage into four classes based on clinical signs is a useful tool for estimating the percentage of acute blood loss. These changes represent a continuum of ongoing hemorrhage and serve only to guide initial therapy. **Subsequent volume replacement is determined by the patient's response to initial therapy.** This classification system is useful in emphasizing the early signs and pathophysiology of the shock state.

Class I hemorrhage is exemplified by the condition of an individual who has donated a unit of blood. **Class II hemorrhage** is uncomplicated hemorrhage for which crystalloid fluid resuscitation is required. **Class III hemorrhage** is a complicated hemorrhagic state in which at least crystalloid infusion is required and perhaps also blood replacement. **Class IV hemorrhage** is considered a preterminal event; unless very aggressive measures are taken, the patient will die within minutes. Table 3.1 outlines the estimated blood loss and other critical measures for patients in each classification of shock.

Several confounding factors profoundly alter the classic hemodynamic response to an acute loss of circulating blood volume, and these must be promptly recognized by all individuals involved in the initial assessment and resuscitation of injured patients who are at risk for hemorrhagic shock. These factors include:

- Patient's age
- Severity of injury, with special attention to type and anatomic location of injury
- Time lapse between injury and initiation of treatment
- Prehospital fluid therapy
- Medications used for chronic conditions

It is dangerous to wait until a trauma patient fits a precise physiologic classification of shock before initiating appropriate volume restoration. Hemorrhage control and balanced fluid resuscitation must be initiated when early signs and symptoms of blood loss are apparent or suspected—not when the blood pressure is falling or absent. Bleeding patients need blood!

Class I Hemorrhage—Up to 15% Blood Volume Loss

The clinical symptoms of volume loss with class I hemorrhage are minimal. In uncomplicated situations, minimal tachycardia occurs. No measurable changes occur in blood pressure, pulse pressure, or respiratory rate. For otherwise healthy patients, this amount of blood loss does not require replacement, because transcapillary refill and other compensatory mechanisms will restore blood volume within 24 hours, usually without the need for blood transfusion.

Class II Hemorrhage—15% to 30% Blood Volume Loss

In a 70-kg male, volume loss with class II hemorrhage represents 750 to 1500 mL of blood. Clinical

■ TABLE 3.1 Estimated Blood Loss[1] Based on Patient's Initial Presentation

	CLASS I	CLASS II	CLASS III	CLASS IV
Blood loss (mL)	Up to 750	750–1500	1500–2000	>2000
Blood loss (% blood volume)	Up to 15%	15%–30%	30%–40%	>40%
Pulse rate (BPM)	<100	100-120	120-140	>140
Systolic b pressure	Normal	Normal	Decreased	Decreased
Pulse pressure (mm Hg)	Normal or increased	Decreased	Decreased	Decreased
Respiratory rate	14–20	20–30	30–40	>35
Urine output (mL/hr)	>30	20–30	5–15	Negligible
CNS/mental status	Slightly anxious	Mildly anxious	Anxious, confused	Confused, lethargic
Initial fluid replacement	Crystalloid	Crystalloid	Crystalloid and blood	Crystalloid and blood

[1] For a 70-kg man.

signs include tachycardia (heart rate above 100 in an adult), tachypnea, and decreased pulse pressure; the latter sign is related primarily to a rise in the diastolic component due to an increase in circulating catecholamines. These agents produce an increase in peripheral vascular tone and resistance. Systolic pressure changes minimally in early hemorrhagic shock; therefore, it is important to evaluate pulse pressure rather than systolic pressure. Other pertinent clinical findings with this amount of blood loss include subtle central nervous system (CNS) changes, such as anxiety, fright, and hostility. Despite the significant blood loss and cardiovascular changes, urinary output is only mildly affected. The measured urine flow is usually 20 to 30 mL/hour in an adult.

Accompanying fluid losses can exaggerate the clinical manifestations of class II hemorrhage. Some patients in this category may eventually require blood transfusion, but most are stabilized initially with crystalloid solutions.

Class III Hemorrhage—30% to 40% Blood Volume Loss

The blood loss with class III hemorrhage (approximately 1500–2000 mL in an adult) can be devastating. Patients almost always present with the classic signs of inadequate perfusion, including marked tachycardia and tachypnea, significant changes in mental status, and a measurable fall in systolic pressure. In an uncomplicated case, this is the least amount of blood loss that consistently causes a drop in systolic pressure. Patients with this degree of blood loss almost always require transfusion. However, the priority of initial management is to stop the hemorrhage, by emergency operation or embolization if necessary. Most patients in this category will require packed red blood cells (pRBCs) and blood product resuscitation in order to reverse the shock state. The decision to transfuse blood is based on the patient's response to initial fluid resuscitation.

Class IV Hemorrhage—More than 40% Blood Volume Loss

The degree of exsanguination with class IV hemorrhage is immediately life-threatening. Symptoms include marked tachycardia, a significant decrease in systolic blood pressure, and a very narrow pulse pressure (or an unobtainable diastolic pressure). Urinary output is negligible, and mental status is markedly depressed. The skin is cold and pale. Patients with class IV hemorrhage frequently require rapid transfusion and immediate surgical intervention. These decisions are based on the patient's response to the initial management techniques described in this chapter. Loss of more than 50% of blood volume results in loss of consciousness and decreased pulse and blood pressure.

CLINICAL USEFULNESS OF CLASSIFICATION SCHEME

The clinical usefulness of this classification scheme is illustrated by the following example: A 70-kg patient with hypotension who arrives at an ED or trauma center has lost an estimated 1470 mL of blood (70 kg × 7% × 30% = 1.47 L, or 1470 mL). Resuscitation will likely require crystalloid, pRBCs, and blood products. Nonresponse to fluid administration almost always indicates persistent blood loss with the need for operative or angiographic control.

FLUID CHANGES SECONDARY TO SOFT TISSUE INJURY

Major soft tissue injuries and fractures compromise the hemodynamic status of injured patients in two ways:

1. First, blood is lost into the site of injury, particularly in cases of major fractures. For example, a fractured tibia or humerus can be associated with the loss of as much as 1.5 units (750 mL) of blood. Twice that amount (up to 1500 mL) is commonly associated with femur fractures, and several liters of blood can accumulate in a retroperitoneal hematoma associated with a pelvic fracture.

2. The second factor to be considered is the edema that occurs in injured soft tissues. The degree of this additional volume loss is related to the magnitude of the soft tissue injury. Tissue injury results in activation of a systemic inflammatory response and production and release of multiple cytokines. Many of these locally active hormones have profound effects on the vascular endothelium, which increases permeability. Tissue edema is the result of shifts in fluid primarily from the plasma into the extravascular, extracellular space due to alterations in endothelial permeability. Such shifts produce an additional depletion in intravascular volume.

Initial Management of Hemorrhagic Shock

? *What can I do about shock?*

The diagnosis and treatment of shock must occur almost simultaneously. For most trauma patients, treatment is instituted as if the patient has hypovolemic shock, unless there is clear evidence that the shock state has a different cause. **The basic management principle is to stop the bleeding and replace the volume loss.**

PHYSICAL EXAMINATION

The physical examination is directed toward the immediate diagnosis of life-threatening injuries and includes assessment of the ABCDEs. Baseline recordings are important to monitor the patient's response to therapy, and measurements of vital signs, urinary output, and level of consciousness are essential. A more detailed examination of the patient follows as the situation permits. See Chapter 1: Initial Assessment and Management.

Airway and Breathing

Establishing a patent airway with adequate ventilation and oxygenation is the first priority. Supplementary oxygen is provided to maintain oxygen saturation at greater than 95%. See Chapter 2: Airway and Ventilatory Management.

Circulation—Hemorrhage Control

Priorities for managing circulation include controlling obvious hemorrhage, obtaining adequate intravenous access, and assessing tissue perfusion. Bleeding from external wounds usually can be controlled by direct pressure to the bleeding site, although massive blood loss from an extremity may require a tourniquet. A sheet or pelvic binder from an extremity may be used to control bleeding from pelvic fractures. The adequacy of tissue perfusion dictates the amount of fluid resuscitation required. Surgical or angiographic control may be required to control internal hemorrhage. The priority is to stop the bleeding, not to calculate the volume of fluid lost.

Disability—Neurologic Examination

A brief neurologic examination will determine the patient's level of consciousness, eye motion and pupillary response, best motor function, and degree of sensation. This information is useful in assessing cerebral perfusion, following the evolution of neurologic disability, and predicting future recovery. Alterations in CNS function in patients who have hypotension as a result of hypovolemic shock do not necessarily imply direct intracranial injury and may reflect inadequate brain perfusion. Restoration of cerebral perfusion and oxygenation must be achieved before ascribing these findings to intracranial injury. See Chapter 6: Head Trauma.

Exposure—Complete Examination

After lifesaving priorities are addressed, the patient must be completely undressed and carefully examined from head to toe to search for associated injuries.

When undressing the patient, it is essential to prevent hypothermia. The use of fluid warmers and external passive and active warming techniques are essential to prevent hypothermia.

Gastric Dilation—Decompression

Gastric dilation often occurs in trauma patients, especially in children, which can cause unexplained hypotension or cardiac dysrhythmia, usually bradycardia from excessive vagal stimulation. **In unconscious patients, gastric distention increases the risk of aspiration of gastric contents, which is a potentially fatal complication.** Gastric decompression is accomplished by intubating the stomach with a tube passed nasally or orally and attaching it to suction to evacuate gastric contents. However, proper positioning of the tube does not completely obviate the risk of aspiration.

Urinary Catheterization

Bladder catheterization allows for assessment of the urine for hematuria (indicating the retroperitoneum may be a significant source of blood loss) and continuous evaluation of renal perfusion by monitoring urinary output. Blood at the urethral meatus or a high-riding, mobile, or nonpalpable prostate in males is an absolute contraindication to the insertion of a transurethral catheter prior to radiographic confirmation of an intact urethra. See Chapter 5: Abdominal and Pelvic Trauma.

VASCULAR ACCESS LINES

Access to the vascular system must be obtained promptly. This is best accomplished by inserting two large-caliber (minimum of 16-gauge in an adult) peripheral intravenous catheters before placement of a central venous line is considered. The rate of flow is proportional to the fourth power of the radius of the cannula and inversely related to its length (Poiseuille's law). Hence, short, large-caliber peripheral intravenous lines are preferred for the rapid infusion of large volumes of fluid. Fluid warmers and rapid infusion pumps are used in the presence of massive hemorrhage and severe hypotension.

The most desirable sites for peripheral, percutaneous intravenous lines in adults are the forearms and antecubital veins. If circumstances prevent the use of peripheral veins, large-caliber, central venous (i.e., femoral, jugular, or subclavian vein) access using the Seldinger technique or saphenous vein cutdown is indicated, depending on the clinician's skill and experience. See Skill Station IV: Shock Assessment and Management, and Skill Station V: Venous Cutdown.

Frequently in an emergency situation, central venous access is not accomplished under tightly controlled or completely sterile conditions. Therefore, these lines should be changed in a more controlled environment as soon as the patient's condition permits. Consideration also must be given to the potential for serious complications related to attempted central venous catheter placement, such as pneumothorax or hemothorax, in patients who may already be unstable.

In children younger than 6 years, the placement of an intraosseous needle should be attempted before inserting a central line. The important determinant for selecting a procedure or route for establishing vascular access is the clinician's experience and skill. Intraosseous access with specially designed equipment is possible in *all age groups,* and is being used with increasing frequency. As in the pediatric population, this access may be used in-hospital until intravenous access is obtained.

As intravenous lines are started, blood samples are drawn for type and crossmatch, appropriate laboratory analyses, toxicology studies, and pregnancy testing for all females of childbearing age. Arterial blood gas (ABG) analysis is performed at this time. A chest x-ray must be obtained after attempts at inserting a subclavian or internal jugular CVP monitoring line to document the position of the line and evaluate for a pneumothorax or hemothorax.

INITIAL FLUID THERAPY

Warmed isotonic electrolyte solutions, such as lactated Ringer's and normal saline, are used for initial resuscitation. This type of fluid provides transient intravascular expansion and further stabilizes the vascular volume by replacing accompanying fluid losses into the interstitial and intracellular spaces.

An initial, warmed fluid bolus is given. The usual dose is 1 to 2 L for adults and 20 mL/kg for pediatric patients. Absolute volumes of resuscitation fluids should be based on patient response. It is important to remember that this initial fluid amount includes any fluid given in the prehospital setting. The patient's response is observed during this initial fluid administration, and further therapeutic and diagnostic decisions are based on this response.

The amount of fluid and blood required for resuscitation is difficult to predict on initial evaluation of the patient. Table 3.1 provides general guidelines for establishing the amount of fluid and blood likely required. **It is most important to assess the patient's response to fluid resuscitation and identify evidence of adequate end-organ perfusion and oxygenation (i.e., via urinary output, level of consciousness, and peripheral perfusion).** If, during resuscitation, the amount of fluid required to restore or maintain adequate organ perfusion greatly exceeds

these estimates, a careful reassessment of the situation and search for unrecognized injuries and other causes of shock are necessary.

The goal of resuscitation is to restore organ perfusion. This is accomplished by the use of resuscitation fluids to replace lost intravascular volume. Note, however, that if blood pressure is raised rapidly before the hemorrhage has been definitively controlled, increased bleeding can occur. **Persistent infusion of large volumes of fluid and blood in an attempt to achieve a normal blood pressure is not a substitute for definitive control of bleeding.** Excessive fluid administration can exacerbate the lethal triad of coagulopathy, acidosis, and hypothermia with activation of the inflammatory cascade.

Fluid resuscitation and avoidance of hypotension are important principles in the initial management of blunt trauma patients, particularly those with traumatic brain injury (TBI). In penetrating trauma with hemorrhage, delaying aggressive fluid resuscitation until definitive control may prevent additional bleeding. Although complications associated with resuscitation injury are undesirable, the alternative of exsanguination is even less so. A careful, balanced approach with frequent reevaluation is required.

Balancing the goal of organ perfusion with the risks of rebleeding by accepting a lower-than-normal blood pressure has been termed "controlled resuscitation," "balanced resuscitation," "hypotensive resuscitation," and "permissive hypotension." The goal is the balance, not the hypotension. Such a resuscitation strategy may be a bridge to, but is not a substitute for, definitive surgical control of bleeding.

PITFALLS

Recognize the source of occult hemorrhage. Remember, "Blood on the floor + four more." Chest, pelvis (retroperitoneum), abdomen, and thigh.

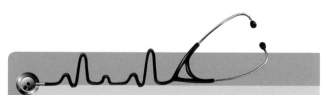

Scenario ■ *continued* The patient's chest x-ray shows a wide mediastinum and several rib fractures on the left side. Her pelvic x-ray is normal. Her FAST exam shows no cardiac abnormalities. There is fluid in Morrison's pouch. Her respiratory rate is 36, pulse 140, and blood pressure 80/palp.

Evaluation of Fluid Resuscitation and Organ Perfusion

? *What is the patient's response?*

The same signs and symptoms of inadequate perfusion that are used to diagnose shock are useful determinants of patient response. The return of normal blood pressure, pulse pressure, and pulse rate are signs that suggest perfusion is returning to normal. However, these observations give no information regarding organ perfusion. Improvements in the CVP status and skin circulation are important evidence of enhanced perfusion, but are difficult to quantitate. The volume of urinary output is a reasonably sensitive indicator of renal perfusion; normal urine volumes generally imply adequate renal blood flow, if not modified by the administration of diuretic agents. For this reason, urinary output is one of the prime monitors of resuscitation and patient response. Changes in CVP can provide useful information, and the risks incurred in the placement of a CVP line are justified for complex cases.

URINARY OUTPUT

Within certain limits, urinary output is used to monitor renal blood flow. Adequate resuscitation volume replacement should produce a urinary output of approximately 0.5 mL/kg/hr in adults, whereas 1 mL/kg/hr is an adequate urinary output for pediatric patients. For children under 1 year of age, 2 mL/kg/hour should be maintained. The inability to obtain urinary output at these levels or a decreasing urinary output with an increasing specific gravity suggests inadequate resuscitation. This situation should stimulate further volume replacement and diagnostic endeavors.

ACID-BASE BALANCE

Patients in early hypovolemic shock have respiratory alkalosis due to tachypnea. Respiratory alkalosis is frequently followed by mild metabolic acidosis in the early phases of shock and does not require treatment. Severe metabolic acidosis can develop from long-standing or severe shock. Metabolic acidosis is caused by anaerobic metabolism, which results from inadequate tissue perfusion and the production of lactic acid. Persistent acidosis is usually caused by inadequate resuscitation or ongoing blood loss and, in normothermic patients in shock, it should be treated with fluids, blood, and consideration of operative intervention to control hemorrhage. Base deficit and/or lactate can be useful in determining the presence and severity of shock. Serial measurement of these parameters can be used to monitor the response to therapy. Sodium bicarbonate should not be used to treat metabolic acidosis secondary to hypovolemic shock.

Therapeutic Decisions Based on Response to Initial Fluid Resuscitation

The patient's response to initial fluid resuscitation is the key to determining subsequent therapy. Having established a preliminary diagnosis and treatment plan based on the initial evaluation, the clinician now modifies the plan based on the patient's response. Observing the response to the initial resuscitation identifies patients whose blood loss was greater than estimated and those with ongoing bleeding who require operative control of internal hemorrhage. Resuscitation in the operating room can accomplish simultaneously the direct control of bleeding by the surgeon and the restoration of intravascular volume. In addition, it limits the probability of overtransfusion or unnecessary transfusion of blood in patients whose initial status was disproportionate to the amount of blood loss.

It is particularly important to distinguish patients who are "hemodynamically stable" from those who are "hemodynamically normal." A hemodynamically stable patient may have persistent tachycardia, tachypnea, and oliguria; this patient is clearly underresuscitated and still in shock. In contrast, hemodynamically normal patients exhibit no signs of inadequate tissue perfusion.

The potential patterns of response to initial fluid administration can be divided into three groups: rapid response, transient response, and minimal or no response. Vital signs and management guidelines for patients in each of these categories are outlined in Table 3.2.

RAPID RESPONSE

Patients in this group, termed "rapid responders," respond rapidly to the initial fluid bolus and remain hemodynamically normal after the initial fluid bolus has been given and the fluids are slowed to maintenance rates. Such patients usually have lost minimal (less than 20%) blood volume. No further fluid bolus or immediate blood administration is indicated for patients in this response group. Typed and crossmatched blood should be kept available. **Surgical consultation and evaluation are necessary during initial assessment and treatment, as operative intervention may still be necessary.**

■ TABLE 3.2 Responses to Initial Fluid Resuscitation[1]

	RAPID RESPONSE	TRANSIENT RESPONSE	MINIMAL OR NO RESPONSE
Vital signs	Return to normal	Transient improvement, recurrence of decreased blood pressure and increased heart rate	Remain abnormal
Estimated blood loss	Minimal (10%–20%)	Moderate and ongoing (20%–40%)	Severe (>40%)
Need for more crystalloid	Low	Low to moderate	Moderate as a bridge to transfusion
Need for blood	Low	Moderate to high	Immediate
Blood preparation	Type and crossmatch	Type-specific	Emergency blood release
Need for operative intervention	Possibly	Likely	Highly likely
Early presence of surgeon	Yes	Yes	Yes

[1]Isotonic crystalloid solution, 2000 mL in adults; 20 mL/kg in children.

TRANSIENT RESPONSE

Patients in the second group, termed "transient responders," respond to the initial fluid bolus. However, they begin to show deterioration of perfusion indices as the initial fluids are slowed to maintenance levels, indicating either an ongoing blood loss or inadequate resuscitation. Most of these patients initially have lost an estimated 20% to 40% of their blood volume. Transfusion of blood and blood products is indicated, but more important is the recognition that this patient requires operative or angiographic control of hemorrhage. A transient response to blood administration should identify patients who are still bleeding and require rapid surgical intervention.

MINIMAL OR NO RESPONSE

Failure to respond to crystalloid and blood administration in the ED dictates the need for immediate, definitive intervention (e.g., operation or angioembolization) to control exsanguinating hemorrhage. On very rare occasions, failure to respond may be due to pump failure as a result of blunt cardiac injury, cardiac tamponade, or tension pneumothorax. Nonhemorrhagic shock always should be considered as a diagnosis in this group of patients. CVP monitoring and cardiac ultrasonography help to differentiate between the various causes of shock.

PITFALLS

- Delay in definitive management can be lethal.
- Do not overlook a source of bleeding.

Blood Replacement

The decision to initiate blood transfusion is based on the patient's response, as described in the previous section. Patients who are transient responders or nonresponders—those with Class III or Class IV hemorrhage—will need pRBCs and blood products as an early part of their resuscitation (■ FIGURE 3-4).

CROSSMATCHED, TYPE-SPECIFIC, AND TYPE O BLOOD

The main purpose of blood transfusion is to restore the oxygen-carrying capacity of the intravascular volume. Fully crossmatched blood is preferable. However, the complete crossmatching process requires approximately 1 hour in most blood banks. For patients who stabilize rapidly, crossmatched blood should be obtained and made available for transfusion when indicated.

Type-specific blood can be provided by most blood banks within 10 minutes. Such blood is compatible with ABO and Rh blood types, but incompatibilities of other antibodies may exist. Type-specific blood is preferred for patients who are transient responders, as described in the previous section. If type-specific blood is required, complete crossmatching should be performed by the blood bank.

If type-specific blood is unavailable, type O packed cells are indicated for patients with exsanguinating hemorrhage. To avoid sensitization and future complications, Rh-negative cells are preferred for females of childbearing age. As soon as it is available, the use of unmatched, type-specific blood is preferred over type O blood. This is true unless multiple, unidentified cas-

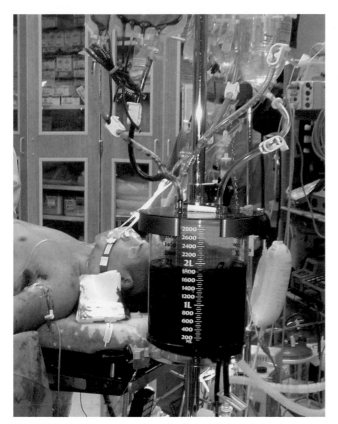

■ **FIGURE 3-4** Massive transfusion of blood products in a trauma patient.

ualties are being treated simultaneously and the risk of inadvertently administering the wrong unit of blood to a patient is great.

WARMING FLUIDS—PLASMA AND CRYSTALLOID

Hypothermia must be prevented and reversed if a patient has hypothermia on arrival at the hospital. The use of blood warmers in the ED is critical, even if cumbersome. The most efficient way to prevent hypothermia in any patient receiving massive volumes of crystalloid is to heat the fluid to $39°C$ ($102.2°$ F) before infusing it. This can be accomplished by storing crystalloids in a warmer or with the use of a microwave oven. Blood products cannot be warmed in a microwave oven, but they can be heated by passage through intravenous fluid warmers.

AUTOTRANSFUSION

Adaptations of standard tube thoracostomy collection devices are commercially available; these allow for sterile collection, anticoagulation (generally with sodium citrate solutions, not heparin), and retransfusion

of shed blood. Collection of shed blood for autotransfusion should be considered for any patient with a major hemothorax.

MASSIVE TRANSFUSION

A small subset of patients with shock will require massive transfusion, most often defined as >10 units of pRBCs within the first 24 hours of admission. Early administration of pRBCs, plasma, and platelets, and minimizing aggressive crystalloid administration in these patients may result in improved survival. This approach has been termed balanced, hemostatic or damage control resuscitation. Concomitant efforts to rapidly control bleeding and reduce the detrimental effects of coagulopathy, hypothermia, and acidosis in these patients are extremely important. A massive transfusion protocol that includes the immediate availability of all blood components should be in place in order to provide optimal resuscitation for these patients, as the resources required are tremendous. These protocols also improve outcome.

COAGULOPATHY

Severe injury and hemorrhage result in the consumption of coagulation factors and early coagulopathy. Such coagulopathy is present in up to 30% of severely injured patients on admission. Massive fluid resuscitation, with the resultant dilution of platelets and clotting factors, along with the adverse effect of hypothermia on platelet aggregation and the clotting cascade, contributes to coagulopathy in injured patients. Prothrombin time, partial thromboplastin time, and platelet count are valuable baseline studies to obtain in the first hour, especially if the patient has a history of coagulation disorders or takes medications that alter coagulation, or a reliable bleeding history cannot be obtained. In patients who do not require massive transfusion, the use of platelets, cryoprecipitate, and fresh-frozen plasma should be guided by these coagulation parameters, including fibrinogen levels.

Patients with major brain injury are particularly prone to coagulation abnormalities. Coagulation parameters need to be closely monitored in these patients; the early administration of plasma and/or platelets improves survival if they are on known anticoagulants or antiplatelet agents.

CALCIUM ADMINISTRATION

Most patients receiving blood transfusions do not need calcium supplements. When necessary, administration should be guided by measurement of ionized calcium. Excessive, supplemental calcium may be harmful.

Special considerations in the diagnosis and treatment of shock include the mistaken equation of blood pressure with cardiac output, advanced age, athletes in shock, pregnancy, patient medications, hypothermia, and the presence of pacemakers.

EQUATING BLOOD PRESSURE WITH CARDIAC OUTPUT

Treatment of hypovolemic (hemorrhagic) shock requires correction of inadequate organ perfusion by increasing organ blood flow and tissue oxygenation. Increasing blood flow requires an increase in cardiac output. Ohm's law ($V = I \times R$) applied to cardiovascular physiology states that blood pressure (V) is proportional to cardiac output (I) and systemic vascular resistance (R) (afterload). **An increase in blood pressure should not be equated with a concomitant increase in cardiac output or the recovery from shock.** An increase in peripheral resistance—for example, with vasopressor therapy—with no change in cardiac output results in increased blood pressure, but no improvement in tissue perfusion or oxygenation.

ADVANCED AGE

Elderly trauma patients require special consideration. The aging process produces a relative decrease in sympathetic activity with respect to the cardiovascular system. This is thought to result from a deficit in the receptor response to catecholamines, rather than from a reduction in catecholamine production. Cardiac compliance decreases with age, and older patients are unable to increase heart rate or the efficiency of myocardial contraction when stressed by blood volume loss, as are younger patients.

Atherosclerotic vascular occlusive disease makes many vital organs extremely sensitive to even the slightest reduction in blood flow. Many elderly patients have preexisting volume depletion resulting from long-term diuretic use or subtle malnutrition. For these reasons, hypotension secondary to blood loss is poorly tolerated by elderly trauma patients. ß-adrenergic blockade can mask tachycardia as an early indicator of shock. Other medications can adversely affect the stress response to injury or block it completely. Because the therapeutic range for volume resuscitation is relatively narrow in elderly patients, it is prudent to consider early invasive monitoring as a means to avoid excessive or inadequate volume restoration.

The reduction in pulmonary compliance, decrease in diffusion capacity, and general weakness of the muscles of respiration limit the ability of elderly patients to meet the increased demands for gas exchange imposed by injury. This compounds the cellular hypoxia already produced by a reduction in local oxygen delivery. Glomerular and tubular senescence in the kidney reduces the ability of elderly patients to preserve volume in response to the release of stress hormones such as aldosterone, catecholamines, vasopressin, and cortisol. The kidney also is more susceptible to the effects of reduced blood flow and nephrotoxic agents such as drugs, contrast agents, and the toxic products of cellular destruction.

For all of these reasons, mortality and morbidity rates increase directly with age and long-term health status for mild and moderately severe injuries. Despite the adverse effects of the aging process, comorbidities from preexisting disease, and a general reduction in the "physiologic reserve" of geriatric patients, the majority of these patients may recover and return to their preinjury status. Treatment begins with prompt, aggressive resuscitation and careful monitoring. See Chapter 11: Geriatric Trauma.

ATHLETES

Rigorous athletic training routines change the cardiovascular dynamics of this group of patients. Blood volume may increase 15% to 20%, cardiac output sixfold, stroke volume 50%, and the resting pulse can average 50. The ability of athletes' bodies to compensate for blood loss is truly remarkable. The usual responses to hypovolemia may not be manifested in athletes, even when significant blood loss has occurred.

PREGNANCY

Physiologic maternal hypervolemia requires a greater blood loss to manifest perfusion abnormalities in the mother, which also may be reflected in decreased fetal perfusion. See Chapter 12: Trauma in Pregnancy and Intimate Partner Voilence.

MEDICATIONS

ß-adrenergic receptor blockers and calcium-channel blockers can significantly alter a patient's hemodynamic response to hemorrhage. Insulin overdosing may be responsible for hypoglycemia and may have contributed to the injury-producing event. Long-term diuretic therapy may explain unexpected hypokalemia, and nonsteroidal antiinflammatory drugs (NSAIDs) may adversely affect platelet function.

HYPOTHERMIA

Patients suffering from hypothermia and hemorrhagic shock do not respond normally to the administration of blood and fluid resuscitation, and coagulopathy may develop or worsen. Body temperature is an important vital sign to monitor during the initial assessment phase. Esophageal or bladder temperature is an accurate clinical measurement of the core temperature. A trauma victim under the influence of alcohol and exposed to cold temperature extremes is more likely to have hypothermia as a result of vasodilation. Rapid rewarming in an environment with appropriate external warming devices, heat lamps, thermal caps, heated respiratory gases, and warmed intravenous fluids and blood will generally correct hypotension and mild to moderate hypothermia. Core rewarming (irrigation of the peritoneal or thoracic cavity with crystalloid solutions warmed to 39°C [102.2°F] or extracorporeal bypass) is indicated for severe hypothermia. Hypothermia is best treated by prevention. See Chapter 9: Thermal Injuries.

PRESENCE OF PACEMAKER

Patients with pacemakers are unable to respond to blood loss in the expected fashion, because cardiac output is directly related to heart rate. In the significant number of patients with myocardial conduction defects who have such devices in place, CVP monitoring is invaluable to guide fluid therapy.

Reassessing Patient Response and Avoiding Complications

Inadequate volume replacement is the most common complication of hemorrhagic shock. Immediate, appropriate, and aggressive therapy that restores organ perfusion minimizes such complications.

CONTINUED HEMORRHAGE

An undiagnosed source of bleeding is the most common cause of poor response to fluid therapy. Patients with this condition are generally included in the transient response category, as defined previously. Immediate surgical intervention may be necessary.

FLUID OVERLOAD AND CVP MONITORING

After a patient's initial assessment and treatment have been completed, the risk of fluid overload is minimized by careful monitoring. Remember, the goal of therapy is restoration of organ perfusion and adequate tissue oxygenation, confirmed by appropriate urinary output, CNS function, skin color, and return of pulse and blood pressure toward normal.

Monitoring the response to resuscitation is best accomplished for some patients in an environment in which sophisticated techniques are used. Early transfer of the patient to an intensive care unit should be considered for elderly patients and patients with non-hemorrhagic causes of shock.

CVP monitoring is a relatively simple procedure used as a standard guide for assessing the ability of the right side of the heart to accept a fluid load. Properly interpreted, the response of the CVP to fluid administration helps evaluate volume replacement. Several points to remember are:

1. The precise measure of cardiac function is the relationship between ventricular end diastolic volume and stroke volume. Right atrial pressure (CVP) and cardiac output (as reflected by evidence of perfusion or blood pressure, or even by direct measurement) are indirect and, at best, insensitive estimates of this relationship. Remembering these facts is important to avoid overdependency on CVP monitoring.

2. The initial CVP level and actual blood volume are not necessarily related. The initial CVP is sometimes high, even with a significant volume deficit, especially in patients with chronic obstructive pulmonary disease, generalized vasoconstriction, and rapid fluid replacement. The initial venous pressure also may be high because of the inappropriate use of exogenous vasopressors.

3. A minimal rise in an initially low CVP with fluid therapy suggests the need for further volume expansion (use an appropriate fluid resuscitation category) and a renewed search for the source of bleeding.

4. A declining CVP suggests ongoing fluid loss and the need for additional fluid or blood replacement (i.e., transient response to fluid resuscitation category).

5. An abrupt or persistent elevation in CVP suggests that volume replacement is adequate or too rapid, or that cardiac function is compromised.

6. Pronounced elevations of CVP may be caused by hypervolemia as a result of overtransfusion, cardiac dysfunction, cardiac tamponade, or increased intrathoracic pressure from a tension pneumothorax. Catheter malposition can produce erroneously high CVP measurements.

Aseptic techniques must be used when central venous lines are placed. Multiple sites provide access to the central circulation, and the decision regarding which route to use is determined by the clinician's skill and experience. The ideal position for the tip of the catheter is in the superior vena cava, just proximal to the right atrium. Techniques for catheter placement are discussed in detail in Skill Station IV: Shock Assessment and Management.

The placement of central venous lines carries the risk of potentially life-threatening complications. Infections, vascular injury, nerve injury, embolization, thrombosis, and pneumothorax can result. CVP monitoring reflects right heart function. It may not be representative of left heart function in patients with primary myocardial dysfunction or abnormal pulmonary circulation.

RECOGNITION OF OTHER PROBLEMS

When a patient fails to respond to therapy, consider undiagnosed bleeding, cardiac tamponade, tension pneumothorax, ventilatory problems, unrecognized fluid loss, acute gastric distention, myocardial infarction, diabetic acidosis, hypoadrenalism, and neurogenic shock. Constant reevaluation, especially when patients' conditions deviate from expected patterns, is the key to recognizing such problems as early as possible.

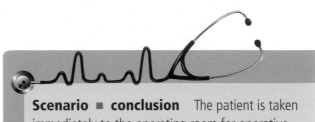

Scenario ■ conclusion   The patient is taken immediately to the operating room for operative control of hemorrhage. Blood and plasma are given, and the massive transfusion protocol is initiated.

Chapter Summary

1 Shock is an abnormality of the circulatory system that results in inadequate organ perfusion and tissue oxygenation. Shock management, based on sound physiologic principles, is usually successful.

2 Hypovolemia is the cause of shock in most trauma patients. Treatment of these patients requires immediate hemorrhage control and fluid or blood replacement. Operative control of the patient's continuing hemorrhage may be necessary.

3 The diagnosis and treatment of shock must occur almost simultaneously. For most trauma patients, treatment is instituted as if the patient has hypovolemic shock, unless there is clear evidence that the shock state has a different cause. The basic management principle is to stop the bleeding and replace the volume loss.

4 Initial assessment of a patient in shock requires careful physical examination, looking for signs of tension pneumothorax, cardiac tamponade, and other causes of the shock state.

5 The management of hemorrhagic shock includes rapid hemostasis and balanced resuscitation with crystalloids and blood. Early identification and control of the source of hemorrhage is essential.

6 The classes of hemorrhage serve as an early guide to appropriate resuscitation. Careful monitoring of physiologic response and the ability to control bleeding will dictate ongoing resuscitation efforts.

7 Blood is administered to resume the oxygen-carrying capacity of the intravascular volume.

8 Challenges in the diagnosis and treatment of shock include equating blood pressure with cardiac output, extremes of age, athletes, pregnancy, medications, hypothermia, and pacemakers.

▶ BIBLIOGRAPHY

1. Abou-Khalil B, Scalea TM, Trooskin SZ, et al. Hemodynamic responses to shock in young trauma patients: need for invasive monitoring. *Crit Care Med* 1994;22(4):633-639.

2. Alam HB, Rhee P. New developments in fluid resuscitation. *Surg Clin North Am* 2007;87(1):55-72,vi.

3. Asensio JA, Murray J, Demetriades D, et al. Penetrating cardiac injuries: a prospective study of variables predicting outcomes. *J Am Coll Surg* 1998;186(1):24-34.

4. Bickell WH, Wall MJ, Pepe PE, et al. Immediate versus delayed fluid resuscitation for hypotensive patients with penetrating torso injuries. *N Engl J Med* 1994;331(17):1105-1109.

5. Brohi K, Cohen MJ, Ganter MT, et al. Acute coagulopathy of trauma: hypoperfusion induces systemic anticoagulation and hyperfibrinolysis. *J Trauma* 2008;64:1211-7.

6. Bruns B, Lindsey M, Rowe K, Brown S, Minei JP, Gentilello LM, Shafi S. Hemoglobin drops within minutes of injuries and predicts need for an intervention to stop hemorrhage. *J Trauma* 2007Aug;63(2):312-5.

7. Bunn F, Roberts I, Tasker R, Akpa E. Hypertonic versus near isotonic crystalloid for fluid resuscitation in critically ill patients. *Cochrane Database Syst Rev* 2004;(3):CD002045.

8. Burris D, Rhee P, Kaufmann C, et al. Controlled resuscitation for uncontrolled hemorrhagic shock. *J Trauma* 1999;46(2):216-223.

9. Carrico CJ, Canizaro PC, Shires GT. Fluid resuscitation following injury: rationale for the use of balanced salt solutions. *Crit Care Med* 1976;4(2):46-54.

10. Chernow B, Rainey TG, Lake CR. Endogenous and exogenous catecholamines. *Crit Care Med* 1982;10:409.

11. Cogbill TH, Blintz M, Johnson JA, et al. Acute gastric dilatation after trauma. *J Trauma* 1987;27(10):1113-1117.

12. Cook RE, Keating JF, Gillespie I. The role of angiography in the management of haemorrhage from major fractures of the pelvis. *J Bone Joint Surg Br* 2002;84(2):178-182.

13. Cooper DJ, Walley KR, Wiggs RB, et al. Bicarbonate does not improve hemodynamics in critically ill patients who have lactic acidosis. *Ann Intern Med* 1990;112:492.

14. Cotton BA, Au BK, Nunez TC, Gunter OL, Robertson AM, Young PP. Predefined massive transfusion protocols are associated with a reduction in organ failure and postinjury complications. *J Trauma* 2009;66:41-9.

15. Cotton BA, Dossett LA, Au BK, Nunez TC, Robertson AM, Young PP. Room for (performance) improvement: provider-related factors associated with poor outcomes in massive transfusion. *J Trauma* 2009;67:1004-1012.

16. Davis JW, Kaups KL, Parks SN. Base deficit is superior to pH in evaluating clearance of acidosis after traumatic shock. *J Trauma* 1998Jan;44(1):114-118.

17. Davis JW, Parks SN, Kaups KL, et al. Admission base deficit predicts transfusion requirements and risk of complications. *J Trauma* 1997Mar;42(3):571-573.

18. Dent D, Alsabrook G, Erickson BA, et al. Blunt splenic injuries: high nonoperative management rate can be achieved with selective embolization. *J Trauma* 2004;56(5):1063-1067.

19. Dutton RP, Mackenzie CF, Scalea TM. Hypotensive resuscitation during active hemorrhage: impact on in-hospital mortality. *J Trauma* 2002;52(6):1141-1146.

20. Dzik WH, Kirkley SA. Citrate toxicity during massive blood transfusion. *Transfus Med Rev* 1988Jun;2(2):76-94.

21. Eastridge BJ, Salinas J, McManus JG, Blackburn L, Bugler EM, Cooke WH, Convertino VA, Wade CE, Holcomb JB. Hypotension begins at 110 mm Hg: redefining "hypotension" with data. *J Trauma* 2007Aug;63(2):291-9.

22. Fangio P, Asehnoune K, Edouard A, Smail N, Benhamou D. Early embolization and vasopressor administration for management of life-threatening hemorrhage from pelvic fracture. *J Trauma* 2005;58(5), 978-984; discussion 984.

23. Ferrara A, MacArthur JD, Wright HK, et al. Hypothermia and acidosis worsen coagulopathy in patients requiring massive transfusion. *Am J Surg* 1990;160:515.

24. Glover JL, Broadie TA. Intraoperative autotransfusion. *World J Surg* 1987;11:60-64.

25. Granger DN. Role of xanthine oxidase and granulocytes in ischemia-reperfusion injury. *Am J Physiol* 1988;255:H1269-H1275.

26. Greaves I, Porter KM, Revell MP. Fluid resuscitation in pre-hospital trauma care: a consensus view. *J R Coll Surg Edinb* 2002;47(2):451-457.

27. Guyton AC, Lindsey AW, Kaufman BN. Effect of mean circulatory filling pressure and other peripheral circulatory factors on cardiac output. *Am J Physiol* 1955;180:463-468.

28. Hak DJ. The role of pelvic angiography in evaluation and management of pelvic trauma. *Orthop Clin North Am* 2004;35(4):439-443,v.

29. Harrigan C, Lucas CE, Ledgerwood AM, et al. Serial changes in primary hemostasis after massive transfusion. *Surgery* 1985;98:836-840.

30. Holcomb JB, Wade CE, Michalek JE, Chisholm GB, Zarzabal LA, Schreiber MA, Gonzalez EA, Pomper GJ, Perkins JG, Spinella PC, Williams KL, Park MS. Increased plasma and platelet to red blood cell ratios improves outcome in 466 massively transfused civilian trauma patients. *Ann Surg* 2008Sep;248(3):447-58.

31. Hoyt DB. Fluid resuscitation: the target from an analysis of trauma systems and patient survival. *J Trauma* 2003;54(5 Suppl):S31-35.

32. Jurkovich QJ. Hypothermia in the trauma patient. In: Maull KI, ed. *Advances in Trauma.* Chicago: Yearbook; 1989:111-140.

33. Kaplan LJ, Kellum JA. Initial pH, base deficit, lactate, anion gap, strong ion difference, and strong ion gap predict outcome from major vascular injury. *Crit Care Med* 2004;32(5):1120-1124.

34. Karmy-Jones R, Nathens A, Jurkovich GJ, et al. Urgent and emergent thoracotomy for penetrating chest trauma. *J Trauma* 2004;56(3):664-668; discussion 668-669.

35. Knudson MM, Maull KI. Nonoperative management of solid organ injuries. Past, present, and future. *Surg Clin North Am* 1999;79(6):1357-1371.

36. Kragh JF Jr, Walters TJ, Baer DG, Fox CJ, Wade CE, Salinas J, Holcomb JB. Survival with emergency tourniquet use to stop bleeding in major limb trauma. *Ann Surg* 2009Jan;249(1):1-7.

37. Kruse JA, Vyskocil JJ, Haupt MT. Intraosseous: a flexible option for the adult or child with delayed, difficult, or impossible conventional vascular access. *Crit Care Med* 1994;22:728-735.

38. Lowry SF, Fong Y. Cytokines and the cellular response to injury and infection. In: Wilmore DW, Brennan MF, Harken AH, et al., eds. *Care of the Surgical Patient.* New York: Scientific American; 1990.

39. Lucas CE, Ledgerwood AM. Cardiovascular and renal response to hemorrhagic and septic shock. In: Clowes GHA Jr, ed. *Trauma, Sepsis and Shock: The Physiological Basis of Therapy.* New York: Marcel Dekker; 1988:87-215.

40. Mandal AK, Sanusi M. Penetrating chest wounds: 24 years' experience. *World J Surg* 2001;25(9):1145-1149.

41. Mansour MA, Moore EE, Moore FA, Read RR. Exigent postinjury thoracotomy analysis of blunt versus penetrating trauma. *Surg Gynecol Obstet* 1992;175(2):97-101.

42. Martin MJ, Fitz Sullivan E, Salim A, et al. Discordance between lactate and base deficit in the surgical intensive care unit: which one do you trust? *Am J Surg* 2006;191(5): 625-630.

43. McManus J, Yershov AL, Ludwig D, Holcomb JB, Salinas J, Dubick MA, Convertino VA, Hinds D, David W, Flanagan T, Duke JH. Radial pulse character relationships to systolic blood pressure and trauma outcomes. *Prehosp Emerg Care* 2005Oct-Dec;9(4):423-8.

44. Mizushima Y, Tohira H, Mizobata Y, Matsuoka T, Yokota J. Fluid resuscitation of trauma patients: how fast is the optimal rate? *Am J Emerg Med* 2005;23(7):833-837.

45. Novak L, Shackford SR, Bourguignon P, et al. Comparison of standard and alternative prehospital resuscitation in uncontrolled hemorrhagic shock and head injury. *J Trauma* 1999;47(5):834-844.

46. Nunez TC, Young PP, Holcomb JB, Cotton BA. Creation, implementation, and maturation of a massive transfusion protocol for the exsanguinating trauma patient. *J Trauma* 2010Jun;68(6):1498-505.

47. Peck KR, Altieri M. Intraosseous infusions: an old technique with modern applications. *Pediatr Nurs* 1988;14(4):296-298.

48. Revell M, Greaves I, Porter K. Endpoints for fluid resuscitation in hemorrhagic shock. *J Trauma* 2003;54(5 Suppl):S63-S67.

49. Riskin DJ, Tsai TC, Riskin L, Hernandez-Boussard T, Purtill M, Maggio PM, Spain DA, Brundage SI. Massive transfusion protocols: the role of aggressive resuscitation versus product ratio in mortality reduction. *J Am Coll Surg* 2009(2):198-205.

50. Roback JD, Caldwell S, Carson J, Davenport R, Drew MJ, Eder A, Fung M, Hamilton M, Hess JR, Luban N, Perkins JG, Sachais BS, Shander A, Silverman T, Snyder E, Tormey C, Waters J, Djulbegovic B. Evidence-based practice guidelines for plasma transfusion. *Transfusion* 2010.

51. Rhodes M, Brader A, Lucke J, et al. A direct transport to the operating room for resuscitation of trauma patients. *J Trauma* 1989;29:907-915.

52. Rohrer MJ, Natale AM. Effect of hypothermia on the coagulation cascade. *Crit Care Med* 1992;20:490.

53. Rotondo MF, Schwab CW, McGonigal MD, et al. "Damage control": an approach for improved survival in exsanguinating penetrating abdominal injury. *J Trauma* 1993;35:375-382.

54. Sadri H, Nguyen-Tang T, Stern R, Hoffmeyer P, Peter R. Control of severe hemorrhage using C-clamp and arterial embolization in hemodynamically unstable patients with pelvic ring disruption. *Arch Orthop Trauma Surg* 2005;125(7):443-447.

55. Sarnoff SJ. Myocardial contractility as described by ventricular function curves: observations on Starling's law of the heart. *Physiol Rev* 1988;35:107-122.

56. Sawyer RW, Bodai BI. The current status of intraosseous infusion. *J Am Coll Surg* 1994;179:353-361.

57. Scalea TM, Hartnett RW, Duncan AO, et al. Central venous oxygen saturation: a useful clinical tool in trauma patients. *J Trauma* 1990;30(12):1539-1543.

58. Thourani VH, Feliciano DV, Cooper WA, et al. Penetrating cardiac trauma at an urban trauma center: a 22-year perspective. *Am Surg* 1999;65(9):811-816; discussion 817-818.

59. Tyburski JG, Astra L, Wilson RF, Dente C, Steffes C. Factors affecting prognosis with penetrating wounds of the heart. *J Trauma* 2000;48(4):587-590; discussion 590-591.

60. von OUO, Bautz P, De GM. Penetrating thoracic injuries: what we have learnt. *Thorac Cardiovasc Surg* 2000;48(1):55-61.

61. Werwath DL, Schwab CW, Scholter JR, et al. Microwave oven: a safe new method of warming crystalloids. *Am J Surg* 1984;12:656-659.

62. Williams JF, Seneff MG, Friedman BC, et al. Use of femoral venous catheters in critically ill adults: prospective study. *Crit Care Med* 1991;19:550-553.

63. York J, Arrilaga A, Graham R, et al. Fluid resuscitation of patients with multiple injuries and severe closed head injury: experience with an aggressive fluid resuscitation strategy. *J Trauma* 2000;48(3):376-379.

Shock Assessment and Management

⏵⏵ INTERACTIVE SKILL PROCEDURES

Note: Accompanying some of the skills in this Skill Station is a series of scenarios for you to review and use to prepare for this station. Tables pertaining to the initial assessment and management of the patient in shock are also provided for your review. Standard precautions are required whenever caring for trauma patients.

THE FOLLOWING PROCEDURES ARE INCLUDED IN THIS SKILL STATION:

⏵⏵ **Skill IV-A:** Peripheral Venous Access

⏵⏵ **Skill IV-B:** Femoral Venipuncture: Seldinger Technique

⏵⏵ **Skill IV-C:** Subclavian Venipuncture: Infraclavicular Approach

⏵⏵ **Skill IV-D:** Internal Jugular Venipuncture: Middle or Central Route

⏵⏵ **Skill IV-E:** Intraosseous Puncture/ Infusion: Proximal Tibial Route

⏵⏵ **Skill IV-F:** Identification and Management of Pelvic Fractures: Application of Pelvic Binder

Objectives

Performance at this skill station will allow the participant to practice techniques necessary to treat a patient in shock, determine the cause of the shock state, perform the initial management of shock, and manage the patient's response to treatment. Specifically, the student will be able to:

1 Recognize the shock state.

2 Identify the causes of the shock state.

3 Identify the surface markings and demonstrate the techniques of vascular access for the following:

• Peripheral venous system

• Femoral vein

• Internal jugular vein

• Subclavian vein

• Intraosseous infusion

4 Identify the appropriate surface landmarks for placing a pelvic binder and successfully place a commercial binder or sheet wrap.

5 Explain the value of the anteroposterior (AP) pelvic x-ray examination to identify the potential for massive blood loss, and describe the maneuvers that can be used to reduce pelvic volume and control bleeding.

6 Select the appropriate equipment for pediatric patients based on age (Broselow™ tape).

7 Use adjuncts in the assessment and management of the shock state, including:

• X-ray examination (chest and pelvic films)

• Diagnostic peritoneal lavage (DPL)

• Focused assessment sonography in trauma (FAST)

• Computed tomography (CT)

8 Identify patients who require definitive hemorrhage control or transfer to an intensive care unit.

9 Identify which additional therapeutic measures are necessary based on the patient's response to treatment and the clinical significance of the responses of patients, as classified by:

• Rapid response

• Transient response

• Nonresponse

▶ SCENARIOS

SCENARIO IV-1

A 42-year-old female was ejected from a vehicle during an automobile collision. En route to the emergency department (ED), prehospital personnel report that her heart rate is 110 beats/min, her blood pressure is 88/46 mm Hg, and her respiratory rate is 30 breaths/min. The patient is confused, and her peripheral capillary refill is reduced. (See Table IV.1.) Her airway is patent. She is in respiratory distress with neck vein distention, absent breath sounds on the right, and tracheal deviation to the left.

SCENARIO IV-2 (Continuation of Previous Scenario)

After needle decompression and chest-tube insertion, the patient's heart rate is 120 beats/min, the blood pressure is 80/46 mm Hg, and the respiratory rate is 30 breaths/min. Her skin is pale, cool, and moist to touch. She moans when stimulated. (See Table IV.2.)

SCENARIO IV-3 (Continuation of previous scenario)

After the initiation of vascular access and infusion of 2000 mL of warmed crystalloid solution, the patient's heart rate has decreased to 90 beats/min; the blood pressure is 110/80 mm Hg and the respiratory rate is 22 breaths/min. The patient is now able to speak, her breathing is less labored, and her peripheral perfusion has improved. (See Table IV.2.)

SCENARIO IV-4 (Continuation of previous scenario)

The patient responds initially to the rapid infusion of 1500 mL of warmed crystalloid solution by a transient increase in blood pressure to 110/80 mm Hg, a decrease in the heart rate to 96 beats/min, and improvements in level of consciousness and peripheral perfusion. Fluid infusion is slowed to maintenance levels. Five minutes later, the assistant reports a deterioration in the blood pressure to 88/60 mm Hg, an increase in the heart rate to 115 beats/min, and a return in the delay of the peripheral capillary refill. (See Table IV.3.)

Alternative Scenario: The rapid infusion of 2000 mL of warmed crystalloid solution produces only a modest increase in the patient's blood pressure to 90/60 mm Hg, and her heart rate remains at 110 beats/min. Her urinary output since the insertion of the urinary catheter has been only 5 mL of very dark urine.

■ TABLE IV.1 INITIAL ASSESSMENT AND SHOCK MANAGEMENT

CONDITION	ASSESSMENT (PHYSICAL EXAMINATION)	MANAGEMENT
Tension pneumothorax	• Tracheal deviation • Distended neck veins • Tympany • Absent breath sounds	• Needle decompression • Tube thoracostomy
Massive hemothorax	• Tracheal deviation • Flat neck veins • Percussion dullness • Absent breath sounds	• Venous access • Volume replacement • Surgical consultation/thoracotomy • Tube thoracostomy
Cardiac tamponade	• Distended neck veins • Muffled heart tones • Ultrasound	• Venous access • Volume replacement • Thoracotomy • Pericardiocentesis
Intraabdominal hemorrhage	• Distended abdomen • Uterine lift, if pregnant • DPL /ultrasonography • Vaginal examination	• Venous access • Volume replacement • Surgical consultation • Displace uterus from vena cava
Obvious external bleeding	• Identify source of obvious external bleeding	• Direct pressure • Splints • Closure of actively bleeding scalp wounds

■ TABLE IV.2 PELVIC FRACTURES

CONDITION	IMAGE FINDINGS	SIGNIFICANCE	INTERVENTION
Pelvic fracture	**Pelvic x-ray** • Pubic ramus fracture	• Less blood loss than other types • Lateral compression mechanism	• Volume replacement • Probable transfusion • Decreased pelvic volume • Pelvic binder • External fixator • Angiography • Skeletal traction • Orthopedic consultation
	• Open book	• Pelvic volume increased • Major source of blood loss	
	• Vertical shear	• Major source of blood loss	
Visceral organ injury	**CT scan** • Intraabdominal hemorrhage	• Potential for continuing blood loss • Performed only in hemodynamically normal patients	• Volume replacement • Possible transfusion • Surgical consultation

■ TABLE IV.3 TRANSIENT RESPONDER

ETIOLOGY	PHYSICAL EXAM	ADDITIONAL DIAGNOSTIC STEPS	INTERVENTION
Underestimation of blood loss or continuing blood loss	• Abdominal distention • Pelvic fracture • Extremity fracture • Obvious external bleeding	• DPL or ultrasonography	• Surgical consultation • Volume infusion • Blood transfusion • Apply appropriate splints
Nonhemorrhagic • Cardiac tamponade	• Distended neck veins • Decreased heart sounds • Normal breath sounds	• Echocardiogram • FAST	• Thoracotomy • Transfer
• Recurrent/persistent tension pneumothorax	• Distended neck veins • Tracheal shift • Absent breath sounds • Hyperresonant chest percussion	• Clinical diagnosis	• Reevaluate chest • Needle decompression • Tube thoracostomy

■ TABLE IV.4 NONRESPONDER

ETIOLOGY	PHYSICAL EXAM	ADDITIONAL DIAGNOSTIC STEPS	INTERVENTION
Massive blood loss (Class III or IV) • Intraabdominal bleeding	• Abdominal distention	• DPL or ultrasonography	• Immediate intervention by surgeon • Volume restoration
Nonhemorrhagic • Tension pneumothorax	• Distended neck veins • Tracheal shift • Absent breath sounds • Hyperresonant chest percussion	• Clinical diagnosis	• Reevaluate chest • Needle decompression • Tube thoracotomy
• Cardiac tamponade	• Distended neck veins • Decreased heart sounds • Normal breath sounds	• FAST • Pericardiocentesis	• Thoracotomy
• Blunt cardiac injury	• Irregular heart rate • Inadequate perfusion	• Ischemic ECG changes • ECG	• Ensure no source of hemorrhage missed • Inotropic support • Invasive monitoring

SCENARIO IV-5

A 42-year-old female, ejected from her vehicle during a crash, arrives in the ED unconscious with a heart rate of 140 beats/min, a blood pressure of 60 mm Hg by palpation, and pale, cool, and pulseless extremities. Endotracheal intubation and assisted ventilation are initiated. The rapid volume infusion of 2000 mL of warmed crystalloid solution does not improve her vital signs, and she does not demonstrate evidence of improved organ perfusion. (See Table IV.4.)

SCENARIO IV-6

An 18-month-old boy is brought to the ED by his mother, who apparently experiences spousal abuse. The child has evidence of multiple soft-tissue injuries about the chest, abdomen, and extremities. His skin color is pale, he has a weak, thready pulse rate of 160 beats/min, and he responds only to painful stimuli with a weak cry.

▶ Skill IV-A: Peripheral Venous Access

STEP 1. Select an appropriate site on an extremity (antecubital, forearm, or saphenous vein).

STEP 2. Apply an elastic tourniquet above the proposed puncture site.

STEP 3. Clean the site with antiseptic solution.

STEP 4. Puncture the vein with a large-caliber, plastic, over-the-needle catheter. Observe for blood return.

STEP 5. Thread the catheter into the vein over the needle.

STEP 6. Remove the needle and tourniquet.

STEP 7. If appropriate, obtain blood samples for laboratory tests.

STEP 8. Connect the catheter to the intravenous infusion tubing and begin the infusion of warmed crystalloid solution.

STEP 9. Observe for possible infiltration of fluids into the tissues.

STEP 10. Secure the catheter and tubing to the skin of the extremity.

▶ Skill IV-B: Femoral Venipuncture: Seldinger Technique

Note: Sterile technique should be used when performing this procedure.

STEP 1. Place the patient in the supine position.

STEP 2. Cleanse the skin around the venipuncture site well and drape the area.

STEP 3. Locate the femoral vein by palpating the femoral artery. The vein lies directly medial to the femoral artery (remember the mnemonic NAVEL, from lateral to medial: nerve, artery, vein, empty space, lymphatic). Keep a finger on the artery to facilitate anatomical location and avoid insertion of the catheter into the artery. Ultrasound can be used as an adjunct for placement of central venous lines.

STEP 4. If the patient is awake, use a local anesthetic at the venipuncture site.

STEP 5. Make a small skin incision at the entry point of wire or dilatation of central vein to insert large bore catheter.

STEP 6. Introduce a large-caliber needle attached to a 12-mL syringe with 0.5 to 1 mL of saline. The needle, directed toward the patient's head, should enter the skin directly over the femoral vein (■ FIGURE IV-1A). Hold the needle and syringe parallel to the frontal plane.

STEP 7. Directing the needle cephalad and posteriorly, slowly advance it while gently withdrawing the plunger of the syringe.

STEP 8. When a free flow of blood appears in the syringe, remove the syringe and occlude the needle with a finger to prevent air embolism. If the vein is not entered, withdraw the needle and redirect it. If two attempts

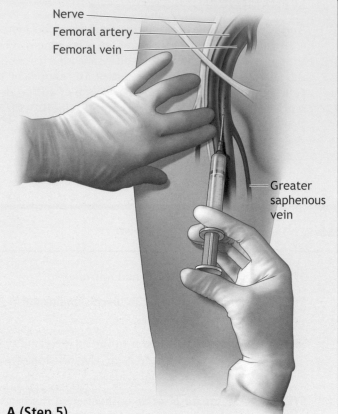

A (Step 5)

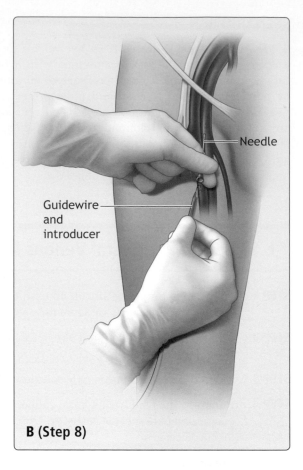

B (Step 8)

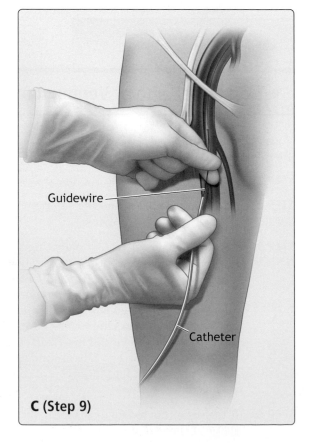

C (Step 9)

■ FIGURE IV-1 Femoral Venipuncture: Seldinger Technique.
(A) Introduce a large-caliber needle attached to a 12-mL
syringe with 0.5 to 1 mL of saline. The needle, directed
toward the patient's head, should enter the skin directly over
the femoral vein. (B) Insert the guidewire and remove the
needle. Use an introducer if required. (C) Insert the catheter
over the guidewire.

are unsuccessful, a more experienced clinician should attempt the procedure, if available.

STEP 9. Insert the guidewire and remove the needle. Use an introducer if required (■ FIGURE IV-1B).

STEP 10. Insert the catheter over the guidewire (■ FIGURE IV-1C).

STEP 11. Remove the guidewire and connect the catheter to the intravenous tubing.

STEP 12. Affix the catheter in place (with a suture), apply antibiotic ointment, and dress the area.

STEP 13. Tape the intravenous tubing in place.

STEP 14. Obtain chest and abdominal x-ray films to confirm the position and placement of the intravenous catheter.

STEP 15. Change the catheter as soon as it is practical.

▶▶ MAJOR COMPLICATIONS OF FEMORAL VENOUS ACCESS

- Deep-vein thrombosis
- Arterial or neurologic injury
- Infection
- Arteriovenous fistula

▶ Skill IV-C: Subclavian Venipuncture: Infraclavicular Approach

Note: Sterile technique should be used when performing this procedure.

STEP 1. Place the patient in the supine position, with the head at least 15 degrees down to distend the neck veins and prevent air embolism. Only if a cervical spine injury has been excluded can the patient's head be turned away from the venipuncture site.

STEP 2. Cleanse the skin around the venipuncture site well and drape the area.

STEP 3. If the patient is awake, use a local anesthetic at the venipuncture site.

STEP 4. Introduce a large-caliber needle, attached to a 12-mL syringe with 0.5 to 1 mL of saline, 1 cm below the junction of the middle and medial one-third of the clavicle. Ultrasound can be used as an adjunct for the placement of central venous lines

STEP 5. After the skin has been punctured, with the bevel of the needle upward, expel the skin plug that can occlude the needle.

STEP 6. Hold the needle and syringe parallel to the frontal plane.

STEP 7. Direct the needle medially, slightly cephalad, and posteriorly behind the clavicle toward the posterior, superior angle of the sternal end of the clavicle (toward the finger placed in the suprasternal notch).

STEP 8. Slowly advance the needle while gently withdrawing the plunger of the syringe.

STEP 9. When a free flow of blood appears in the syringe, rotate the bevel of the needle caudally, remove the syringe, and occlude the needle with a finger to prevent air embolism. If the vein is not entered, withdraw the needle and redirect it. If two attempts are unsuccessful, a more experienced clinician should attempt the procedure, if available.

STEP 10. Insert the guidewire while monitoring the electrocardiogram for rhythm abnormalities.

STEP 11. Remove the needle while holding the guidewire in place.

STEP 12. Insert the catheter over the guidewire to a predetermined depth (the tip of the catheter should be above the right atrium for fluid administration).

STEP 13. Connect the catheter to the intravenous tubing.

STEP 14. Affix the catheter securely to the skin (with a suture), apply antibiotic ointment, and dress the area.

STEP 15. Tape the intravenous tubing in place.

STEP 16. Obtain a chest x-ray film to confirm the position of the intravenous line and identify a possible pneumothorax.

▶ Skill IV-D: Internal Jugular Venipuncture: Middle or Central Route

Note: This procedure is frequently difficult to perform in injured patients because they are often immobilized to protect the cervical spine. Sterile technique should be used when performing this procedure.

STEP 1. Place the patient in the supine position, with the head at least 15 degrees down to distend the neck veins and prevent an air embolism. Only if the cervical spine has been cleared radiographically can the patient's head be turned away from the venipuncture site.

STEP 2. Cleanse the skin around the venipuncture site well and drape the area.

STEP 3. If the patient is awake, use a local anesthetic at the venipuncture site.

STEP 4. Introduce a large-caliber needle, attached to a 12-mL syringe with 0.5 to 1 mL of saline, into the center of the triangle formed by the two lower heads of the sternomastoid and the clavicle. Ultrasound can be used as an adjunct for the placement of central venous lines.

STEP 5. After the skin has been punctured, with the bevel of the needle upward, expel the skin plug that can occlude the needle.

STEP 6. Direct the needle caudally, parallel to the sagittal plane, at an angle 30 degrees posterior to the frontal plane.

STEP 7. Slowly advance the needle while gently withdrawing the plunger of the syringe.

STEP 8. When a free flow of blood appears in the syringe, remove the syringe and occlude the needle with a finger to prevent air embolism. If the vein is not entered, withdraw the needle and redirect it 5 to 10 degrees laterally.

STEP 9. Insert the guidewire while monitoring the electrocardiogram (ECG) for rhythm abnormalities.

STEP 10. Remove the needle while securing the guidewire and advance the catheter over the wire. Connect the catheter to the intravenous tubing.

STEP 11. Affix the catheter in place to the skin with suture, apply antibiotic ointment, and dress the area.

STEP 12. Tape the intravenous tubing in place.

STEP 13. Obtain a chest film to confirm the position of the intravenous line and identify a possible pneumothorax.

▶▶ COMPLICATIONS OF CENTRAL VENOUS PUNCTURE

- Pneumothorax or hemothorax
- Venous thrombosis
- Arterial or neurologic injury
- Arteriovenous fistula
- Chylothorax
- Infection
- Air embolism

▶ Skill IV-E: Intraosseous Puncture/Infusion: Proximal Tibial Route

Note: Sterile technique should be used when performing this procedure.

This procedure is appropriate for all ages when venous access is impossible because of circulatory collapse or when percutaneous peripheral venous cannulation has failed on two attempts. Intraosseous infusions (blood and crystalloids) should be limited to emergency resuscitation discontinued as soon as other venous access has been obtained.

Methylene blue dye can be mixed with the saline or water for demonstration purposes on chicken or turkey bones only. When the needle is properly placed within the medullary canal, the methylene blue dye/saline solution seeps from the upper end of the chicken or turkey bone when the solution is injected (see Step 8). Swelling around the intraosseous needle should prompt discontinuation of fluid infusion and removal of the intraosseous device.

STEP 1. Place the patient in the supine position. Select an uninjured lower extremity, place sufficient padding under the knee to effect approximate 30-degree flexion of the knee, and allow the patient's heel to rest comfortably on the gurney or stretcher.

STEP 2. Identify the puncture site—the anteromedial surface of the proximal tibia, approximately one fingerbreadth (1 to 3 cm) below the tubercle.

STEP 3. Cleanse the skin around the puncture site well and drape the area.

STEP 4. If the patient is awake, use a local anesthetic at the puncture site.

STEP 5. Initially at a 90-degree angle, introduce a short (threaded or smooth), large-caliber, bone-marrow aspiration needle (or a short, 18-gauge spinal needle with stylet) into the skin and periosteum, with the needle bevel directed toward the foot and away from the epiphyseal plate.

STEP 6. After gaining purchase in the bone, direct the needle 45 to 60 degrees away from the epiphyseal plate (■ FIGURE IV-2). Using a gentle twisting or boring motion, advance the needle through the bone cortex and into the bone marrow.

STEP 7. Remove the stylet and attach to the needle a 12-mL syringe with approximately 6 mL of sterile saline. Gently draw on the plunger

STEP 8. of the syringe. Aspiration of bone marrow into the syringe signifies entrance into the medullary cavity.

STEP 8. Inject the saline into the needle to expel any clot that can occlude the needle. If the saline flushes through the needle easily and there is no evidence of swelling, the needle is likely located in the appropriate place. If bone marrow was not aspirated as outlined in Step 7, but the needle flushes easily when injecting the saline and there is no evidence of swelling, the needle is likely in the appropriate place. In addition, proper placement of the needle is indicated if the needle remains upright without support and intravenous solution flows freely without evidence of subcutaneous infiltration.

STEP 9. Connect the needle to the large-caliber intravenous tubing and begin fluid infusion. Carefully screw the needle further into the medullary cavity until the needle hub rests on the patient's skin and free flow continues. If a smooth needle is used, it should be stabilized at a 45- to 60-degree angle to the anteromedial surface of the patient's leg.

STEP 10. Apply antibiotic ointment and a 3×3 sterile dressing. Secure the needle and tubing in place.

STEP 11. Routinely reevaluate the placement of the intraosseous needle, ensuring that it remains through the bone cortex and in the medullary canal. Remember, intraosseous infusion should be limited to emergency resuscitation of the patient and discontinued as soon as other venous access has been obtained.

▶▶ COMPLICATIONS OF INTRAOSSEOUS PUNCTURE

- Infection
- Through-and-through penetration of the bone
- Subcutaneous or subperiosteal infiltration
- Pressure necrosis of the skin
- Physeal plate injury
- Hematoma

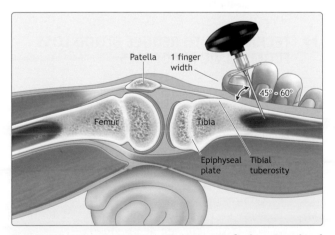

■ **FIGURE IV-2 Intraosseous Puncture/Infusion: Proximal Tibial Route.** After gaining purchase in the bone, direct the needle 45 to 60 degrees away from the epiphyseal plate.

▶ Skill IV-F: Identification and Management of Pelvic Fractures: Application of Pelvic Binder

STEP 1. Identify the mechanism of injury, which can suggest the possibility of a pelvic fracture—for example, ejection from a motor vehicle, crushing injury, pedestrian-vehicle collision, or motorcycle collision.

STEP 2. Inspect the pelvic area for ecchymosis, perineal or scrotal hematoma, and blood at the urethral meatus.

STEP 3. Inspect the legs for differences in length or asymmetry in rotation of the hips.

STEP 4. Perform a rectal examination, noting the position and mobility of the prostate gland, any palpable fracture, or the presence of gross or occult blood in the stool.

STEP 5. Perform a vaginal examination, noting palpable fractures, the size and consistency of the uterus, or the presence of blood. Remember, females of childbearing age may be pregnant.

STEP 6. If Steps 2 through 5 are abnormal, or if the mechanism of injury suggests a pelvic fracture, obtain an AP x-ray film of the patient's pelvis. (Note: The mechanism of injury may suggest the type of fracture.)

STEP 7. If Steps 2 through 5 are normal, palpate the bony pelvis to identify painful areas.

STEP 8. Determine pelvic stability by gently applying anterior-posterior compression and lateral-to-medial compression over the anterosuperior iliac crests. Test for axial mobility by gently pushing and pulling on the legs to determine stability in a cranial-caudal direction. Immobilize the pelvis properly by using a sheet and/or a commercially available binder (e.g., T-pod).

STEP 9. Cautiously insert a urinary catheter, if not contraindicated, or perform retrograde urethrography if a urethral injury is suspected.

STEP 10. Interpret the pelvic x-ray film, giving special consideration to fractures that are frequently associated with significant blood loss—for example, fractures that increase the pelvic volume.

A. Confirm the patient's identification on the film.

B. Systematically evaluate the film for:

- Width of the symphysis pubis—greater than a 1-cm separation may signify significant pelvic injury
- Integrity of the superior and inferior pubic rami bilaterally
- Integrity of the acetabula, as well as femoral heads and necks
- Symmetry of the ilium and width of the sacroiliac joints
- Symmetry of the sacral foramina by evaluating the arcuate lines
- Fracture(s) of the transverse processes of L5

C. Remember, the bony pelvis is a ring that rarely sustains an injury in only one location. Displacement of ringed structures implies two fracture sites.

D. Remember, fractures that increase the pelvic volume—for example, vertical shear and open-book fractures, are often associated with massive blood loss.

▶▶ TECHNIQUES TO REDUCE BLOOD LOSS FROM PELVIC FRACTURES

STEP 1. Avoid excessive and repeated manipulation of the pelvis.

STEP 2. Internally rotate the lower legs to close an open-book type fracture. Pad bony prominences and tie the rotated legs together. This maneuver can reduce a displaced symphysis, decrease the pelvic volume, and serve as a temporary measure until definitive treatment can be provided.

STEP 3. Apply a pelvic external fixation device (early orthopedic consultation).

STEP 4. Apply skeletal limb traction (early orthopedic consultation).

STEP 5. Embolize pelvic vessels via angiography.

STEP 6. Obtain early surgical and orthopedic consultation to determine priorities.

STEP 7. Place sandbags under each buttock if there is no indication of spinal injury and other techniques to close the pelvis are not available.

STEP 8. Apply a pelvic binder.

STEP 9. Arrange for transfer to a definitive-care facility if local resources are not available to manage this injury.

Venous Cutdown (Optional Station)

▶▶ INTERACTIVE SKILL PROCEDURES

Note: Accompanying some of the skills in this Skill Station is a series of scenarios for you to review and use to prepare for this station. Tables pertaining to the initial assessment and management of the patient in shock are also provided for your review. Standard precautions are required whenever caring for trauma patients.

THE FOLLOWING PROCEDURE IS INCLUDED IN THIS SKILL STATION:

▶▶ **Skill IV-A:** Venous Cutdown

Objectives

Performance at this skill station will allow the participant to practice and demonstrate on a live, anesthetized animal or a fresh, human cadaver the technique of peripheral venous cutdown. Specifically, the student will be able to:

1 Identify and describe the surface markings and structures necessary to perform a peripheral venous cutdown.

2 Describe the indications and contraindications for a peripheral venous cutdown.

Anatomic Considerations for Venous Cutdown

■ The primary site for a peripheral venous cutdown is the greater saphenous vein at the ankle, which is located at a point approximately 2 cm anterior and superior to the medial malleolus. (See ■ FIGURE V-1A.)

■ A secondary site is the antecubital medial basilic vein, located 2.5 cm lateral to the medial epicondyle of the humerus at the flexion crease of the elbow.

▶ Skill V-A: Venous Cutdown

STEP 1. Cleanse the skin around the venipuncture site well and drape the area.

STEP 2. If the patient is awake, use a local anesthetic at the venipuncture site.

STEP 3. Make a full-thickness, transverse skin incision through the anesthetized area to a length of 2.5 cm.

STEP 4. By blunt dissection, using a curved hemostat, identify the vein and dissect it free from any accompanying structures.

STEP 5. Elevate and dissect the vein for a distance of approximately 2 cm to free it from its bed.

STEP 6. Ligate the distal mobilized vein, leaving the suture in place for traction.

STEP 7. Pass a tie around the vein in a cephalad direction.

STEP 8. Make a small, transverse venotomy and gently dilate the venotomy with the tip of a closed hemostat.

STEP 9. Introduce a plastic cannula through the venotomy and secure it in place by tying the upper ligature around the vein and cannula (■ FIGURE V-1B). The cannula should be inserted an adequate distance to prevent dislodging.

STEP 10. Attach the intravenous tubing to the cannula and close the incision with interrupted sutures.

STEP 11. Apply a sterile dressing with a topical antibiotic ointment.

▶▶ COMPLICATIONS OF PERIPHERAL VENOUS CUTDOWN

- Cellulitis
- Hematoma
- Phlebitis
- Perforation of the posterior wall of the vein
- Venous thrombosis
- Nerve transection
- Arterial transaction

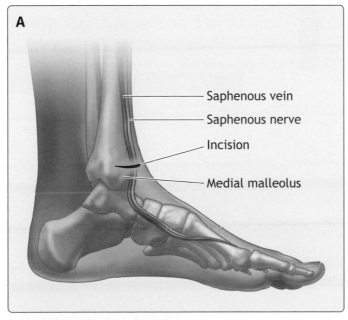

A

Saphenous vein
Saphenous nerve
Incision
Medial malleolus

B

Saphenous nerve
Vein
Catheter

■ FIGURE V-1 Venous Cutdown

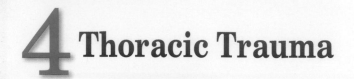

4 Thoracic Trauma

Thoracic injury is common in the poly-trauma patient and can pose life-threatening problems if not promptly identified during the primary survey.

Outline

Scenario A 27-year-old male was the unrestrained driver in a high-speed, frontal-impact collision. Vital signs are: blood pressure 90/70; heart rate 110; and respiratory rate 36. Initial assessment reveals a Glasgow Coma Scale (GCS) score of 15 and a patent airway.

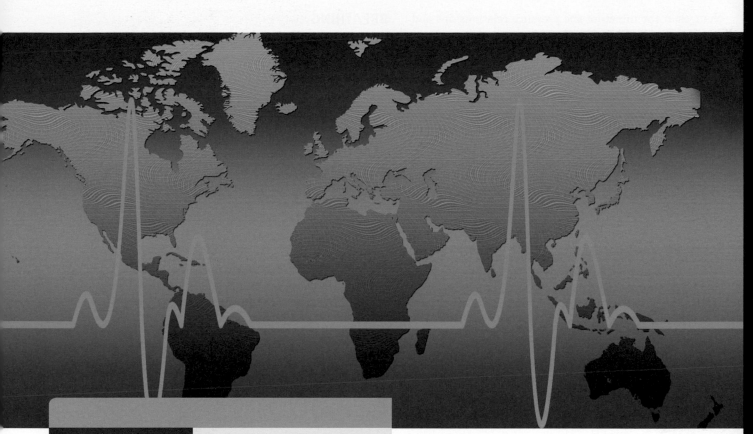

Objectives

1 Identify and initiate treatment of the following injuries during the primary survey:

A E
- Airway obstruction
- Tension pneumothorax
B E
- Open pneumothorax
- Flail chest and pulmonary contusion
C E
- Massive hemothorax
- Cardiac tamponade

things that can kill if don't deal c right away

2 Identify and initiate treatment of the following potentially life-threatening injuries during the secondary survey:

- Simple pneumothorax
- Hemothorax
- Pulmonary contusion
- Tracheobronchial tree injury
- Blunt cardiac injury
- Traumatic aovrtic disruption
- Traumatic diaphragmatic injury
- Blunt esophageal rupture

potential to kill if Ø dealt c at some point.

3 Describe the significance and treatment of the following injuries:

- Subcutaneous emphysema
- Thoracic crush injuries
- Sternal, rib, and clavicular fractures

? *What are the immediately life-threatening chest injuries?*

Thoracic trauma is a significant cause of mortality. Many patients with thoracic trauma die after reaching the hospital; however, many of these deaths could be prevented with prompt diagnosis and treatment. Less than 10% of blunt chest injuries and only 15% to 30% of penetrating chest injuries require operative intervention (typically thoracoscopy or thoracotomy). In fact, most patients who sustain thoracic trauma can be treated by technical procedures within the capabilities of clinicians who take this course. Many of the principles outlined in this chapter also apply to iatrogenic thoracic injuries, such as hemothorax or pneumothorax with central line placement and esophageal injury during endoscopy.

Hypoxia, hypercarbia, and acidosis often result from chest injuries. Tissue hypoxia results from the inadequate delivery of oxygen to the tissues because of hypovolemia (blood loss), pulmonary ventilation/perfusion mismatch (e.g., contusion, hematoma, and alveolar collapse), and changes in the intrathoracic pressure relationships (e.g., tension pneumothorax and open pneumothorax). This hypoperfusion leads to metabolic acidosis. Hypercarbia with resultant respiratory acidosis most often follows inadequate ventilation caused by changes in the intrathoracic pressure relationships and depressed level of consciousness. The initial assessment and treatment of patients with thoracic trauma consists of the primary survey, resuscitation of vital functions, detailed secondary survey, and definitive care. Because hypoxia is the most serious aspect of chest injury, the goal of early intervention is to prevent or correct hypoxia. Injuries that are an immediate threat to life are treated as quickly and simply as is possible. Most life-threatening thoracic injuries can be treated with airway control or an appropriately placed chest tube or needle. The secondary survey is influenced by the history of the injury and a high index of suspicion for specific injuries.

Primary Survey: Life-Threatening Injuries

? *What are the pathophysiologic consequences of these chest injuries?*

The primary survey of patients with thoracic injuries begins with the airway, followed by breathing and then circulation. **Major problems should be corrected as they are identified.**

AIRWAY

It is necessary to recognize and address major injuries affecting the airway during the primary survey. Airway patency and air exchange should be assessed by listening for air movement at the patient's nose, mouth, and lung fields; inspecting the oropharynx for foreign-body obstruction; and observing for intercostal and supraclavicular muscle retractions.

Laryngeal injury can accompany major thoracic trauma. Although the clinical presentation is occasionally subtle, acute airway obstruction from laryngeal trauma is a life-threatening injury. See Chapter 2: Airway and Ventilatory Management.

Injury to the upper chest can create a palpable defect in the region of the sternoclavicular joint, with posterior dislocation of the clavicular head, which causes upper airway obstruction. Identification of this injury is made by listening for upper airway obstruction (stridor) or a marked change in the expected voice quality, if the patient is able to talk. Management consists of a closed reduction of the injury, which can be performed by extending the shoulders or grasping the clavicle with a pointed instrument, such as a towel clamp, and manually reducing the fracture. Once reduced, this injury is usually stable if the patient remains in the supine position.

Other injuries affecting the airway are addressed in Chapter 2: Airway and Ventilatory Management.

BREATHING

The patient's chest and neck should be completely exposed to allow for assessment of breathing and the neck veins. This may require temporarily releasing the front of the cervical collar following blunt trauma. In this case, cervical spine immobilization should always be actively maintained by holding the patient's head while the collar is loose. Respiratory movement and quality of respirations are assessed by observing, palpating, and listening.

Important, yet often subtle, signs of chest injury or hypoxia include an increased respiratory rate and change in the breathing pattern, which is often manifested by progressively shallower respirations. Cyanosis is a late sign of hypoxia in trauma patients. However, the absence of cyanosis does not necessarily indicate adequate tissue oxygenation or an adequate airway. The major thoracic injuries that affect breathing and that must be recognized and addressed during the primary survey include tension pneumothorax, open pneumothorax (sucking chest wound), flail chest and pulmonary contusion, and massive hemothorax.

PITFALLS

After intubation, one of the common reasons for loss of breath sounds in the left thorax is a right mainstem intubation. During the reassessment, be sure to check the position of the endotracheal tube before assuming that the change in physical examination is due to a pneumothorax or hemothorax.

✶Tension Pneumothorax (think when BLUNT trauma)

A tension pneumothorax develops when a "one-way valve" air leak occurs from the lung or through the chest wall (■ FIGURE 4-1). Air is forced into the pleural space without any means of escape, eventually completely collapsing the affected lung. The mediastinum is displaced to the opposite side, decreasing venous return and compressing the opposite lung. Shock results from the marked decrease in venous return causing a reduction in cardiac output and is often classified as obstructive shock.

The most common cause of tension pneumothorax is mechanical ventilation with positive-pressure ventilation in patients with visceral pleural injury. However, a tension pneumothorax can complicate a simple pneumothorax following penetrating or blunt chest trauma in which a parenchymal lung injury fails to seal, or after a misguided attempt at subclavian or internal jugular venous catheter insertion. Occasionally, traumatic defects in the chest wall also can cause a tension pneumothorax if incorrectly covered with occlusive dressings

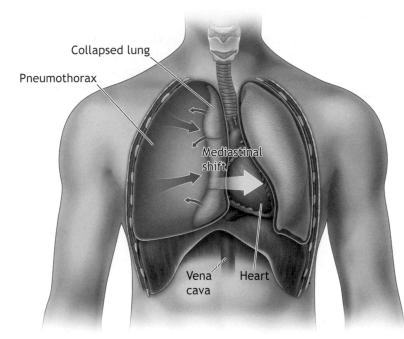

Collapsed lung

Pneumothorax

Mediastinal shift

Vena cava

Heart

■ **FIGURE 4-1 Tension Pneumothorax.** A tension pneumothorax develops when a "one-way valve" air leak occurs from the lung or through the chest wall. Air is forced into the pleural space, eventually completely collapsing the affected lung.

or if the defect itself constitutes a flap-valve mechanism. Tension pneumothorax rarely occurs from markedly displaced thoracic spine fractures.

Tension pneumothorax is a clinical diagnosis reflecting air under pressure in the affected pleural space. Treatment should not be delayed to wait for radiologic confirmation. Tension pneumothorax is characterized by some or all of the following signs and symptoms:

- Chest pain (pleuritic)
- Air hunger
- Respiratory distress
- Tachycardia
- Hypotension
- Tracheal deviation away from the side of injury
- Unilateral absence of breath sounds
- Elevated hemithorax without respiratory movement
- Neck vein distinction
- Cyanosis (late manifestation)

Because of the similarity in their signs, tension pneumothorax can be confused initially with cardiac tamponade. Differentiation is made by a hyperresonant note on percussion, deviated trachea, and absent breath sounds over the affected hemithorax, which are signs of tension pneumothorax.

Tension pneumothorax requires immediate decompression and may be managed initially by rapidly

inserting a large-caliber needle into the second intercostal space in the midclavicular line of the affected hemithorax (■ **FIGURE 4-2**). However, due to variable thickness of the chest wall, kinking of the catheter and other technical or anatomic complications, this maneuver may not be successful. See <u>Skill Station VII: Chest Trauma Management</u>, <u>Skill VII-A: Needle Thoracentesis</u>. When successful, this maneuver converts the injury to a simple pneumothorax; however, the possibility of subsequent pneumothorax as a result of

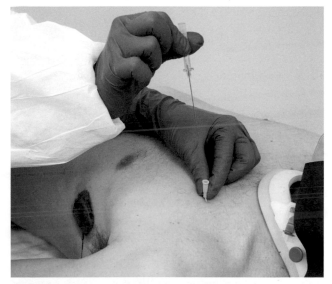

■ **FIGURE 4-2 Needle Decompression.** Tension pneumothorax may be managed initially by rapidly inserting a large-caliber needle into the second intercostal space in the midclavicular line of the affected hemithorax.

★ 5cm needle works >50% of time
☆ 8 cm needle works >90% of time

the needle stick now exists, so repeated reassessment of the patient is necessary.

Chest wall thickness influences the likelihood of success with needle decompression. Recent evidence suggests that a 5 cm needle will reach the pleural space >50% of the time, whereas an 8 cm needle will reach the pleural space >90% of the time. Even with a needle of the appropriate size, the maneuver will not always be successful. Definitive treatment requires the insertion of a chest tube into the fifth intercostal space (usually at the nipple level), just anterior to the midaxillary line.

Open Pneumothorax (Sucking Chest Wound)

Large defects of the chest wall that remain open can result in an open pneumothorax, which is also known as a sucking chest wound (■ FIGURE 4-3). Equilibration between intrathoracic pressure and atmospheric pressure is immediate. Air tends to follow the path of least resistance; as such, if the opening in the chest wall is approximately two-thirds of the diameter of the trachea or greater, air passes preferentially through the chest wall defect with each respiratory effort. Effective ventilation is thereby impaired, leading to hypoxia and hypercarbia.

Initial management of an open pneumothorax is accomplished by promptly closing the defect with a sterile occlusive dressing. The dressing should be large enough to overlap the wound's edges and then taped securely on three sides in order to provide a flutter-type valve effect (■ FIGURE 4-4). As the patient breathes in, the dressing occludes the wound, preventing air from

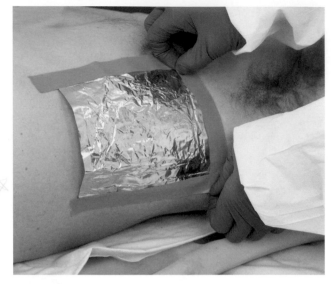

■ **FIGURE 4-4 Dressing for Treatment of Open Pneumothorax.** Promptly close the defect with a sterile occlusive dressing that is large enough to overlap the wound's edges. Tape it securely on three sides to provide a flutter-type valve effect.

entering. During exhalation, the open end of the dressing allows air to escape from the pleural space. A chest tube remote from the wound should be placed as soon as possible. Securely taping all edges of the dressing can cause air to accumulate in the thoracic cavity, resulting in a tension pneumothorax unless a chest tube is in place. Any occlusive dressing (e.g., plastic wrap or pet-

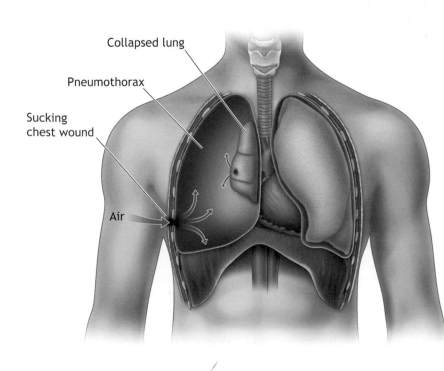

■ **FIGURE 4-3 Open Pneumothorax.** Large defects of the chest wall that remain open can result in an open pneumothorax, or sucking chest wound.

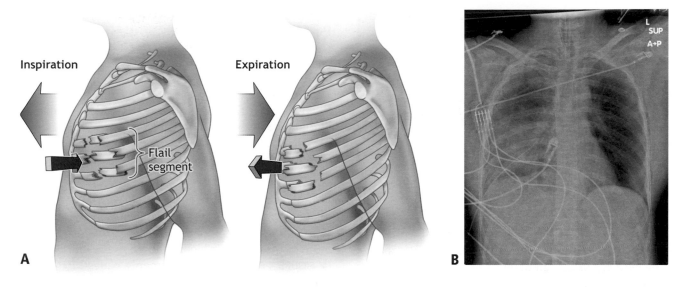

■ **FIGURE 4-5 Flail Chest. (A)** The presence of a flail chest segment results in disruption of normal chest wall movement. Although chest wall instability can lead to paradoxical motion of the chest wall during inspiration and expiration, this defect alone does not cause hypoxia. **(B)** Radiograph view of flail chest.

rolatum gauze) may be used as a temporary measure so that rapid assessment can continue. Subsequent definitive surgical closure of the defect is frequently required. See Skill Station VII: Chest Trauma Management, Skill VII-B: Chest Tube Insertion.

Flail Chest and Pulmonary Contusion

A flail chest occurs when a segment of the chest wall does not have bony continuity with the rest of the thoracic cage (■ **FIGURE 4-5**). This condition usually results from trauma associated with multiple rib fractures—that is, two or more adjacent ribs fractured in two or more places.

The presence of a flail chest segment results in disruption of normal chest wall movement. Although chest wall instability can lead to paradoxical motion of the chest wall during inspiration and expiration, this defect alone does not cause hypoxia. The major difficulty in flail chest stems from the injury to the underlying lung (pulmonary contusion). If the injury to the underlying lung is significant, serious hypoxia can result. Restricted chest wall movement associated with pain and underlying lung injury are major causes of hypoxia.

Flail chest may not be apparent initially if a patient's chest wall has been splinted, in which case he or she will move air poorly, and movement of the thorax will be asymmetrical and uncoordinated. Palpation of abnormal respiratory motion and crepitation of rib or cartilage fractures can aid the diagnosis. A satisfactory chest x-ray may suggest multiple rib fractures, but may not show costochondral separation.

Initial treatment of flail chest includes adequate ventilation, administration of humidified oxygen, and fluid resuscitation. In the absence of systemic hypotension, the administration of crystalloid intravenous solutions should be carefully controlled to prevent volume overload, which can further compromise the patient's respiratory status.

The definitive treatment is to ensure adequate oxygenation, administer fluids judiciously, and provide analgesia to improve ventilation. The latter can be achieved with intravenous narcotics or local anesthetic administration, which avoids the potential respiratory depression common with systemic narcotics. The options for administration of local anesthetics include intermittent intercostal nerve block(s) and intrapleural, extrapleural, or epidural anesthesia. When used properly, local anesthetic agents can provide excellent analgesia and prevent the need for intubation. However, prevention of hypoxia is of paramount importance for trauma patients, and a short period of intubation and ventilation may be necessary until diagnosis of the entire injury pattern is complete. A careful assessment of the respiratory rate, arterial oxygen tension, and work of breathing will indicate appropriate timing for intubation and ventilation.

Massive Hemothorax

Accumulation of blood and fluid in a hemithorax can significantly compromise respiratory efforts by compressing the lung and preventing adequate ventilation. Such massive acute accumulations of blood more dramatically present as hypotension and shock (see page 100).

PITFALLS

Both tension pneumothorax and massive hemothorax are associated with decreased breath sounds on auscultation. Differentiation on physical examination can be made by percussion; hyperresonance supports a pneumothorax, whereas dullness suggests a massive hemothorax. The trachea is often deviated in a tension pneumothorax, and the affected hemithorax can appear elevated without respiratory movement.

CIRCULATION

The patient's pulse should be assessed for quality, rate, and regularity. In patients with hypovolemia, the radial and dorsalis pedis pulses may be absent because of volume depletion. Blood pressure and pulse pressure are measured and the peripheral circulation is assessed by observing and palpating the skin for color and temperature. Neck veins should be assessed for distention, however, keep in mind that neck veins may not be distended in patients with concomitant hypovolemia and either cardiac tamponade, tension pneumothorax, or a traumatic diaphragmatic injury.

A cardiac monitor and pulse oximeter should be attached to the patient. Patients who sustain thoracic trauma especially in the area of the sternum or from a rapid deceleration injury, are also susceptible to myocardial injury, which can lead to dysrhythmias. Hypoxia and acidosis enhance this possibility. Dysrhythmias

should be managed according to standard protocols. Pulseless electric activity (PEA) is manifested by an electrocardiogram (ECG) that shows a rhythm while the patient has no identifiable pulse. PEA can be present in cardiac tamponade, tension pneumothorax, profound hypovolemia, and cardiac rupture.

The major thoracic injuries that affect circulation and should be recognized and addressed during the primary survey are tension pneumothorax, massive hemothorax, and cardiac tamponade.

Massive Hemothorax

Massive hemothorax results from the rapid accumulation of more than 1500 mL of blood or one-third or more of the patient's blood volume in the chest cavity (■ FIGURE 4-6). It is most commonly caused by a penetrating wound that disrupts the systemic or hilar vessels. However, massive hemothorax can also result from blunt trauma.

In patients with massive hemothorax, the neck veins may be flat as a result of severe hypovolemia, or they may be distended if there is an associated tension pneumothorax. Rarely will the mechanical effects of massive intrathoracic blood shift the mediastinum enough to cause distended neck veins. A massive hemothorax is suggested when shock is associated with the absence of breath sounds or dullness to percussion on one side of the chest. This blood loss is complicated by hypoxia.

Massive hemothorax is initially managed by the simultaneous restoration of blood volume and decompression of the chest cavity. Large-caliber intravenous

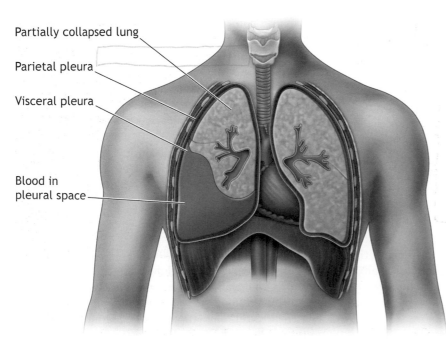

Partially collapsed lung

Parietal pleura

Visceral pleura

Blood in pleural space

■ FIGURE 4-6 Massive Hemothorax. This condition results from the rapid accumulation of more than 1500 mL of blood or one-third or more of the patient's blood volume in the chest cavity.

lines and a rapid crystalloid infusion are begun, and type-specific blood is administered as soon as possible. Blood from the chest tube should be collected in a device suitable for autotransfusion. A single chest tube (36 or 40 French) is inserted, usually at the nipple level, just anterior to the midaxillary line, and rapid restoration of volume continues as decompression of the chest cavity is completed. When massive hemothorax is suspected, prepare for autotransfusion. If 1500 mL of fluid is immediately evacuated, early thoracotomy is almost always required.

Patients who have an initial output of less than 1500 mL of fluid, but continue to bleed, may also require thoracotomy. This decision is not based solely on the rate of continuing blood loss (200 mL/hr for 2 to 4 hours), but also on the patient's physiologic status. The persistent need for blood transfusions is an indication for thoracotomy. During patient resuscitation, the volume of blood initially drained from the chest tube and the rate of continuing blood loss must be factored into the amount of intravenous fluid required for replacement. The color of the blood (indicating an arterial or venous source) is a poor indicator of the necessity for thoracotomy.

Penetrating anterior chest wounds medial to the nipple line and posterior wounds medial to the scapula should alert the practitioner to the possible need for thoracotomy because of potential damage to the great vessels, hilar structures, and the heart, with the associated potential for cardiac tamponade. **Thoracotomy is not indicated unless a surgeon, qualified by training and experience, is present.**

Cardiac Tamponade (think PENETRATING trauma)

Cardiac tamponade most commonly results from penetrating injuries. However, blunt injury also can cause the pericardium to fill with blood from the heart, great vessels, or pericardial vessels (■ FIGURE 4-7). The human pericardial sac is a fixed fibrous structure; a relatively small amount of blood can restrict cardiac activity and interfere with cardiac filling. Cardiac tamponade may develop slowly, allowing for a less urgent evaluation, or may occur rapidly, requiring rapid diagnosis and treatment. The diagnosis of cardiac tamponade can be difficult in the setting of a busy trauma or emergency room.

Cardiac tamponade is indicated by the presence of the classic diagnostic Beck's triad: venous pressure elevation, decline in arterial pressure, and muffled heart tones. However, muffled heart tones are difficult to assess in the noisy exam area, and distended neck veins may be absent due to hypovolemia. Additionally, tension pneumothorax, particularly on the left side, can mimic cardiac tamponade. Kussmaul's sign (a rise in venous pressure with inspiration when breathing spontaneously) is a true paradoxical venous

— Jugular venous distention
— ↓ BP
— Muffled ♡ sounds

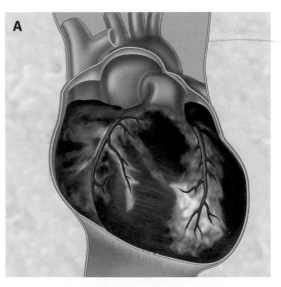

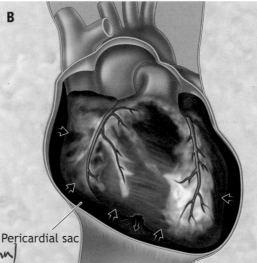

Pericardial sac

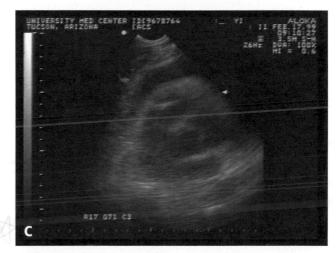

■ **FIGURE 4-7 Cardiac Tamponade. (A)** Normal heart. **(B)** Pericardial tamponade can result from penetrating or blunt injuries that cause the pericardium to fill with blood from the heart, great vessels, or pericardial vessels. **(C)** Ultrasound image showing cardiac tamponade.

pressure abnormality associated with tamponade. PEA is suggestive of cardiac tamponade, but can have other causes, as listed above. Insertion of a central venous line with measurement of central venous pressure (CVP) may aid diagnosis, but CVP can be elevated for a variety of reasons.

Additional diagnostic methods include echocardiogram, focused assessment sonography in trauma (FAST), or pericardial window. In hemodynamically abnormal patients with blunt or penetrating trauma and suspected cardiac tamponade an examination of the pericardial sac for the presence of fluid should be obtained as part of a focused ultrasound examination performed by a properly trained provider in the emergency department (ED). FAST is a rapid and accurate method of imaging the heart and pericardium. It is 90–95% accurate for the presence of pericardial fluid for the experienced operator. Concomitant hemothorax may account for both false positive and false negative ultrasound exams. See Chapter 5: Abdominal and Pelvic Trauma.

Prompt diagnosis and evacuation of pericardial blood is indicated for patients who do not respond to the usual measures of resuscitation for hemorrhagic shock and in whom cardiac tamponade is suspected. The diagnosis can usually be made with the FAST exam. If a qualified surgeon is present, surgery should be performed to relieve the tamponade. This is best performed in the operating room if the patient's condition allows. **If surgical intervention is not possible, pericardiocentesis can be diagnostic as well as therapeutic, but it is not definitive treatment for cardiac tamponade.** See Skill Station VII: Chest Trauma Management, Skill VII-C: Pericardiocentesis.

Although cardiac tamponade may be strongly suspected, the initial administration of intravenous fluid will raise the venous pressure and improve cardiac output transiently while preparations are made for surgery. If subxyphoid pericardiocentesis is used as a temporizing maneuver, the use of a plastic-sheathed needle or the Seldinger technique for insertion of a flexible catheter is ideal, but the urgent priority is to aspirate blood from the pericardial sac. If ultrasound imaging is available, it can facilitate accurate insertion of the needle into the pericardial space.

Because of the propensity of injured myocardium to self-seal, aspiration of pericardial blood alone may temporarily relieve symptoms. However all patients with acute tamponade and a positive pericardiocentesis will require surgery to examine the heart and repair the injury. Pericardiocentesis may not be diagnostic or therapeutic when the blood in the pericardial sac has clotted. Preparation to transfer such a patient to an appropriate facility for definitive care is always necessary. Pericardiotomy via thoracotomy is indicated only when a qualified surgeon is available.

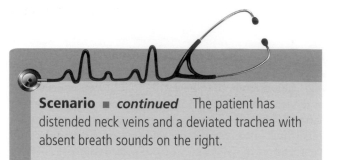

Scenario ■ *continued* The patient has distended neck veins and a deviated trachea with absent breath sounds on the right.

Resuscitative Thoracotomy

Closed heart massage for cardiac arrest or PEA is ineffective in patients with hypovolemia. Patients with penetrating thoracic injuries who arrive pulseless, but with myocardial electrical activity, may be candidates for immediate resuscitative thoracotomy. **A qualified surgeon must be present at the time of the patient's arrival to determine the need and potential for success of a resuscitative thoracotomy in the emergency department (ED).** Restoration of intravascular volume should be continued, and endotracheal intubation and mechanical ventilation are essential.

A patient who has sustained a penetrating wound and required cardiopulmonary resuscitation (CPR) in the prehospital setting should be evaluated for any signs of life. If there are none, and no cardiac electrical activity is present, no further resuscitative effort should be made. Patients who sustain blunt injuries and arrive pulseless but with myocardial electrical activity (PEA) are not candidates for emergency department resuscitative thoracotomy. Signs of life include reactive pupils, spontaneous movement, or organized ECG activity.

The therapeutic maneuvers that can be effectively accomplished with a resuscitative thoracotomy are:

■ Evacuation of pericardial blood causing tamponade

■ Direct control of exsanguinating intrathoracic hemorrhage

■ Open cardiac massage

■ Cross-clamping of the descending aorta to slow blood loss below the diaphragm and increase perfusion to the brain and heart

Despite the value of these maneuvers, multiple reports confirm that thoracotomy in the ED for patients with blunt trauma and cardiac arrest is rarely effective.

Once these and other immediately life-threatening injuries have been treated, attention may be directed to the secondary survey.

Secondary Survey: Potentially Life-Threatening Injuries

? *What adjunctive tests are used during the secondary survey to allow complete evaluation for potentially life-threatening thoracic injuries?*

The secondary survey involves further, in-depth physical examination, an upright chest x-ray examination if the patient's condition permits, arterial blood gas (ABG) measurements, and pulse oximetry and ECG monitoring. In addition to lung expansion and the presence of fluid, the chest film should be examined for widening of the mediastinum, a shift of the midline, and loss of anatomic detail. Multiple rib fractures and fractures of the first or second rib(s) suggest that a significant force has been delivered to the chest and underlying tissues. Ultrasound has been used to detect both pneumothoraces and hemothoraces. However, other potentially life-threatening injuries are not well-visualized on ultrasound, making the chest radiograph a necessary part of any evaluation after traumatic injury. See Skill Station VI: X-Ray Identification of Thoracic Injuries.

The following eight lethal injuries are described below:

- Simple pneumothorax
- Hemothorax
- Pulmonary contusion
- Tracheobronchial tree injury
- Blunt cardiac injury
- Traumatic aortic disruption
- Traumatic diaphragmatic injury
- Blunt esophageal rupture

Unlike immediately life-threatening conditions that are recognized during the primary survey, these injuries are often not obvious on physical examination.

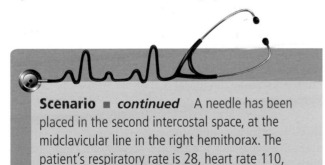

Scenario ■ *continued* A needle has been placed in the second intercostal space, at the midclavicular line in the right hemithorax. The patient's respiratory rate is 28, heart rate 110, and blood pressure 110/70.

Diagnosis requires a high index of suspicion and appropriate use of adjunctive studies. These injuries are more often missed than diagnosed during the initial posttraumatic period; however, if overlooked, lives can be lost.

SIMPLE PNEUMOTHORAX

Pneumothorax results from air entering the potential space between the visceral and parietal pleura (■ FIGURE 4-8). Both penetrating and nonpenetrating trauma can cause this injury. Lung laceration with air leakage is the most common cause of pneumothorax resulting from blunt trauma.

The thorax is normally completely filled by the lung, being held to the chest wall by surface tension between the pleural surfaces. Air in the pleural space disrupts the cohesive forces between the visceral and parietal pleura, which allows the lung to collapse. A ventilation/perfusion defect occurs because the blood that perfuses the nonventilated area is not oxygenated.

When a pneumothorax is present, breath sounds are often decreased on the affected side, and percussion may demonstrate hyperresonance. The finding of hyperresonance is extremely difficult to determine in a busy resuscitation bay. An upright, expiratory x-ray of the chest aids in the diagnosis.

Any pneumothorax is best treated with a chest tube placed in the fourth or fifth intercostal space, just anterior to the midaxillary line. Observation and aspiration of a small, asymptomatic pneumothorax may be appropriate, but the choice should be made by a qualified doctor; otherwise, placement of a chest tube should be performed. Once a chest tube is inserted and connected to an underwater seal apparatus with or without suction, a chest x-ray examination is necessary to confirm reexpansion of the lung. **Neither general anesthesia nor positive-pressure ventilation should be administered in a patient who has sustained a traumatic pneumothorax or who is at risk for unexpected intraoperative tension pneumothorax until a chest tube has been inserted.** A simple pneumothorax can readily convert to a life-threatening tension pneumothorax, particularly if it is initially unrecognized and positive-pressure ventilation is applied.

The patient with a pneumothorax should also undergo chest decompression before transport via air ambulance due to the expansion of the pneumothorax at altitude, even in a pressurized cabin.

PITFALLS

A simple pneumothorax in a trauma patient should not be ignored or overlooked. It may progress to a tension pneumothorax.

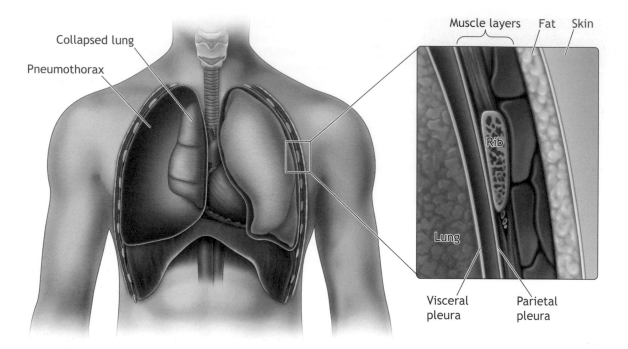

Collapsed lung
Pneumothorax

Muscle layers   Fat   Skin

Rib

Lung

Visceral pleura   Parietal pleura

■ **FIGURE 4-8 Simple Pneumothorax.** Pneumothorax results from air entering the potential space between the visceral and parietal pleura.

N.B. Massive HEMOTHORAX = >1500 mL blood

HEMOTHORAX

The primary cause of hemothorax (<1500 mL blood) is lung laceration or laceration of an intercostal vessel or internal mammary artery due to either penetrating or blunt trauma. Thoracic spine fractures may also be associated with a hemothorax. Bleeding is usually self-limited and does not require operative intervention.

An acute hemothorax large enough to appear on a chest x-ray film is best treated with a large-caliber (36 or 40 French) chest tube. The chest tube evacuates blood, reduces the risk of a clotted hemothorax, and, importantly, provides a method for continuous monitoring of blood loss. Evacuation of blood and fluid also facilitates a more complete assessment of potential diaphragmatic injury. Although many factors are involved in the decision to operate on a patient with a hemothorax, the patient's physiologic status and the volume of blood drainage from the chest tube are major factors. As a guideline, if 1500 mL of blood is obtained immediately through the chest tube, if drainage of more than 200 mL/hr for 2 to 4 hours occurs,

or if blood transfusion is required, operative exploration should be considered. The ultimate decision for operative intervention is based on the patient's hemodynamic status.

PULMONARY CONTUSION   *✗ Judicious fluids*

Pulmonary contusion can occur without rib fractures or flail chest, particularly in young patients without completely ossified ribs. However, in adults it is most commonly seen with concomitant rib fractures, and it is the most common potentially lethal chest injury. The resultant respiratory failure can be subtle, developing over time rather than occurring instantaneously. The plan for definitive management may change with time and patient response, warranting careful monitoring and reevaluation of the patient.

Patients with significant hypoxia (i.e., PaO2 <65 mm Hg [8.6 kPa] or SaO2 <90%) on room air may require intubation and ventilation within the first hour after injury. Associated medical conditions, such as chronic obstructive pulmonary disease and renal failure, increase the likelihood of needing early intubation and mechanical ventilation.

Pulse oximetry monitoring, ABG determinations, ECG monitoring, and appropriate ventilatory equipment are necessary for optimal treatment. Any patient with the aforementioned preexisting conditions who needs to be transferred should undergo intubation and ventilation. (See Figure 4-8.)

PITFALLS

A simple hemothorax that is not fully evacuated can result in a retained, clotted hemothorax with lung entrapment or, if infected, it can develop into an empyema.

BLUNT CARDIAC INJURY

Blunt cardiac injury can result in myocardial muscle contusion, cardiac chamber rupture, coronary artery dissection and/or thrombosis, or valvular disruption. Cardiac rupture typically presents with cardiac tamponade and should be recognized during the primary survey. However, occasionally the signs and symptoms of tamponade are slow to develop with an atrial rupture. Early use of FAST can facilitate diagnosis.

Patients with blunt myocardial injury may report chest discomfort, but this symptom is often attributed to chest wall contusion or fractures of the sternum and/or ribs. The true diagnosis of blunt myocardial injury can be established only by direct inspection of the injured myocardium. Clinically important sequelae are hypotension, dysrhythmias, and/or wall-motion abnormality on two-dimensional echocardiography. The electrocardiographic changes are variable and may even indicate frank myocardial infarction. Multiple premature ventricular contractions, unexplained sinus tachycardia, atrial fibrillation, bundle-branch block (usually right), and ST-segment changes are the most common ECG findings. Elevated central venous pressure in the absence of an obvious cause may indicate right ventricular dysfunction secondary to contusion. It also is important to remember that the traumatic event may have been precipitated by a myocardial ischemic episode.

The presence of cardiac troponins can be diagnostic of myocardial infarction. However, their use in diagnosing blunt cardiac injury is inconclusive and offers no additional information beyond that available from ECG. Patients with a blunt injury to the heart diagnosed by conduction abnormalities (an abnormal ECG) are at risk for sudden dysrhythmias and should be monitored for the first 24 hours. After this interval, the risk of a dysrhythmia appears to decrease substantially. Those without ECG abnormalities do not require further monitoring.

TRAUMATIC AORTIC DISRUPTION

Traumatic aortic rupture is a common cause of sudden death after an automobile collision or fall from a great height (■ FIGURE 4-9). For survivors, recovery is frequently possible if aortic rupture is promptly identified and treated immediately.

Patients with aortic rupture who have a chance of survival tend to have an incomplete laceration near the ligamentum arteriosum of the aorta. Continuity is maintained by an intact adventitial layer or contained mediastinal hematoma and prevents immediate exsanguination and death. Blood may escape into the mediastinum, but one characteristic shared by all survivors is that they have a contained hematoma. Persistent

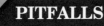

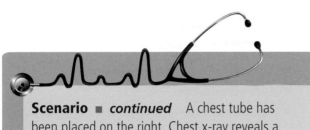

Scenario ■ *continued* A chest tube has been placed on the right. Chest x-ray reveals a wide mediastinum with multiple rib fractures on the right with a pulmonary contusion.

TRACHEOBRONCHIAL TREE INJURY

Injury to the trachea or major bronchus is an unusual and potentially fatal condition that is often overlooked on initial assessment. In blunt trauma the majority of such injuries occur within 1 inch (2.54 cm) of the carina. Most patients with this injury die at the scene. Those who reach the hospital alive have a high mortality rate from associated injuries or delay in diagnosis of the airway injury.

If tracheobronchial injury is suspected, immediate surgical consultation is warranted. Such patients typically present with hemoptysis, subcutaneous emphysema, or tension pneumothorax. Incomplete expansion of the lung after placement of a chest tube suggests a tracheobronchial injury, and placement of more than one chest tube often is necessary to overcome a significant air leak. Bronchoscopy confirms the diagnosis.

Temporary intubation of the opposite mainstem bronchus may be required to provide adequate oxygenation. However, intubation of patients with tracheobronchial injuries is frequently difficult because of anatomic distortion from paratracheal hematoma, associated oropharyngeal injuries, and/or the tracheobronchial injury itself. For such patients, immediate operative intervention is indicated. In more stable patients, operative treatment of tracheobronchial injuries may be delayed until the acute inflammation and edema resolve.

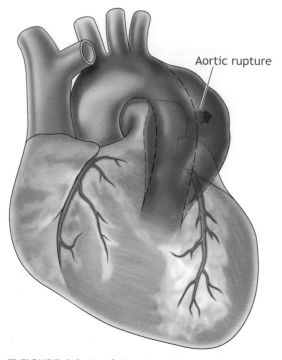

■ FIGURE 4-9 Aortic Rupture. Traumatic aortic rupture is a common cause of sudden death after an automobile collision or fall from a great height.

or recurrent hypotension is usually due to a separate, unidentified bleeding site. Although free rupture of a transected aorta into the left chest does occur and can cause hypotension, it usually is fatal unless the patient undergoes repair within a few minutes.

Specific signs and symptoms of traumatic aortic disruption are frequently absent. A high index of suspicion prompted by a history of decelerating force and characteristic findings on chest x-ray films should be maintained, and the patient should be further evaluated. Adjunctive radiologic signs on chest x-ray, which may or may not be present, indicate the likelihood of major vascular injury in the chest and include:

 PITFALLS

Penetrating objects that traverse the mediastinum may injure the major mediastinal structures, such as the heart, great vessels, tracheobronchial tree, and esophagus. The diagnosis is made when careful examination and a chest x-ray film reveal an entrance wound in one hemithorax and an exit wound or a missile lodged in the contralateral hemithorax. Wounds in which metallic fragments from the missile are in proximity to mediastinal structures also should raise suspicion of a mediastinal traversing injury. Such wounds warrant careful consideration, and surgical consultation is mandatory.

- Widened mediastinum
- Obliteration of the aortic knob
- Deviation of the trachea to the right
- Depression of the left mainstem bronchus
- Elevation of the right mainstem bronchus
- Obliteration of the space between the pulmonary artery and the aorta (obscuration of the aortopulmonary window)
- Deviation of the esophagus (nasogastric tube) to the right
- Widened paratracheal stripe
- Widened paraspinal interfaces
- Presence of a pleural or apical cap
- Left hemothorax
- Fractures of the first or second rib or scapula

False positive and false negative findings can occur with each x-ray sign, and, infrequently (1%–13%), no mediastinal or initial chest x-ray abnormality is present in patients with great-vessel injury. If there is even a slight suspicion of aortic injury, the patient should be evaluated at a facility capable of repairing a diagnosed injury.

Helical contrast-enhanced computed tomography (CT) of the chest has been shown to be an accurate screening method for patients with suspected blunt aortic injury. CT scanning should be performed liberally, because the findings on chest x-ray, especially the supine view, are unreliable. If the results are equivocal, aortography should be performed. In general, patients who are hemodynamically abnormal should not be placed in a CT scanner. The sensitivity and specificity of helical contrast-enhanced CT have been shown to be close to 100%, but this result is very technology-dependent. If enhanced helical CT of the chest is negative for mediastinal hematoma and aortic rupture, no further diagnostic imaging of the aorta is necessary. When the CT is positive for blunt aortic rupture, the extent of the injury may be further defined with CT angiogram or aortography. Transesophageal echocardiography (TEE) also appears to be a useful, less invasive diagnostic tool. The trauma surgeon caring for the patient is in the best position to determine which, if any, other diagnostic tests are warranted.

In hospitals that lack the capability to care for cardiothoracic injuries, the decision to transfer patients with potential aortic injury may be difficult. A properly performed and interpreted helical CT that is normal may obviate the need for transfer to a higher level of care to exclude thoracic aortic injury.

A qualified surgeon should treat patients with blunt traumatic aortic injury and assist in the diagnosis. The treatment is either primary repair or resection

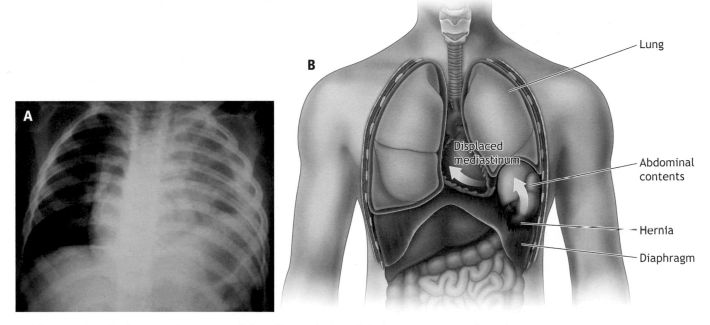

■ **FIGURE 4-10 Diaphragmatic Rupture. (A)** Radiograph view. **(B)** Blunt trauma produces large radial tears that lead to herniation, whereas penetrating trauma produces small perforations that can take time, sometimes even years, to develop into diaphragmatic hernias.

PITFALLS

Delayed or extensive evaluation of the wide mediastinum without cardiothoracic surgery capabilities can result in an early in-hospital rupture of the contained hematoma and rapid death from exsanguination. All patients with a mechanism of injury and simple chest x-ray findings suggestive of aortic disruption should be transferred to a facility capable of rapid definitive diagnosis and treatment of this injury.

---

of the torn segment and replacement with an interposition graft. Endovascular repair is now an acceptable alternative approach.

TRAUMATIC DIAPHRAGMATIC INJURY

Traumatic diaphragmatic ruptures are more commonly diagnosed on the left side, perhaps because the liver obliterates the defect or protects it on the right side of the diaphragm, whereas the appearance of displaced bowel, stomach, and nasogastric (NG) tube is more easily detected in the left chest. Blunt trauma produces large radial tears that lead to herniation (■ **FIGURE 4-10**), whereas penetrating trauma produces small perforations that can take time, sometimes even years, to develop into diaphragmatic hernias.

Diaphragmatic injuries are frequently missed initially when the chest film is misinterpreted as showing an elevated diaphragm, acute gastric dilatation, loculated hemopneumothorax, or subpulmonary hematoma. The appearance of an elevated right diaphragm on chest x-ray may be the only finding of a right-sided injury. If a laceration of the left diaphragm is suspected, a gastric tube should be inserted. When the gastric tube appears in the thoracic cavity on the chest film, the need for special contrast studies is eliminated. Occasionally, the condition is not identified on the initial x-ray film or subsequent CT scan. An upper gastrointestinal contrast study should be performed if the diagnosis is not clear. The appearance of peritoneal lavage fluid in the chest tube drainage also confirms the diagnosis. Minimally invasive endoscopic procedures (e.g., laparoscopy or thoracoscopy) may be helpful in evaluating the diaphragm in indeterminate cases.

Operation for other abdominal injuries often reveals a diaphragmatic tear. Treatment is by direct repair.

PITFALLS

Diaphragm injuries may be missed during the initial trauma evaluation. An undiagnosed diaphragm injury can result in pulmonary compromise or entrapment and strangulation of peritoneal contents.

BLUNT ESOPHAGEAL RUPTURE

Esophageal trauma most commonly results from penetrating injury. Blunt esophageal trauma, although very rare, can be lethal if unrecognized. Blunt injury of the esophagus is caused by the forceful expulsion of gastric contents into the esophagus from a severe blow to the upper abdomen. This forceful ejection produces a linear tear in the lower esophagus, allowing leakage into the mediastinum. The resulting mediastinitis and immediate or delayed rupture into the pleural space cause empyema.

The clinical picture of patients with blunt esophageal rupture is identical to that of postemetic esophageal rupture. Esophageal injury should be considered in any patient who has a left pneumothorax or hemothorax without a rib fracture; received a severe blow to the lower sternum or epigastrium and is in pain or shock out of proportion to the apparent injury; and has particulate matter in the chest tube after the blood begins to clear. The presence of mediastinal air also suggests the diagnosis, which often can be confirmed by contrast studies and/or esophagoscopy.

Treatment consists of wide drainage of the pleural space and mediastinum with direct repair of the injury via thoracotomy, if feasible. Repairs performed within a few hours of injury lead to a much better prognosis.

Other Manifestations of Chest Injuries

Other significant thoracic injuries, including subcutaneous emphysema; crushing injury (traumatic asphyxia); and rib, sternum, and scapular fractures, should be detected during the secondary survey. Although these injuries may not be immediately life-threatening, they have the potential to do significant harm.

SUBCUTANEOUS EMPHYSEMA

Subcutaneous emphysema can result from airway injury, lung injury, or, rarely, blast injury. Although it does not require treatment, the underlying injury must be addressed. If positive-pressure ventilation is required, tube thoracostomy should be considered on the side of the subcutaneous emphysema in anticipation of a tension pneumothorax developing.

CRUSHING INJURY TO THE CHEST (TRAUMATIC ASPHYXIA)

Findings associated with a crush injury to the chest include upper torso, facial, and arm plethora with petechiae secondary to acute, temporary compression of the superior vena cava. Massive swelling and even cerebral edema may be present. Associated injuries must be treated.

RIB, STERNUM, AND SCAPULAR FRACTURES

The ribs are the most commonly injured component of the thoracic cage, and injuries to the ribs are often significant. Pain on motion typically results in splinting of the thorax, which impairs ventilation, oxygenation, and effective coughing. The incidence of atelectasis and pneumonia rises significantly with preexisting lung disease.

The upper ribs (1 to 3) are protected by the bony framework of the upper limb. The scapula, humerus, and clavicle, along with their muscular attachments, provide a barrier to rib injury. Fractures of the scapula, first or second rib, or the sternum suggest a magnitude of injury that places the head, neck, spinal cord, lungs, and great vessels at risk for serious associated injury. Because of the severity of the associated injuries, mortality may be as high as 35%.

Sternal and scapular fractures are generally the result of a direct blow. Pulmonary contusion may accompany sternal fractures, and blunt cardiac injury should be considered with all such fractures. Operative repair of sternal and scapular fractures occasionally is indicated. Rarely, posterior sternoclavicular dislocation results in mediastinal displacement of the clavicular heads with accompanying superior vena caval obstruction. Immediate reduction is required.

The middle ribs (4 to 9) sustain the majority of blunt trauma. Anteroposterior compression of the thoracic cage will bow the ribs outward with a fracture in the midshaft. Direct force applied to the ribs tends to fracture them and drive the ends of the bones into the thorax, increasing the potential for intrathoracic injury, such as a pneumothorax or hemothorax.

As a general rule, a young patient with a more flexible chest wall is less likely to sustain rib fractures. Therefore, the presence of multiple rib fractures in young patients implies a greater transfer of force than in older patients. Fractures of the lower ribs (10 to 12) should increase suspicion for hepatosplenic injury.

Localized pain, tenderness on palpation, and crepitation are present in patients with rib injury. A palpable or visible deformity suggests rib fractures. A chest x-ray film should be obtained primarily to exclude other intrathoracic injuries and not just to identify rib fractures. Fractures of anterior cartilages or separation of costochondral junctions have the same significance as rib fractures, but will not be seen on the x-ray examinations. Special rib-technique x-rays are not considered useful because they may not detect all rib injuries and add nothing to treatment decisions, whereas they are expensive and require painful positioning of the patient. See Skill Station VI: X-Ray Identification of Thoracic Injuries.

The presence of rib fractures in the elderly should raise significant concern, as the incidence of pneumonia and mortality is double that in younger patients See Chapter 11: Geriatric Trauma. Taping, rib belts, and external splints are contraindicated. Relief of pain is important to enable adequate ventilation. Intercostal block, epidural anesthesia, and systemic analgesics are effective and may be necessary. Early and aggressive pain control, including the use of systemic narcotics and local or regional anesthesia, improves outcome in this population.

Increased use of CT has resulted in the identification of injuries not previously known or diagnosed, such as minimal aortic injuries and occult pneumothoraces and hemothoraces. Appropriate treatment of these occult injuries should be discussed with the relative specialty consultant.

PITFALLS

Underestimating the severe pathophysiology of rib fractures is a common pitfall, particularly in patients at the extremes of age. Aggressive pain control without respiratory depression is the key management principle.

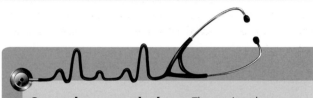

Scenario ▪ conclusion   The patient has an aortic injury diagnosed by chest CT. He receives an intravenous narcotic for pain control and 1 liter of crystalloid solution prior to operation for his aortic injury.

Chapter Summary

1 Thoracic injury is common in the poly-trauma patient and can pose life-threatening problems if not promptly identified and treated during the primary survey. These patients can usually be treated or their conditions temporarily relieved by relatively simple measures, such as intubation, ventilation, tube thoracostomy, and fluid resuscitation. The ability to recognize these important injuries and the skill to perform the necessary procedures can be lifesaving. The primary survey includes management of the following conditions:

▶ Airway obstruction

▶ Tension pneumothorax

▶ Open pneumothorax

▶ Flail chest and pulmonary contusion

▶ Massive hemothorax

▶ Cardiac tamponade

2 The secondary survey includes identification and initial treatment of the following potentially life-threatening injuries, utilizing adjunctive studies, such as x-rays, laboratory tests, and ECG:

▶ Simple pneumothorax

▶ Hemothorax

▶ Pulmonary contusion

▶ Tracheobronchial tree injury

▶ Blunt cardiac injury

▶ Traumatic aortic disruption

▶ Traumatic diaphragmatic injury

▶ Blunt esophageal rupture

3 Several manifestations of thoracic trauma are indicative of a greater risk of associated injuries:

▶ Subcutaneous emphysema

▶ Crush injuries of the chest

▶ Injuries to the upper ribs (1–3), scapula, and sternum

BIBLIOGRAPHY

1. Ball CG, Kirkpatrick AW, Laupland KB, et al. Incidence, risk factors, and outcomes for occult pneumothoraces in victims of major trauma. *J Trauma* 2005;59(4):917-924; discussion 924-925.

2. Ball CG, Williams BH, Wyrzykowski AD, Nicholas JM, Rozycki GS, Feliciano DV. A caveat to the performance of pericardial ultrasound in patients with penetrating cardiac wounds. *J Trauma* 2009;67(5):1123-4.

3. Brasel KJ, Stafford RE, Weigelt JA, Tenquist JE, Borgstrom DC. Treatment of occult pneumothoraces from blunt trauma. *J Trauma* 1999; 46(6), 987-990; discussion 990-991.

4. Bulger EM, Edwards T, Klotz P, Jurkovich GJ. Epidural analgesia improves outcome after multiple rib fractures. *Surgery* 2004;136(2):426-430.

5. Callaham M. Pericardiocentesis in traumatic and nontraumatic cardiac tamponade. *Ann Emerg Med* 1984;13(10):924-945.

6. Cook J, Salerno C, Krishnadasan B, Nicholls S, Meissner M, Karmy-Jones R. The effect of changing presentation and management on the outcome of blunt rupture of the thoracic aorta. *J Thorac Cardiovasc Surg* 2006;131(3):594-600.

7. Demetriades D, Velmahos G, et al. Diagnosis and treatment of blunt aortic injuries: changing perspectives. *J Trauma* 2008;64:1415-1419.

8. Demetriades D, Velmahos G, et al. Operative repair or endovascular stent graft in blunt traumatic thoracic aortic injuries: results of an American Association for the Surgery of Trauma multicenter study. *J Trauma* 2008;64:561-571.

9. Dulchavsky SA, Schwarz KL, Kirkpatrick AW, et al. Prospective evaluation of thoracic ultrasound in the detection of pneumothorax. *J Trauma* 2001; (Feb50):201-5.

10. Dunham CM, Barraco RD, Clark DE, et al. Guidelines for emergency tracheal intubation immediately following traumatic injury: an EAST Practice Management Guidelines Workgroup. *J Trauma* 2003;55:162-179.

11. Dyer DS, Moore EE, Ilke DN, McIntyre RC, Bernstein SM, Durham JD, Mestek MF, Heinig MJ, Russ PD, Symonds DL, Honigman B, Kumpe DA, Roe EJ, Eule J Jr. Thoracic aortic injury: how predictive is mechanism and is chest computed tomography a reliable screening tool? A prospective study of 1,561 patients. *J Trauma* 2000;48(4):673-82; discussion 682-3.

12. Ekeh AP, Peterson W, et al. Is chest x-ray an adequate screening tool for the diagnosis of blunt thoracic aortic injury? *J Trauma* 2008;65:1088-1092.

13. Flagel B, Luchette FA, Reed RL, et al. Half a dozen ribs: the breakpoint for mortality. *Surgery* 2005;138:717-725.

14. Graham JG, Mattox KL, Beall AC Jr. Penetrating trauma of the lung. *J Trauma* 1979;19:665.

15. Harcke HT, Pearse LA, Levy AD, Getz JM, Robinson SR. Chest wall thickness in military personnel: implications for needle thoracentesis in tension pneumothorax. *Mil Med* 2007;172(120):1260-1263.

16. Heniford BT, Carrillo EG, Spain DA, et al. The role of thoracoscopy in the management of retained thoracic collections after trauma. *Ann Thorac Surg* 1997;63(4):940-943.

17. Hershberger RC, Bernadette A, et al. Endovascualar grafts for treatment of traumatic injury to the aortic arch and great vessels. *J Trauma* 2009;67(3):660-671.

18. Hopson LR, Hirsh E, Delgado J, Domeier RM, McSwain NE, Krohmer J. Guidelines for withholding or termination of resuscitation in prehospital traumatic cardiopulmonary arrest: a joint position paper from the National Association of EMS Physicians Standards and Clinical Practice Committee and the American College of Surgeons Committee on Trauma. *Prehosp Emerg Care* 2003;7(1):141-146.

19. Hopson LR, Hirsh E, Delgado J, et al. Guidelines for withholding or termination of resuscitation in prehospital traumatic cardiopulmonary arrest. *J Am Coll Surg* 2003;196(3),475-481.

20. Kenji Inaba, MD, FRCSC, FACS, Bernardino C. Branco, MD, Marc Eckstein, MD, David V. Shatz, MD, Matthew J. Martin, MD, Donald J. Green, MD, Thomas T. Noguchi, MD, and Demetrios Demetriades, MD, PhD. *Optimal Positioning for Emergent Needle Thoracostomy: A Cadaver-Based Study. J Trauma* 2011;71:1099-1103.

21. Hunt PA, Greaves I, Owens WA. Emergency thoracotomy in thoracic trauma—a review. *Injury* 2006;37(1):1-19.

22. Karalis DG, Victor MF, Davis GA, et al. The role of echocardiography in blunt chest trauma: a transthoracic and transesophageal echocardiography study. *J Trauma* 1994;36(1):53-58.

23. Karmy-Jones R, Jurkovich GJ, Nathens AB, Shatz DV, Brundage S, Wall MJ Jr, Engelhardt S, Hoyt DB, Holcroft J, Knudson MM. Timing of urgent thoracotomy for hemorrhage after trauma: a multicenter study. *Archives of Surgery* 2001;136(5):513-8.

24. Lang-Lazdunski L, Mourox J, Pons F, et al. Role of videothoracoscopy in chest trauma. *Ann Thorac Surg* 1997;63(2):327-333.

25. Lockey D, Crewdson K, Davies G. Traumatic cardiac arrest: who are the survivors? *Ann Emerg Med* 2006;48(3):240-244.

26. Marnocha KE, Maglinte DDT, Woods J, et al. Blunt chest trauma and suspected aortic rupture: reliability of chest radiograph findings. *Ann Emerg Med* 1985;14(7):644-649.

27. Meyer DM, Jessen ME, Wait MA. Early evacuation of traumatic retained hemothoraces using thoracoscopy: A prospective randomized trial. *Ann Thorac Surg* 1997;64(5):1396-1400.

28. Mirvis SE, Shanmugantham K, Buell J, et al. Use of spiral computed tomography for the assessment of blunt trauma patients with potential aortic injury. *J Trauma* 1999;45:922-930.

29. Moon MR, Luchette FA, Gibson SW, et al. Prospective, randomized comparison of epidural versus parenteral opioid analgesia in thoracic trauma. *Ann Surg* 1999;229:684-692.

30. Powell DW, Moore EE, Cothren CC, et al. Is emergency department resuscitative thoracotomy futile

care for the critically injured patient requiring pre-hospital cardiopulmonary resuscitation? *J Am Coll Surg* 2004;199(2):211-215.

31. Ramzy AI, Rodriguez A, Turney SZ. Management of major tracheobronchial ruptures in patients with multiple system trauma. *J Trauma* 1988;28:914-920.

32. Reed AB, Thompson JK, Crafton CJ, et al. Timing of endovascular repair of blunt traumatic thoracic aortic transections. *J Vasc Surg* 2006;43(4):684-688.

33. Rhee PM, Acosta J, Bridgeman A, Wang D, Jordan M, Rich N. Survival after emergency department thoracotomy: review of published data from the past 25 years. *J Am Coll Surg* 2000;190(3):288-298.

34. Richardson JD, Adams L, Flint LM. Selective management of flail chest and pulmonary contusion. *Ann Surg* 1982;196(4):481-487.

35. Rosato RM, Shapiro MJ, Keegan MJ, et al. Cardiac injury complicating traumatic asphyxia. *J Trauma* 1991;31(10):1387-1389.

36. Rozycki GS, Feliciano DV, Oschner MG, et al. The role of ultrasound in patients with possible penetrating cardiac wounds: a prospective multicenter study. *J Trauma* 1999;46(4):542-551.

37. Simon B, Cushman J, Barraco R, et al. Pain management in blunt thoracic trauma: an EAST Practice Management Guidelines Workgroup. *J Trauma* 2005;59:1256-1267.

38. Sisley AC, Rozyycki GS, Ballard RB, Namias N, Salomone JP, Feliciano DV. Rapid detection of traumatic effusion using surgeon-performed ultrasonography. *J Trauma* 1998;44:291-7.

39. Smith MD, Cassidy JM, Souther S, et al. Transesophageal echocardiography in the diagnosis of traumatic rupture of the aorta. *N Engl J Med* 1995;332:356-362.

40. Søreide K, Søiland H, Lossius HM, et al. Resuscitative emergency thoracotomy in a Scandinavian trauma hospital—is it justified? *Injury* 2007;38(1):34-42.

41. Stafford RE, Linn J, Washington L. Incidence and management of occult hemothoraces. *Am J Surg* 2006;192(6):722-726.

42. Swaaenburg JC, Klaase JM, DeJongste MJ, et al. Troponin I, troponin T, CKMB-activity and CKMG-mass as markers for the detection of myocardial contusion in patients who experienced blunt trauma. *Clin Chim Acta* 1998;272(2):171-181.

43. Tehrani HY, Peterson BG, Katariya K, et al. Endovascular repair of thoracic aortic tears. *Ann Thorac Surg* 2006;82(3):873-877.

44. Weiss RL, Brier JA, O'Connor W, et al. The usefulness of transesophageal echocardiography in diagnosing cardiac contusions. *Chest* 1996;109(1):73-77.

45. Wilkerson RG, Stone MB. Sensitivity of bedside ultrasound and supine anteroposterior chest radiographs for the identification of pneumothorax after blunt trauma. [Review] [24 refs] *Acad Emerg Med* 2010;17(1):11-7.

46. Woodring JH. A normal mediastinum in blunt trauma rupture of the thoracic aorta and brachiocephalic arteries. *J Emerg Med* 1990;8:467-476.

X-Ray Identification of Thoracic Injuries

▶▶ INTERACTIVE SKILL PROCEDURES

Note: This Skill Station includes a systematic method for evaluating chest x-ray films. A series of x-rays with related scenarios is shown to students for their evaluation and management decisions based on the findings. Standard precautions are required whenever caring for trauma patients.

THE FOLLOWING PROCEDURE IS INCLUDED IN THIS SKILL STATION:

> ▶▶ **Skill VI-A:** Process for Initial Review of Chest X-Rays

Objectives

Performance at this skill station will allow the participant to:

1 Describe the process for viewing a chest x-ray film for the purpose of identifying life-threatening and potentially life-threatening thoracic injuries.

2 Identify various thoracic injuries by using the following seven specific anatomic guidelines for examining a series of chest x-rays:

- Trachea and bronchi
- Pleural spaces and lung parenchyma
- Mediastinum
- Diaphragm
- Bony thorax
- Soft tissues
- Tubes and lines

3 Given a series of x-rays:

- Diagnose fractures
- Diagnose a pneumothorax and a hemothorax
- Identify a widened mediastinum
- Delineate associated injuries
- Identify other areas of possible injury

▶ THORAX X-RAY SCENARIOS

PATIENT VI-1

X-ray film of a 33-year-old bicyclist who was hit by a car.

PATIENT VI-2

X-ray film of a young female with a small stab wound above the nipple on the right side with ipsilateral diminished breath sounds.

PATIENT VI-3

X-ray film of a 56-year-old truck driver who hit an abutment and reported left-sided chest pain and respiratory distress.

PATIENT VI-4

X-ray film of a 22-year-old male in distress after a fight in a bar (stab wound in the back, fourth intercostal space on left).

PATIENT VI-5

X-ray film of a 42-year-old male in respiratory distress after sustaining a gunshot wound in a jewelry shop robbery.

PATIENT VI-6

X-ray film of a motorcyclist with severe head trauma on admission.

PATIENT VI-7

X-ray film of a 36-year-old male after treatment of an obvious pneumothorax on the right side, still desaturated.

PATIENT VI-8

X-ray film of a 45-year-old male motorcyclist who hit a tree at high speed. He was intubated by emergency medical services (EMS) and presents as hemodynamically normal.

PATIENT VI-9

X-ray film of a 56-year-old motorcyclist who sustained a collision with a truck. He was intubated and received a thorax drain in the prehospital setting.

PATIENT VI-10

X-ray film of an 18-year-old gang leader who was assaulted. He has multiple contusions, an altered level of consciousness, and a small entrance wound on the right hemithorax. He has received initial resuscitation.

PATIENT VI-11

X-ray film of a 56-year-old male who fell off a ladder (6 m or approximately 20 feet) with severe head injury.

▶ Skill VI-A: Process for Initial Review of Chest X-Rays

▶▶ I. OVERVIEW

STEP 1. Confirm that the film being viewed is of your patient.

STEP 2. Quickly assess for suspected pathology.

STEP 3. Use the patient's clinical findings to focus the review of the chest x-ray film, and use the x-ray findings to guide further physical evaluation (Table VI.1).

▶▶ II. TRACHEA AND BRONCHI

STEP 1. Assess the position of the tube in cases of endotracheal intubation.

STEP 2. Assess for the presence of interstitial or pleural air that can represent tracheobronchial injury.

STEP 3. Assess for tracheal lacerations that can present as pneumomediastinum, pneumothorax, subcutaneous and interstitial emphysema of the neck, or pneumoperitoneum.

■ TABLE VI.1 CHEST X-RAY SUGGESTIONS

FINDINGS	DIAGNOSES TO CONSIDER
Respiratory distress without x-ray findings	Central nervous system (CNS) injury, aspiration, traumatic asphyxia
Any rib fracture	Pneumothorax, pulmonary contusion
Fracture of first three ribs or sternoclavicular fracture–dislocation	Airway or great vessel injury
Fracture of lower ribs 9 to 12	Abdominal injury
Two or more rib fractures in two or more places	Flail chest, pulmonary contusion
Scapular fracture	Great vessel injury, pulmonary contusion, brachial plexus injury
Mediastinal widening	Great vessel injury, sternal fracture, thoracic spine injury
Persistent large pneumothorax or air leak after chest tube insertion	Bronchial tear
Mediastinal air	Esophageal disruption, tracheal injury, pneumoperitoneum
Gastrointestinal (GI) gas pattern in the chest (loculated air)	Diaphragmatic rupture
NG tube in the chest	Diaphragmatic rupture or ruptured esophagus
Air fluid level in the chest	Hemopneumothorax or diaphragmatic rupture
Disrupted diaphragm	Abdominal visceral injury
Free air under the diaphragm	Ruptured hollow abdominal viscus

STEP 4. Assess for bronchial disruption that can present as a free pleural communication and produce a massive pneumothorax with a persistent air leak that is unresponsive to tube thoracostomy.

▶▶ III. PLEURAL SPACES AND LUNG PARENCHYMA

STEP 1. Assess the pleural space for abnormal collections of fluid that can represent a hemothorax.

STEP 2. Assess the pleural space for abnormal collections of air that can represent a pneumothorax—usually seen as an apical lucent area without bronchial or vascular markings.

STEP 3. Assess the lung fields for infiltrates that can suggest pulmonary contusion, hematoma, aspiration, and so on. Pulmonary contusion appears as air-space consolidation that can be irregular and patchy, homogeneous, diffuse, or extensive.

STEP 4. Assess the parenchyma for evidence of laceration. Lacerations appear as hematomas, vary according to the magnitude of injury, and appear as areas of consolidation.

▶▶ IV. MEDIASTINUM

STEP 1. Assess for air or blood that can displace mediastinal structures, blur the demarcation between tissue planes, or outline them with radiolucency.

STEP 2. Assess for radiologic signs associated with cardiac or major vascular injury.

   A. Air or blood in the pericardium can result in an enlarged cardiac silhouette. Progressive changes in cardiac size can represent an expanding pneumopericardium or hemopericardium.

   B. Aortic rupture can be suggested by:
   - A widened mediastinum—most reliable finding
   - Fractures of the first and second ribs
   - Obliteration of the aortic knob
   - Deviation of the trachea to the right
   - Presence of a pleural cap
   - Elevation and rightward shift of the right mainstem bronchus
   - Depression of the left mainstem bronchus
   - Obliteration of the space between the pulmonary artery and aorta
   - Deviation of the esophagus (nasogastric [NG] tube) to the right

▶▶ V. DIAPHRAGM

Note: Diaphragmatic rupture requires a high index of suspicion, based on the mechanism of injury, signs and symptoms, and x-ray findings. Initial chest x-ray examination may not clearly identify a diaphragmatic injury. Sequential films or additional studies may be required.

STEP 1. Carefully evaluate the diaphragm for:

    A. Elevation (may rise to fourth intercostal space with full expiration)

    B. Disruption (stomach, bowel gas, or NG tube above the diaphragm)

    C. Poor identification (irregular or obscure) due to overlying fluid or soft-tissue masses

STEP 2. X-ray changes suggesting injury include:

    A. Elevation, irregularity, or obliteration of the diaphragm—segmental or total

    B. A mass-like density above the diaphragm that can be due to a fluid-filled bowel, omentum, liver, kidney, spleen, or pancreas (may appear as a "loculated pneumothorax")

    C. Air or contrast-containing stomach or bowel above the diaphragm

    D. Contralateral mediastinal shift

    E. Widening of the cardiac silhouette if the peritoneal contents herniate into the pericardial sac

    F. Pleural effusion

STEP 3. Assess for associated injuries, such as splenic, pancreatic, renal, and liver.

▶▶ VI. BONY THORAX

STEP 1. Assess the clavicle for evidence of:

    A. Fracture

    B. Associated injury, such as great-vessel injury

STEP 2. Assess the scapula for evidence of:

    A. Fracture

    B. Associated injury, such as airway or great-vessel injury, pulmonary contusion

STEP 3. Assess ribs 1 through 3 for evidence of:

    A. Fracture

    B. Associated injury, such as pneumothorax, major airway, or great-vessel injury

STEP 4. Assess ribs 4 through 9 for evidence of:

    A. Fracture, especially in two or more contiguous ribs in two places (flail chest)

    B. Associated injury, such as pneumothorax, hemothorax, pulmonary contusion

STEP 5. Assess ribs 9 through 12 for evidence of:

    A. Fracture, especially in two or more places (flail chest)

    B. Associated injury, such as pneumothorax, pulmonary contusion, spleen, liver, and/or kidney

STEP 6. Assess the sternomanubrial junction and sternal body for evidence of fracture or dislocation. (Sternal fractures can be mistaken on the anteroposterior [AP] film for a mediastinal hematoma. After the patient is stabilized, a coned-down view, over-penetrated film, lateral view, or computed tomography [CT] may be obtained to better identify suspected sternal fracture.)

STEP 7. Assess the sternum for associated injuries, such as myocardial contusion and great-vessel injury (widened mediastinum), although these combinations are relatively infrequent.

▶▶ VII. SOFT TISSUES

STEP 1. Assess for:

    A. Displacement or disruption of tissue planes

    B. Evidence of subcutaneous air

▶▶ VIII. TUBES AND LINES

STEP 1. Assess for placement and positioning of:

    A. Endotracheal tube

    B. Chest tubes

    C. Central access lines

    D. NG tube

    E. Other monitoring devices

▶▶ IX. X-RAY REASSESSMENT

The patient's clinical findings should be correlated with the x-ray findings, and vice versa. After careful, systematic evaluation of the initial chest film, additional x-rays or radiographic and/or imaging studies may be necessary as historical facts and physical findings dictate. Remember, neither the physical examination nor the chest x-ray film should be viewed in isolation. Findings on the physical examination should be used to focus the review of the chest x-ray film, and findings on the chest x-ray film should be used to guide the physical examination and direct the use of ancillary di-agnostic procedures. For example, review of the previous x-ray film and repeat chest films may be indicated if significant changes occur in the patient's status. Thoracic CT, thoracic arteriography, or pericardial ul-trasonography/echocardiography may be indicated for specificity of diagnosis.

Chest Trauma Management

▶▶ INTERACTIVE SKILL PROCEDURES

Note: Standard precautions are required whenever caring for trauma patients.

THE FOLLOWING PROCEDURES ARE INCLUDED IN THIS SKILL STATION:

> ▶▶ **Skill VII-A:** Needle Thoracentesis

> ▶▶ **Skill VII-B:** Chest Tube Insertion

> ▶▶ **Skill VII-C:** Pericardiocentesis (Optional)

Objectives

Performance at this skill station will allow the student to practice and demonstrate on a live, anesthetized animal; a fresh, human cadaver; or an anatomic human body manikin the techniques of needle thoracic decompression of a tension pneumothorax, chest tube insertion for the emergency management of hemopneumothorax, and, if indicated by the course director, pericardiocentesis. Specifically, the student also will be able to:

1 Identify the surface markings and techniques for pleural decompression with needle thoracentesis, chest tube insertion, and needle pericardiocentesis.

2 Describe the underlying pathophysiology of tension pneumothorax and cardiac tamponade as a result of trauma.

3 Describe the complications of needle thoracentesis, chest tube insertion, and pericardiocentesis.

▶ Skill VII-A : Needle Thoracentesis

Note: This procedure is appropriate for patients in critical condition with rapid deterioration who have a life-threatening tension pneumothorax and in whom placement of an expeditious chest tube is not possible. Success rate in the presence of a tension pneumothorax is 50–75% due to length of needle and catheter, size of chest wall, and kinking of the catheter. If this technique is used and the patient does not have a tension pneumothorax, a pneumothorax and/or damage to the lung may occur.

STEP 1. Assess the patient's chest and respiratory status.

STEP 2. Administer high-flow oxygen and apply ventilation as necessary.

STEP 3. Identify the second intercostal space, in the midclavicular line on the side of the tension pneumothorax.

STEP 4. Surgically prepare the chest.

STEP 5. Locally anesthetize the area if the patient is conscious and if time permits.

STEP 6. Place the patient in an upright position if a cervical spine injury has been excluded.

STEP 7. Keeping the Luer-Lok in the distal end of the catheter, insert an over-the-needle catheter (2 in. [5 cm] long) into the skin and direct the needle just over (i.e., superior to) the rib into the intercostal space.

STEP 8. Puncture the parietal pleura.

STEP 9. Remove the Luer-Lok from the catheter and listen for the sudden escape of air when the needle enters the parietal pleura, indicating that the tension pneumothorax has been relieved.

STEP 10. Remove the needle and replace the Luer-Lok in the distal end of the catheter. Leave the plastic catheter in place and apply a bandage or small dressing over the insertion site.

STEP 11. Prepare for a chest tube insertion. The chest tube is typically inserted at the nipple level just anterior to the midaxillary line of the affected hemithorax.

STEP 12. Connect the chest tube to an underwater-seal device or a flutter-type valve apparatus and remove the catheter used to relieve the tension pneumothorax initially.

STEP 13. Obtain a chest x-ray film.

▶ Skill VII-B: Chest Tube Insertion

▶▶ COMPLICATIONS OF NEEDLE THORACENTESIS

- Local hematoma
- Pneumothorax
- Lung laceration

STEP 1. Determine the insertion site, usually at the nipple level (fifth intercostal space), just anterior to the midaxillary line on the affected side. A second chest tube may be used for a hemothorax.

STEP 2. Surgically prepare and drape the chest at the predetermined site of the tube insertion.

STEP 3. Locally anesthetize the skin and rib periosteum.

STEP 4. Make a 2- to 3-cm transverse (horizontal) incision at the predetermined site and bluntly dissect through the subcutaneous tissues, just over the top of the rib.

STEP 5. Puncture the parietal pleura with the tip of a clamp and put a gloved finger into the incision to avoid injury to other organs and to clear any adhesions, clots, and so on. Once the tube in the proper place, remove the clamp from the tube.

STEP 6. Clamp the proximal end of the thoracostomy tube and advance it into the pleural space to the desired length. The tube should be directed posteriorly along the inside of the chest wall.

STEP 7. Look for "fogging" of the chest tube with expiration or listen for air movement.

STEP 8. Connect the end of the thoracostomy tube to an underwater-seal apparatus.

STEP 9. Suture the tube in place.

STEP 10. Apply an occlusive dressing and tape the tube to the chest.

STEP 11. Obtain a chest x-ray film.

STEP 12. Obtain arterial blood gas values and/or institute pulse oximetry monitoring as necessary.

▶▶ COMPLICATIONS OF CHEST TUBE INSERTION

- Laceration or puncture of intrathoracic and/or abdominal organs, which can be prevented by using the finger technique before inserting the chest tube
- Introduction of pleural infection—for example, thoracic empyema
- Damage to the intercostal nerve, artery, or vein:
  - Converting a pneumothorax to a hemopneumothorax
  - Resulting in intercostal neuritis/ neuralgia
- Incorrect tube position, extrathoracic or intrathoracic
- Chest tube kinking, clogging, or dislodging from the chest wall, or disconnection from the underwater-seal apparatus
- Persistent pneumothorax:
  - Large primary leak
  - Leak at the skin around the chest tube; suction on tube too strong
  - Leaky underwater-seal apparatus
- Subcutaneous emphysema, usually at tube site
- Recurrence of pneumothorax upon removal of chest tube; seal of thoracostomy wound not immediate
- Lung fails to expand because of plugged bronchus; bronchoscopy required
- Anaphylactic or allergic reaction to surgical preparation or anesthetic

▶ Skill VII-C: Pericardiocentesis (Optional)

STEP 1. Monitor the patient's vital signs and electrocardiogram (ECG) before, during, and after the procedure.

STEP 2. Surgically prepare the xiphoid and subxiphoid areas, if time allows.

STEP 3. Locally anesthetize the puncture site, if necessary.

STEP 4. Using a 16- to 18-gauge, 6-in. (15-cm) or longer over-the-needle catheter, attach a 35-mL empty syringe with a three-way stopcock.

STEP 5. Assess the patient for any mediastinal shift that may have caused the heart to shift significantly.

STEP 6. Puncture the skin 1 to 2 cm inferior to the left of the xiphochondral junction, at a 45-degree angle to the skin.

STEP 7. Carefully advance the needle cephalad and aim toward the tip of the left scapula.

STEP 8. If the needle is advanced too far (i.e., into the ventricular muscle), an injury pattern known as the "current of injury" appears on the ECG monitor (e.g., extreme ST-T wave changes or widened and enlarged QRS complex). This pattern indicates that the pericardiocentesis needle should be withdrawn until the previous baseline ECG tracing reappears. Premature ventricular contractions also can occur, secondary to irritation of the ventricular myocardium.

STEP 9. When the needle tip enters the blood-filled pericardial sac, withdraw as much nonclotted blood as possible.

STEP 10. During the aspiration, the epicardium approaches the inner pericardial surface again, as does the needle tip. Subsequently, an ECG current of injury pattern may reappear. This indicates that the pericardiocentesis needle should be withdrawn slightly. Should this injury pattern persist, withdraw the needle completely.

STEP 11. After aspiration is completed, remove the syringe and attach a three-way stopcock, leaving the stopcock closed. Secure the catheter in place.

STEP 12. *Option:* Applying the Seldinger technique, pass a flexible guidewire through the needle into the pericardial sac, remove the needle, and pass a 14-gauge flexible catheter over the guidewire. Remove the guidewire and attach a three-way stopcock.

STEP 13. Should the cardiac tamponade symptoms persist, the stopcock may be opened and the pericardial sac reaspirated. This may be repeated as the symptoms of tamponade recur, prior to definitive treatment. The plastic pericardiocentesis catheter can be sutured or taped in place and covered with a small dressing to allow for continued decompression en route to surgery or transfer to another care facility.

▶▶ COMPLICATIONS OF PERICARDIOCENTESIS

- Aspiration of ventricular blood instead of pericardial blood
- Laceration of ventricular epicardium/ myocardium
- Laceration of coronary artery or vein
- New hemopericardium, secondary to lacerations of the coronary artery or vein, and/or ventricular epicardium/ myocardium
- Ventricular fibrillation
- Pneumothorax, secondary to lung puncture
- Puncture of great vessels with worsening of pericardial tamponade
- Puncture of esophagus with subsequent mediastinitis
- Puncture of peritoneum with subsequent peritonitis or false positive aspirate

5 Abdominal and Pelvic Trauma

Unrecognized abdominal and pelvic injuries continue to be a cause of preventable death.

Scenario   A 35-year-old male passenger was in a high-speed motor vehicle collision. His vital signs are: blood pressure 105/80 mm Hg; heart rate 110; and respiratory rate: 18. Glasgow Coma Scale (GCS) score is 15. The patient is complaining of pain in the chest, abdomen, and pelvis.

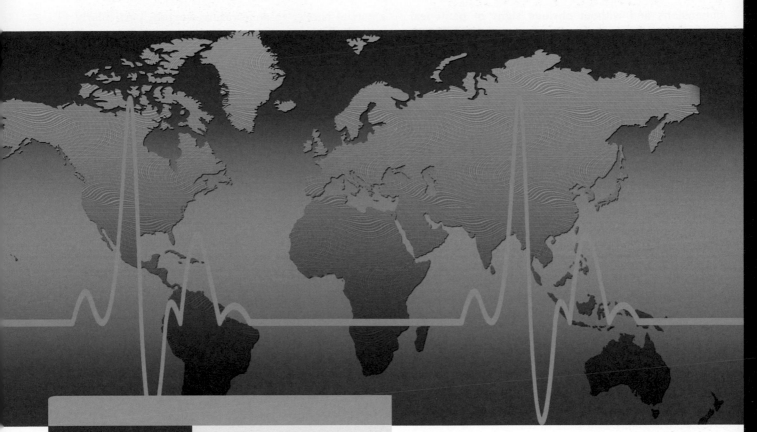

Objectives

1. Identify the key anatomic regions of the abdomen.

2. Recognize a patient at risk for abdominal and pelvic injuries based on the mechanism of injury.

3. Apply the appropriate diagnostic procedures to identify ongoing hemorrhage and injuries that can cause delayed morbidity and mortality.

4. Identify patients who require surgical consultation and possible laparotomy.

5. Describe the acute management of abdominal and pelvic injuries.

? *What priority is abdominal and pelvic trauma in the management of multiply injured patients?*

Evaluation of the abdomen and pelvis is a challenging component of the initial assessment of injured patients. **The assessment of circulation during the primary survey includes early evaluation of the possibility of hemorrhage in the abdomen and pelvis in any patient who has sustained blunt trauma.** Penetrating torso wounds between the nipple and perineum also must be considered as potential causes of intraperitoneal injury. The mechanism of injury, injury forces, location of injury, and hemodynamic status of the patient determine the priority and best method of abdominal and pelvic assessment.

Unrecognized abdominal and pelvic injury continues to be a cause of preventable death after truncal trauma. Rupture of a hollow viscus, bleeding from a solid organ, and bleeding from the bony pelvis may not be easily recognized, and patient assessment is often compromised by alcohol intoxication, use of illicit drugs, injury to the brain or spinal cord, and injury to adjacent structures such as the ribs and spine. **Significant blood loss can be present in the abdominal cavity without any dramatic change in appearance or**

dimensions and without obvious signs of peritoneal irritation. Any patient who has sustained significant blunt torso injury from a direct blow, deceleration, or a penetrating injury must be considered to have an abdominal visceral, vascular, or pelvic injury until proven otherwise.

Anatomy of the Abdomen

The anatomy of the abdomen is illustrated below in ■ FIGURE 5-1.

The abdomen is partially enclosed by the lower thorax. The *anterior abdomen* is defined as the area between the costal margins superiorly, the inguinal ligaments and symphysis pubis inferiorly, and the anterior axillary lines laterally. The majority of the hollow viscera may be involved when there is an injury to the anterior abdomen.

The *thoraco-abdomen* is the area inferior to the trans-nipple line anteriorly and the infra-scapular line posteriorly, and superior to the costal margins. This area, although somewhat protected by the bony thorax, includes the diaphragm, liver, spleen, and stomach. Because the diaphragm rises to the fourth intercostal space during full expiration, fractures of the lower ribs or penetrating wounds below the nipple line can injure abdominal viscera.

The *flank* is the area between the anterior and posterior axillary lines from the sixth intercostal space to the iliac crest. The thick musculature of the abdominal wall in this location, rather than the much thinner aponeurotic sheath of the anterior abdomen, acts as a partial barrier to penetrating wounds, particularly stab wounds.

The *back* is the area located posterior to the posterior axillary lines from the tip of the scapulae to the iliac crests. Similar to the abdominal wall muscles in the flank, the thick back and paraspinal muscles act as a partial barrier to penetrating wounds. The flank and back contain the *retroperitoneal organs*. This potential space is the area posterior to the peritoneal lining of the abdomen. It contains the abdominal aorta; inferior vena cava; most of the duodenum, pancreas, kidneys and ureters; the posterior aspects of the ascending and descending colons; and the retroperitoneal components of the pelvic cavity. **Injuries to the retroperitoneal visceral structures are difficult to recognize because the area is remote from physical examination, and injuries may not initially present with signs or symptoms of peritonitis.** In addition, this space is not sampled by diagnostic peritoneal lavage (DPL) or well visualized with focused assessment sonography in trauma (FAST).

The *pelvic cavity,* surrounded by the pelvic bones, is essentially the lower part of the retroperitoneal and intraperitoneal spaces. It contains the rectum, bladder, iliac vessels, and, in females, internal reproductive organs. **Significant blood loss can occur from either intrapelvic organs or the bony pelvis itself.**

PITFALL

Delay in recognizing intraabdominal or pelvic injury can lead to early death from hemorrhage or delayed death from visceral injury.

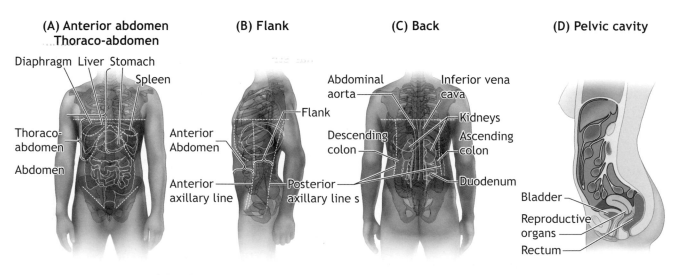

(A) Anterior abdomen Thoraco-abdomen   **(B) Flank**   **(C) Back**   **(D) Pelvic cavity**

■ **FIGURE 5-1** Anatomy of the abdomen.

Mechanism of Injury

? Why is the mechanism of injury important?

Understanding the mechanism of injury facilitates the early identification of potential injuries. This information directs what studies might be necessary for evaluation and the potential need for patient transfer. See Biomechanics of Injury (electronic version only).

BLUNT TRAUMA

A *direct blow*, such as contact with the lower rim of a steering wheel or an intruded door in a motor vehicle crash, can cause compression and crushing injuries to abdominal viscera and pelvis. Such forces deform solid and hollow organs and can cause rupture, with secondary hemorrhage, contamination by visceral contents, and associated peritonitis.

Shearing injuries are a form of crushing injury that can result when a restraint device is worn improperly (■ FIGURE 5-2A). Patients injured in motor vehicle crashes may sustain *deceleration injuries,* in which there is a differential movement of fixed and nonfixed parts of the body. Examples include lacerations of the liver and spleen, both movable organs, at the sites of their fixed supporting ligaments. Bucket handle injuries to the small bowel are also examples of deceleration injuries (■ FIGURE 5-2B).

In patients who sustain blunt trauma, the organs most frequently injured are the spleen (40% to 55%), liver (35% to 45%), and small bowel (5% to 10%). Additionally, there is a 15% incidence of retroperitoneal hematoma in patients who undergo laparotomy for blunt trauma. Although restraint devices prevent more major injuries, they can produce specific patterns of injury, as shown in Table 5.1 on page 126. **Airbag deployment does not preclude abdominal injury.**

PENETRATING TRAUMA

Stab wounds and low-velocity gunshot wounds cause tissue damage by lacerating and cutting. High-velocity gunshot wounds transfer more kinetic energy to abdominal viscera. These wounds can cause increased damage surrounding the track of the missile due to temporary cavitation.

Stab wounds (■ FIGURE 5-3) traverse adjacent abdominal structures and most commonly involve the liver (40%), small bowel (30%), diaphragm (20%), and colon (15%).

Gunshot wounds may cause additional intraabdominal injuries based upon the trajectory, cavitation

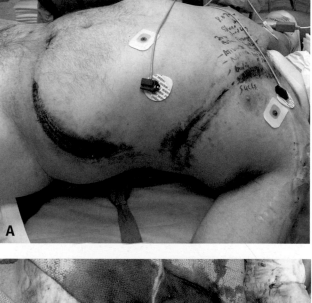

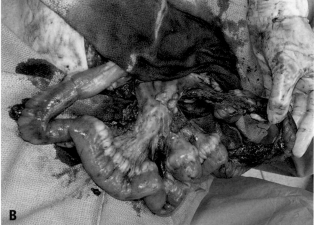

■ **FIGURE 5-2 Lap Belt and Bucket Handle Injuries.** **(A)** Injuries can result when a restraint device is worn improperly. **(B)** Small bowel bucket handle injury.

effect, and possible bullet fragmentation. Gunshot wounds most commonly involve the small bowel (50%), colon (40%), liver (30%), and abdominal vascular structures (25%). Injuries incurred by shotgun blast are affected by the type of shot used and the distance from the gun to the patient.

Explosive devices cause injuries through several mechanisms, including penetrating fragment wounds and blunt injuries from the patient being thrown or struck. Combined penetrating and blunt mechanisms must be considered by the treating clinician. Patients close to the source of the explosion can incur additional pulmonary and hollow viscus injuries related to blast overpressure, which may have delayed presentation. **The potential for overpressure injury should not distract the clinician from a systematic approach to identification and treatment of the common blunt and penetrating injuries.**

■ TABLE 5.1 Truncal and Cervical Injuries from Restraint Devices

RESTRAINT DEVICE	INJURY
Lap Seat Belt • Compression • Hyperflexion	• Tear or avulsion of mesentery (Bucket Handle) • Rupture of small bowel or colon • Thrombosis of iliac artery or abdominal aorta • Chance fracture of lumbar vertebrae • Pancreatic or duodenal injury
Shoulder Harness • Sliding under the seat belt ("submarining") • Compression	• Intimal tear or thrombosis in innominate, carotid, subclavian, or vertebral arteries • Fracture or dislocation of cervical spine • Rib fractures • Pulmonary contusion • Rupture of upper abdominal viscera
Air Bag • Contact • Contact/deceleration • Flexion (unrestrained) • Hyperextension (unrestrained)	• Corneal abrasions • Abrasions of face, neck, and chest • Cardiac rupture • Cervical spine • Thoracic spine fracture

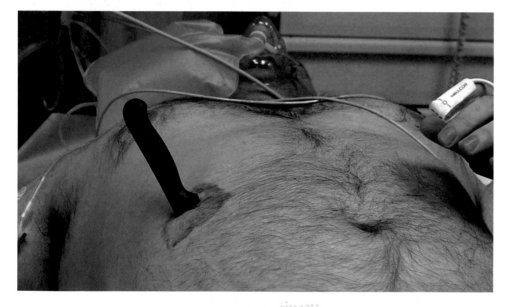

■ **FIGURE 5-3** Stab wounds most commonly injure the liver, small bowel, diaphragm, and colon.

PITFALL

Failure to understand the mechanism leads to lowered index of suspicion and missed injuries, such as:

■ Underestimation of energy delivered to abdomen in blunt trauma

■ Visceral and vascular injuries caused by small external low-velocity wounds, especially stab and fragment wounds

■ Underestimation of the amount of energy delivered in high-velocity wounds, leading to missed injuries tangential to the path of the missile

Scenario ■ *continued*   The patient has left-sided lower chest tenderness with abrasions of his left chest, left abdomen, and left flank. He is tender in the left upper quadrant and has pain with pelvic rock. His pelvis is stable.

Assessment

? How do I know if shock is the result of an intraabdominal or pelvic injury?

In hypotensive patients, the goal is to rapidly determine if an abdominal or pelvic injury is present and whether it is the cause of hypotension. The patient history may predict, and the physical exam, along with rapidly available diagnostic tools, may confirm the presence of abdominal and pelvic injuries that require urgent hemorrhage control. **Hemodynamically normal patients without signs of peritonitis may undergo a more detailed evaluation to determine whether specific injuries that can cause delayed morbidity and mortality are present.** This may include repeated examination to determine whether signs of bleeding or peritonitis develop over time.

HISTORY

When assessing a patient injured in a motor vehicle crash, pertinent historical information includes speed of the vehicle, type of collision (e.g., frontal impact, lateral impact, sideswipe, rear impact, or rollover), vehicle intrusion into the passenger compartment, types of restraints, deployment of air bags, patient's position in the vehicle, and status of passengers, if any. For patients injured by falling, the height of the fall is important to determine due to the potential for deceleration injury from greater heights. Historical information can be provided by the patient, other passengers, the police, or emergency medical personnel. Information about vital signs, obvious injuries, and response to prehospital treatment should also be provided by the prehospital care providers.

When assessing a patient who has sustained penetrating trauma, pertinent historical information includes the time of injury, type of weapon (e.g., knife, handgun, rifle, or shotgun), distance from the assailant (particularly important with shotgun wounds, as the likelihood of major visceral injuries decreases beyond the 10-foot or 3-meter range), number of stab wounds or shots sustained, and the amount of external bleeding from the patient noted at the scene. If possible, important additional information to obtain from the patient includes the magnitude and location of any abdominal pain.

When injuries are caused by an explosive device, the likelihood of visceral overpressure injuries is increased if the explosion occurred in an enclosed space and with decreasing distance of the patient from the explosion.

>10 feet (3 meters) from shot gun, less likely to sustain major visceral injury

PHYSICAL EXAMINATION

? How do I determine if there is an abdominal or pelvic injury?

The abdominal examination should be conducted in a meticulous, systematic fashion in the standard sequence: inspection, auscultation, percussion, and palpation. This is followed by assessment of pelvic stability; urethral, perineal, and rectal exam; vaginal exam; and gluteal exam. The findings, whether positive or negative, should be documented carefully in the patient's medical record.

Inspection

In most circumstances, the patient must be fully undressed to allow for a thorough inspection. The anterior and posterior abdomen, as well as the lower chest and perineum, should be inspected for abrasions, contusions from restraint devices, lacerations, penetrating wounds, impaled foreign bodies, evisceration of omentum or small bowel, and the pregnant state. The patient should be cautiously log rolled to facilitate a complete examination.

The flank, scrotum, and perianal area should be inspected quickly for blood at the urethral meatus; swelling or bruising; or laceration of the perineum, vagina, rectum, or buttocks, which is suggestive of an open pelvic fracture.

At the conclusion of the rapid physical exam, the patient should be covered with warmed blankets to help prevent hypothermia.

PITFALL

Hypothermia contributes to coagulopathy and ongoing bleeding.

Auscultation

in bowel sounds important → present and then becomes absent ↓ think ileus

Auscultation of the abdomen may be difficult in a noisy emergency department, but it can be used to confirm the presence or absence of bowel sounds. Free intraperitoneal blood or gastrointestinal contents may produce an ileus, resulting in the loss of bowel sounds; however, this finding is nonspecific, as ileus can also be caused by extraabdominal injuries. **These findings are most useful when they are normal initially and then change over time.**

Percussion and Palpation

Percussion causes slight movement of the peritoneum and may elicit signs of peritoneal irritation. **When present, no additional evidence of rebound tenderness should be sought, as it may cause the patient further unnecessary pain.**

Voluntary guarding by the patient may make the abdominal examination unreliable. In contrast, involuntary muscle guarding is a reliable sign of peritoneal irritation. Palpation may also elicit and distinguish superficial (abdominal wall) and deep tenderness. The presence of a pregnant uterus, as well as estimation of fetal age, also can be determined.

Palpation of a high-riding prostate gland is a sign of a significant pelvic fracture.

Assessment of Pelvic Stability

Major pelvic hemorrhage occurs rapidly, and the diagnosis must be made quickly so that appropriate resuscitative treatment can be initiated. Unexplained hypotension may be the only initial indication of major pelvic disruption with instability in the posterior ligamentous complex. Mechanical instability of the pelvic ring should be assumed in patients who have pelvic fractures with hypotension and no other source of blood loss. Physical exam findings suggestive of pelvic fracture include evidence of ruptured urethra (high-riding prostate, scrotal hematoma, blood at the urethral meatus), limb length discrepancy, or a rotational deformity of the leg without obvious fracture. In these patients, manual manipulation of the pelvis can be detrimental, as it may dislodge a blood clot that has already formed, thereby precipitating further hemorrhage.

When necessary, mechanical instability of the pelvic ring may be tested by manual manipulation of the pelvis. **This procedure should be performed *only once* during the physical examination, as testing for pelvic instability can result in further hemorrhage. It should not be performed in patients with shock and an obvious pelvic fracture.** The unstable hemipelvis migrates cephalad because of muscular forces and rotates outward secondary to the effect of gravity on the unstable hemipelvis. Because the unstable pelvis is able to rotate externally, the pelvis can be closed by manually pushing on the iliac crests at the level of the anterior superior iliac spine (■ FIGURE 5-4). Motion can be felt if the iliac crests are grasped and the unstable hemipelvis is pushed/rotated inward (internally) and then outward (externally), which is referred to as the compression distraction maneuver.

With posterior ligamentous disruption, the involved hemipelvis can be pushed cephalad as well as pulled caudally. This translational motion can be felt by palpating the posterior iliac spine and tubercle while pushing and pulling the unstable hemipelvis.

The identification of neurologic abnormalities or open wounds in the flank, perineum, and rectum may be evidence of pelvic ring instability. When appropriate, an anteroposterior (AP) x-ray of the pelvis confirms the clinical examination. See Skill Station IV: Shock Assessment and Management.

> **PITFALL**
>
> Repeated manipulation of a fractured pelvis can aggravate hemorrhage. GET ORTHO TO DO IT.

Urethral, Perineal, and Rectal Examination

The presence of blood at the urethral meatus strongly suggests a urethral injury. Inspect the scrotum and perineum for ecchymosis or hematoma, also suggestive of urethral injury. In patients who have sustained blunt trauma, goals of the rectal examination are to assess sphincter tone and rectal mucosal integrity, determine the position of the prostate (high-riding prostate indicates urethral disruption), and identify any fractures of the pelvic bones. In patients with penetrating wounds, the rectal examination is used to assess sphincter tone and look for gross blood from a bowel perforation. **Foley**

■ FIGURE 5-4 **Evaluation of Pelvic Stability.** Gentle pressure over the iliac wings in a downward and medial fashion may reveal laxity or instability.

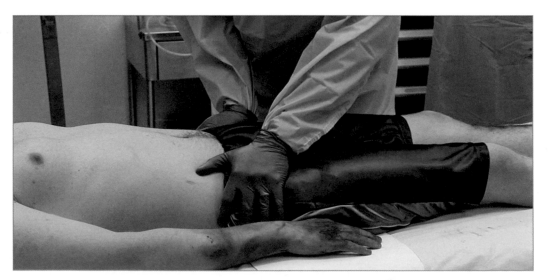

catheters should not be placed in patients with a perineal hematoma or high-riding prostate.

Vaginal Examination

Laceration of the vagina can occur from bony fragments from pelvic fracture(s) or from penetrating wounds. Vaginal exam should be performed when injury is suspected (e.g., in the presence of complex perineal laceration, pelvic fracture, or trans-pelvic gunshot wound).

Gluteal Examination

The gluteal region extends from the iliac crests to the gluteal folds. Penetrating injuries to this area are associated with up to a 50% incidence of significant intraabdominal injuries, including rectal injuries below the peritoneal reflection. Gunshot and stab wounds are associated with intraabdominal injuries; these wounds mandate a search for such injuries.

ADJUNCTS TO PHYSICAL EXAMINATION

Gastric and urinary catheters are frequently inserted as part of the resuscitation phase, once problems with the airway, breathing, and circulation are diagnosed and treated.

Gastric Tube

The therapeutic goals of inserting gastric tubes early in the resuscitation process are to relieve acute gastric dilation, decompress the stomach before performing a DPL, and remove gastric contents. Gastric tubes may reduce the incidence of aspiration in these cases; however, in an awake patient with an active gag reflex they may actually promote vomiting. The presence of blood in the gastric contents suggests an injury to the esophagus or upper gastrointestinal tract if nasopharyngeal and/or oropharyngeal sources are excluded. **If severe facial fractures exist or basilar skull fracture is suspected, the gastric tube should be inserted through the mouth to prevent passage of the tube through the cribriform plate into the brain.**

> ### PITFALL
> Avoid a nasal gastric tube in midface injury. Use the oral gastric route.

Urinary Catheter

The goals of inserting urinary catheters early in the resuscitation process are to relieve retention, decompress the bladder before performing DPL, and allow for monitoring of urinary output as an index of tissue perfusion. Gross hematuria is a sign of trauma to the genitourinary tract and nonrenal intraabdominal organs. **The absence of hematuria, however, does not rule out an injury to the genitourinary tract. The inability to void, unstable pelvic fracture, blood at the meatus, scrotal hematoma or perineal ecchymoses, or a high-riding prostate on rectal examination mandate a retrograde urethrogram to confirm an intact urethra before inserting a urinary catheter.** A disrupted urethra detected during the primary or secondary survey may require the insertion of a suprapubic tube by an experienced doctor.

> ### PITFALL
> A single physical exam or adjunct should not allay clinical suspicion based on the mechanism of injury. Repeated exams and complementary adjuncts may be necessary.

Other Studies

With preparation and an organized team approach, the physical examination can be performed very quickly. **In patients with hemodynamic abnormalities, rapid evaluation is necessary; this can be done with either focused assessment sonography in trauma (FAST) or DPL.** The only contraindication to performing these studies is an existing indication for laparotomy. In addition, hemodynamically normal patients with any of the following signs require additional studies:

- Change in sensorium (potential brain injury, alcohol intoxication, or use of illicit drugs)
- Change in sensation (potential injury to spinal cord)
- Injury to adjacent structures, such as lower ribs, pelvis, lumbar spine
- Equivocal physical examination
- Prolonged loss of contact with patient anticipated, such as general anesthesia for extraabdominal injuries or lengthy x-ray studies
- Lap-belt sign (abdominal wall contusion) with suspicion of bowel injury

When intraabdominal injury is suspected, a number of studies can provide useful information; however, these studies should not delay the transfer of a patient to definitive care.

X-Rays for Abdominal Trauma   An AP chest x-ray is recommended in the assessment of patients with multisystem blunt trauma. Hemodynamically abnormal patients with penetrating abdominal wounds do not require screening x-rays in the emergency department (ED). If the patient is hemodynamically normal and has penetrating trauma above the umbilicus or a suspected thoracoabdominal injury, an upright chest x-ray is useful to exclude an associated hemothorax or pneumothorax, or to document the presence of intraperitoneal air. With marker rings or clips applied to all entrance and exit wound sites, a supine abdominal x-ray may be obtained in hemodynamically normal patients to determine the track of the missile or presence of retroperitoneal air. An anteroposterior pelvic x-ray may be helpful in establishing the source of blood loss in hemodynamically abnormal patients and in patients with pelvic pain or tenderness. The alert, awake patient without pain or tenderness does not need a pelvic radiograph.

Focused Assessment Sonography in Trauma   FAST is one of two rapid studies utilized to identify hemorrhage. In FAST, ultrasound technology is used by properly trained individuals to detect the presence of hemoperitoneum (■ FIGURE 5-5). With specific equipment and in experienced hands, ultrasound has a sensitivity, specificity, and accuracy in detecting intraabdominal fluid comparable to DPL. Thus, ultrasound provides a rapid, noninvasive, accurate, and inexpensive means of diagnosing hemoperitoneum that can be repeated frequently.

Ultrasound scanning can be done at the bedside in the resuscitation room while simultaneously performing other diagnostic or therapeutic procedures. The indications for the procedure are the same as for DPL. See Skill Station VIII: Focused Assessment Sonography in Trauma (FAST).

Furthermore, ultrasound can detect one of the nonhypovolemic reasons for hypotension: pericardial tamponade. Scans are obtained of the pericardial sac (1), hepatorenal fossa (2), splenorenal fossa (3), and pelvis (4) or pouch of Douglas (■ FIGURE 5-6A). After the initial scan is completed, a second scan may be performed after an interval of 30 minutes. This scan can detect progressive hemoperitoneum (■ FIGURE 5-6B).

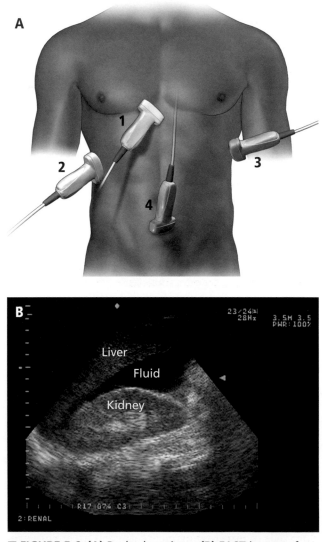

■ FIGURE 5-6 **(A)** Probe locations. **(B)** FAST image of the right upper quadrant showing the liver, kidney, and free fluid.

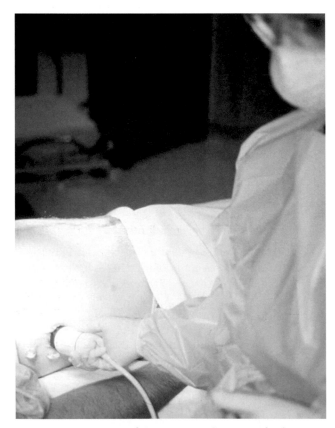

■ FIGURE 5-5 **Focused Assessment Sonography in Trauma (FAST).** In FAST, ultrasound technology is used to detect the presence of hemoperitoneum.

Diagnostic Peritoneal Lavage DPL is another rapid study to identify hemorrhage. Although invasive, it also allows investigation of possible hollow viscus injury. DPL can significantly alter subsequent examinations of the patient and is considered 98% sensitive for intraperitoneal bleeding (■ FIGURE 5-7). It should be performed by a surgical team caring for a patient with hemodynamic abnormalities and multiple blunt injuries, and may also be useful in penetrating trauma.

DPL also is indicated in hemodynamically normal patients with blunt injury when ultrasound or computed tomography (CT) is not available. In settings with either or both of these modalities available, DPL is rarely used, as it is invasive and requires some surgical expertise.

Relative contraindications to DPL include previous abdominal operations, morbid obesity, advanced cirrhosis, and preexisting coagulopathy. Either an open or closed (Seldinger) infraumbilical technique is acceptable in the hands of trained clinicians. In patients with pelvic fractures, an open supraumbilical approach is preferred to avoid entering a pelvic hematoma. In patients with advanced pregnancy, an open suprafundal approach should be used to avoid damaging the enlarged uterus. **Free aspiration of blood, gastrointestinal contents, vegetable fibers, or bile through the lavage catheter in patients with hemodynamic abnormalities mandates laparotomy.**

If gross blood (>10 mL) or gastrointestinal contents are not aspirated, lavage is performed with 1000 mL of warmed isotonic crystalloid solution (10 mL/kg in a child).

After ensuring adequate mixing of peritoneal contents with the lavage fluid by compressing the abdomen and moving the patient by logrolling or tilting him or her into head-down and head-up positions, the effluent is sent to the laboratory for quantitative analysis if gastrointestinal contents, vegetable fibers, or bile are not obviously present. A positive test is indicated by >100,000 red blood cells (RBC)/mm³, 500 white blood cells (WBC)/mm³, or a Gram stain with bacteria present. See Skill Station IX: Diagnostic Peritoneal Lavage.

Computed Tomography CT is a diagnostic procedure that requires transport of the patient to the scanner, administration of contrast, and scanning of the upper and lower abdomen, as well as the lower chest

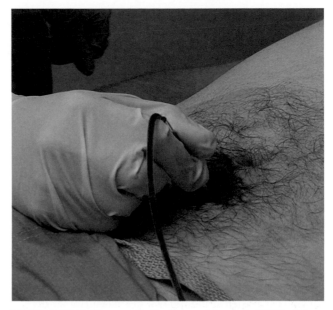

■ FIGURE 5-7 Diagnostic Peritoneal Lavage (DPL). DPL is a rapidly performed, invasive procedure that is considered 98% sensitive for intraperitoneal bleeding.

and pelvis. **It is a time-consuming procedure that should be used *only in hemodynamically normal patients* in whom there is no apparent indication for an emergency laparotomy.** The CT scan provides information relative to specific organ injury and its extent, and can diagnose retroperitoneal and pelvic organ injuries that are difficult to assess with a physical examination, FAST, and peritoneal lavage. Relative contraindications to the use of CT include delay until the scanner is available, an uncooperative patient who cannot be safely sedated, and allergy to the contrast agent when nonionic contrast is not available. **CT can miss some gastrointestinal, diaphragmatic, and pancreatic injuries. In the absence of hepatic or splenic injuries, the presence of free fluid in the abdominal cavity suggests an injury to the gastrointestinal tract and/or its mesentery, and many trauma surgeons find this to be an indication for early operative intervention.**

Contrast Studies A number of contrast studies can aid in the diagnosis of specifically suspected injuries, but they should not delay the care of patients who are hemodynamically abnormal. These include:

- Urethrography
- Cystography
- Intravenous pyelogram
- Gastrointestinal contrast studies

Urethrography should be performed before inserting an indwelling urinary catheter when a urethral injury is suspected. The urethrogram is performed with an 8 French urinary catheter secured in the meatal fossa by balloon inflation to 1.5 to 2 mL. Approximately 30 to 35 mL of undiluted contrast material is instilled with gentle pressure. In males, a radiograph is taken with an anterior-posterior projection and with slight stretching of the penis toward one of the patient's shoulders. An adequate study shows reflux of contrast into the bladder.

An intraperitoneal or extraperitoneal bladder rupture is best diagnosed with a cystogram or CT *cystography*. A syringe barrel is attached to the indwelling bladder catheter, held 40 cm above the patient, and 350 mL of water-soluble contrast is allowed to flow into the bladder until (1) flow stops, (2) the patient voids spontaneously, or (3) the patient is in discomfort. This is followed by instillation of an additional 50 mL of contrast to ensure bladder distension. Anterior-posterior and postdrainage views are essential to definitively exclude injury. CT evaluation of the bladder and pelvis (CT cystogram) is an alternative study that is particularly useful in providing additional information about the kidneys and pelvic bones.

Suspected urinary system injuries are best evaluated by contrast-enhanced CT scan. If CT is not available, *intravenous pyelogram (IVP)* provides an alternative. A high-dose, rapid injection of renal contrast ("screening IVP") is best performed using the recommended dosage of 200 mg of iodine/kg body weight. This involves a bolus injection of 100 mL (standard 1.5 mL/kg for a 70-kg individual) of a 60% iodine solution performed through two 50 mL syringes over 30 to 60 seconds. If only 30% iodine solution is available, the ideal dose is 3.0 mL/kg. Visualization of the calyces of the kidneys on a flat plate x-ray of the abdomen should appear 2 minutes after the injection is completed. Unilateral nonfunction indicates an absent kidney, thrombosis, avulsion of the renal

artery, or massive parenchymal disruption. Nonfunction warrants further radiologic evaluation with a contrast-enhanced CT or renal arteriogram, or surgical exploration, depending on mechanism of injury and local availability or expertise.

Isolated injuries to retroperitoneal gastrointestinal structures (e.g., duodenum, ascending or descending colon, rectum, biliary tract, and pancreas) may not cause peritonitis and may not be detected on DPL. When injury to one of these structures is suspected, CT with contrast, specific upper and lower *gastrointestinal contrast studies*, and pancreatico-biliary imaging studies can be useful. However, these studies should be guided by the surgeon who will ultimately care for the patient.

EVALUATION OF ABDOMINAL TRAUMA

If there is early or obvious evidence that the patient will be transferred to another facility, time-consuming tests, including abdominal CT, should *not* be performed. Table 5.2 compares the use of DPL, FAST, and CT, including their advantages and disadvantages, in the evaluation of blunt trauma.

Scenario ■ *continued* The patient has fractures of the lower ribs on the left side identified on chest x-ray and fractures of the left superior and inferior rami identified on pelvic x-ray. Because of these findings, as well as his abdominal tenderness, the patient undergoes an abdominopelvic CT scan.

■ TABLE 5.2 Comparison of DPL, FAST, and CT in Blunt Abdominal Trauma

	DPL	FAST	CT SCAN
Advantages	• Early diagnosis • Performed rapidly • 98% sensitive • Detects bowel injury • Transport: No	• Early diagnosis • Noninvasive • Performed rapidly • Repeatable • 86%–97% sensitive • Transport: No	• Most specific for injury • 92%–98% sensitive • Non-invasive
Disadvantages	• Invasive • Specificity: Low • Misses injuries to diaphragm and retroperitoneum	• Operator-dependent • Bowel gas and subcutaneous air distortion • Misses diaphragm, bowel, and pancreatic injuries	• Cost and time • Misses diaphragm, bowel, and some pancreatic injuries • Transport: Required
Indications	• Unstable blunt trauma • Penetrating trauma	• Unstable blunt trauma	• Stable blunt trauma • Penetrating back/flank trauma

The evaluation of penetrating trauma involves special consideration to address penetrating wounds to the abdomen and thoracoabdominal region. Options include serial physical examination or DPL in thoracoabdominal or anterior abdominal stab wounds. Double- or triple-contrast CT scans are useful in flank and back injuries. Surgery may be required for immediate diagnosis and treatment.

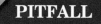

PITFALL

Evaluations should not delay the transfer of the patient to a more appropriate level of care for severe injuries that have already been identified.

Most gunshot wounds to the abdomen are managed by exploratory laparotomy, as the incidence of significant intraperitoneal injury approaches 98% when peritoneal penetration is present. Stab wounds to the abdomen may be managed more selectively, but approximately 30% do cause intraperitoneal injury. Thus, indications for laparotomy in patients with penetrating abdominal wounds include:

- Any hemodynamically abnormal patient

- Gunshot wound with a transperitoneal trajectory

- Signs of peritoneal irritation

- Signs of fascia penetration

PITFALL

Tangential gunshot wounds often are not truly tangential, and concussive and blast injuries can cause intraperitoneal injury without peritoneal penetration.

Thoracoabdominal Wounds

Diagnostic options in asymptomatic patients with possible injuries to the diaphragm and upper abdominal structures include serial physical examinations, serial chest x-rays, DPL, thoracoscopy, laparoscopy, and CT (for right thoracoabdominal wounds).

Local Wound Exploration and Serial Physical Abdominal Examination

Approximately 55% to 60% of all patients with stab wounds that penetrate the anterior peritoneum have hypotension, peritonitis, or evisceration of omentum or small bowel. These patients require an emergency laparotomy. In the remaining patients, in whom anterior peritoneal penetration can be confirmed or strongly suspected by local wound exploration, approximately 50% eventually require operation. Laparotomy remains a reasonable option for all such patients. Less invasive diagnostic options for relatively asymptomatic patients (who may have pain at the site of the stab wound) include serial physical examinations over a 24-hour period, DPL, or diagnostic laparoscopy.

Although a positive FAST may be helpful in this situation, a negative FAST does not exclude the possibility of a significant intraabdominal injury producing small volumes of fluid. Serial physical examinations are labor intensive, but have an overall accuracy rate of 94%. DPL may allow for earlier diagnosis of injury in relatively asymptomatic patients. The accuracy rate is greater than 96% when specific cell counts, rather than gross inspection of the fluid, are used. Use of lower thresholds for penetrating trauma increases sensitivity and decreases specificity. Diagnostic laparoscopy can confirm or exclude peritoneal penetration, but it is less useful in identifying specific injuries.

Serial Physical Examinations Versus Double- or Triple-Contrast CT Scans in Flank and Back Injuries

The thickness of the flank and back muscles protects the underlying viscera from injury from many stab wounds and some gunshot wounds to these areas. Although laparotomy is a reasonable option for all such patients, less invasive diagnostic options in patients who are initially asymptomatic include serial physical examinations, double- or triple-contrast CT scans, and DPL. Serial physical examination in patients who are initially asymptomatic and then become symptomatic is very accurate in detecting retroperitoneal and intraperitoneal injuries with wounds posterior to the anterior axillary line.

Double- (intravenous and oral) or triple- (intravenous, oral, and rectal) contrast enhanced CT is time consuming and may more fully evaluate the retroperitoneal colon on the side of the wound. The accuracy is comparable to that of serial physical examinations, but should allow for earlier diagnosis of injury in relatively asymptomatic patients when the CT is performed properly.

On rare occasions, these retroperitoneal injuries can be missed by serial examinations and contrast CT. Early outpatient follow-up is mandatory after the 24-hour period of inhospital observation because of the subtle presentation of certain colonic injuries.

DPL also can be used in such patients as an early screening test. A positive DPL is an indication for an urgent laparotomy.

PITFALLS

These evaluations are seeking to prove there is no injury in the hemodynamically normal patient. They should not delay a laparotomy in hemodynamically abnormal patients who likely have an abdominal source or in patients with obvious peritonitis.

Scenario ■ continued The CT scan further delineates the rib fractures and pelvic fractures and shows a Grade III (moderately severe) splenic injury with a small amount of free intraperitoneal fluid. The patient's blood pressure remains normal; his heart rate is 110, his base deficit is 3.2, and his lactate is 1.7 mmol/L.

- Blunt abdominal trauma with hypotension with a positive FAST or clinical evidence of intraperitoneal bleeding

- Blunt or penetrating abdominal trauma with a positive DPL

- Hypotension with a penetrating abdominal wound

- Gunshot wounds traversing the peritoneal cavity or visceral/vascular retroperitoneum

- Evisceration

- Bleeding from the stomach, rectum, or genitourinary tract from penetrating trauma

- Peritonitis

- Free air, retroperitoneal air, or rupture of the hemidiaphragm

- Contrast-enhanced CT that demonstrates ruptured gastrointestinal tract, intraperitoneal bladder injury, renal pedicle injury, or severe visceral parenchymal injury after blunt or penetrating trauma

Indications for a Laparotomy in Adults

? Which patients warrant a laparotomy?

In individual patients, surgical judgment is required to determine the timing and need for laparotomy (■ FIGURE 5-8). The following indications are commonly used to facilitate the decision-making process in this regard.

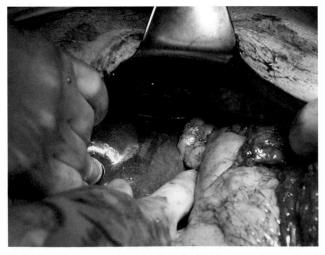

■ **FIGURE 5-8 Laparotomy.** Surgical judgment is required to determine the timing and need for laparotomy.

Specific Diagnoses

The liver, spleen, and kidney are the organs predominantly involved after blunt trauma, although the relative incidence of hollow visceral perforation, lumbar spinal injuries, and uterine rupture increases with incorrect seat belt usage (see Table 5.1). Difficulties in diagnosis can occur with injuries to the diaphragm, duodenum, pancreas, genitourinary system, or small bowel. Most penetrating injuries are diagnosed at laparotomy.

DIAPHRAGM INJURIES

Blunt tears can occur in any portion of either diaphragm; however, the left hemidiaphragm is more commonly injured. The most common injury is 5 to 10 cm in length and involves the posterolateral left hemidiaphragm. Abnormalities on the initial chest x-ray include elevation or "blurring" of the hemidiaphragm, hemothorax, an abnormal gas shadow that obscures the hemidiaphragm, or the gastric tube positioned in the chest. However, the initial chest x-ray can be normal in a small percentage of patients. The diagnosis should be suspected with any wound of the thoracoabdomen and may be confirmed with laparotomy, thoracoscopy, or laparoscopy.

DUODENAL INJURIES

Duodenal rupture is classically encountered in unrestrained drivers involved in frontal-impact motor vehicle collisions and patients who sustain direct blows to the abdomen, such as from bicycle handlebars. A bloody gastric aspirate or retroperitoneal air on a flat plate x-ray of the abdomen or abdominal CT should raise suspicion for this injury. An upper gastrointestinal x-ray series or double-contrast CT is indicated for high-risk patients.

PANCREATIC INJURIES

Pancreatic injuries most often result from a direct epigastric blow that compresses the organ against the vertebral column. **An early normal serum amylase level does not exclude major pancreatic trauma. Conversely, the amylase level can be elevated from nonpancreatic sources.** However, persistently elevated or rising serum amylase levels should prompt further evaluation of the pancreas and other abdominal viscera. Double-contrast CT may not identify significant pancreatic trauma in the immediate postinjury period (up to 8 hours); it should be repeated later if pancreatic injury is suspected. Should there be concern after an equivocal CT, surgical exploration of the pancreas is warranted.

GENITOURINARY INJURIES

Direct blows to the back or flank that result in contusions, hematomas, or ecchymoses are markers of potential underlying renal injury and warrant an evaluation (CT or IVP) of the urinary tract. Additional indications for evaluating the urinary tract include gross hematuria or microscopic hematuria in patients with (1) a penetrating abdominal wound, (2) an episode of hypotension (systolic blood pressure less than 90 mm Hg) in patients with blunt abdominal trauma, and (3) associated intraabdominal injuries in patients with blunt trauma. Gross hematuria and microscopic hematuria in patients with an episode of shock indicate they are at risk for nonrenal abdominal injuries. An abdominal CT scan with IV contrast can document the presence and extent of a blunt renal injury, 95% of which can be treated nonoperatively. Thrombosis of the renal artery or disruption of the renal pedicle secondary to deceleration is a rare upper tract injury in which hematuria may be absent, although the patient can have severe abdominal pain. With either injury, an IVP, CT, or renal arteriogram can be useful in diagnosis.

An anterior pelvic fracture usually is present in patients with urethral injuries. Urethral disruptions are divided into those above (posterior) or below (anterior) the urogenital diaphragm. A posterior urethral injury usually occurs in patients with multisystem injuries and pelvic fractures. In contrast, an anterior urethral injury results from a straddle impact and can be an isolated injury.

HOLLOW VISCUS INJURIES

Blunt injury to the intestines generally results from sudden deceleration with subsequent tearing near a fixed point of attachment, especially if the patient's seat belt was applied incorrectly. The appearance of transverse, linear ecchymoses on the abdominal wall (seat-belt sign) or the presence of a lumbar distraction fracture (Chance fracture) on x-ray should alert the clinician to the possibility of intestinal injury. **Although some patients have early abdominal pain and tenderness, diagnosis can be difficult in others, especially because injured intestinal structures may only produce minimal hemorrhage.**

SOLID ORGAN INJURIES

Injuries to the liver, spleen, and kidney that result in shock, hemodynamic instability, or evidence of continuing bleeding are indications for urgent laparotomy. Solid organ injury in hemodynamically normal patients can often be managed nonoperatively. Such patients should be admitted to the hospital for careful observation, and evaluation by a surgeon is essential. **Concomitant hollow viscus injury occurs in less than 5% of patients initially thought to have isolated solid organ injuries.**

PELVIC FRACTURES AND ASSOCIATED INJURIES

Patients with hypotension and pelvic fractures have a high mortality, and sound decision making is crucial. Pelvic fractures associated with hemorrhage commonly exhibit disruption of the posterior osseous ligamentous (sacroiliac, sacrospinous, sacrotuberous, and the fibromuscular pelvic floor) complex from a sacroiliac fracture and/or dislocation, or from a sacral fracture. Disruption of the pelvic ring tears the pelvic venous plexus and occasionally disrupts the internal iliac arterial system (anteroposterior compression injury). Vertical displacement of the sacroiliac joint may also cause disruption of the iliac vasculature that can cause uncontrolled hemorrhage. Pelvic ring injury may be caused by motorcycle crashes and pedestrian-vehicle collisions, direct crushing injury to the pelvis, and falls from heights greater than 12 feet (3.6 meters). Mortality in patients with all types of pelvic fractures is approximately one in six (5%–30%). Mortality rises to approximately one in four (10%–42%) in patients with closed pelvic fractures and hypotension, and to approximately 50% in patients with open pelvic fractures. Hemorrhage is the major potentially reversible contributing factor to mortality.

In motor vehicle collisions, a common mechanism of pelvic fracture is force applied to the lateral aspect of the pelvis that tends to rotate the involved hemipelvis internally, closing down the pelvic volume and reducing tension on the pelvic vascular system (lateral compression injury). This rotational motion drives the pubis into the lower genitourinary system, potentially creating injury to the bladder and/or urethra. Hemorrhage from this injury, or its sequelae, rarely results in death. See Skill Station XIII: Musculoskeletal Trauma: Assessment and Management, Skill XIII-F: Identification and Management of Pelvic Fractures.

Mechanism of Injury/Classification

The four patterns of force leading to pelvic fractures include (1) AP compression, (2) lateral compression, (3) vertical shear, and (4) complex (combination) pattern. An AP compression injury can be caused by an auto-pedestrian collision or motorcycle crash, a direct crushing injury to the pelvis, or a fall from a height greater than 12 feet (3.6 meters). With disruption of the symphysis pubis, there often is tearing of the posterior osseous ligamentous complex, represented by a sacroiliac fracture and/or dislocation or sacral fracture. With opening of the pelvic ring, there can be hemorrhage from the posterior pelvic venous complex and, occasionally, branches of the internal iliac artery.

Lateral compression injuries often result from motor vehicle crashes and lead to internal rotation of the involved hemipelvis. The pelvic volume is actually compressed in such an injury, so life-threatening hemorrhage is not common.

A high-energy shear force applied in a vertical plane across the anterior and posterior aspects of the ring disrupts the sacrospinous and sacrotuberous ligaments and leads to major pelvic instability. This commonly results from a fall. ■ FIGURE 5-9 illustrates types of pelvic fractures.

Management

Initial management of a major pelvic disruption associated with hemorrhage requires hemorrhage control and fluid resuscitation. Hemorrhage control is achieved through mechanical stabilization of the pelvic ring and external counterpressure. Patients with these injuries may be initially assessed and treated in hospitals that do not have the resources to definitively manage the degree of associated hemorrhage. In such cases, simple techniques can be used to stabilize the pelvis before transferring the patient. Longitudinal traction applied through the skin or the skeleton is a first-line method. Because these injuries externally rotate the hemipelvis, internal rotation of the lower limbs also reduces the pelvic volume. This procedure may be supplemented by applying a support directly to the pelvis. **A sheet, pelvic binder, or other device can apply sufficient stability for the unstable pelvis at the level of the greater trochanters of the femur (■ FIGURE 5-10).**

■ FIGURE 5-9 **Pelvic Fractures. (A)** Closed fracture. **(B)** Open book fracture. **(C)** Vertical shear fracture.

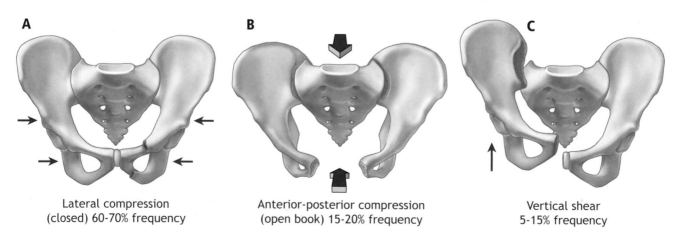

A

Lateral compression
(closed) 60-70% frequency

B

Anterior-posterior compression
(open book) 15-20% frequency

C

Vertical shear
5-15% frequency

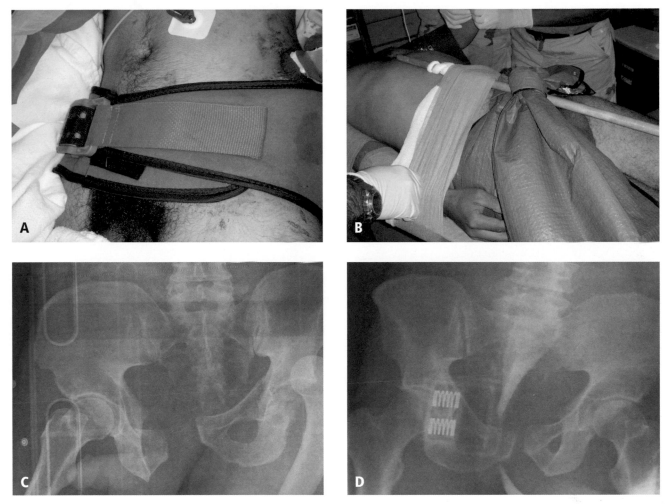

■ **FIGURE 5-10 Pelvic Stabilization. (A)** Pelvic binder. **(B)** Pelvic stabilization using a sheet. **(C)** Before application of pelvic binder. **(D)** After application of pelvic binder.

These temporary methods are suitable to gain early pelvic stabilization. The binders are only a temporary procedure, and caution is necessary, as tight binders can cause skin breakdown and ulceration over the bony prominences. As a result, patients with pelvic binders need to be carefully monitored.

Definitive care of patients with hemodynamic abnormalities demands the cooperative efforts of a team that includes a trauma surgeon, an interventional radiologist if available, and an orthopedic surgeon. Angiographic embolization is often the best option for definitive management of patients with ongoing hemorrhage related to pelvic fractures.

Although definitive management of patients with pelvic fractures varies, one treatment algorithm based on the hemodynamic status for emergency patients is shown in ■ FIGURE 5-11. Since significant resources are required to care for patients with severe pelvic fractures, early consideration of transfer to a trauma center is essential.

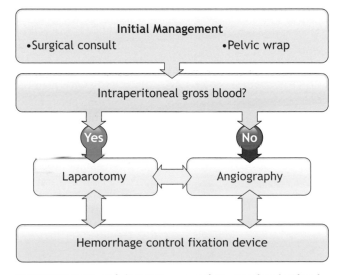

■ **FIGURE 5-11 Pelvic Fractures and Hemorrhagic Shock Management Algorithm**

PITFALL

- Delay in stabilization of the pelvis allows continued hemorrhage.
- The pressure caused by pelvic binders over bony prominences is sufficient to cause skin breakdown and ulceration.

Scenario ■ conclusion   The patient is admitted to the intensive care unit for monitoring, pain control, and respiratory care; his hemodynamics remain normal for 24 hours, after which he is transferred to the ward. He is discharged on hospital day 5.

Chapter Summary

1 The three distinct regions of the abdomen are the peritoneal cavity, retroperitoneal space, and pelvic cavity. The pelvic cavity contains components of both the peritoneal cavity and retroperitoneal space.

2 Early consultation with a surgeon is necessary whenever a patient with possible intraabdominal injuries is brought to the ED. Once the patient's vital functions have been restored, evaluation and management varies depending on the mechanism of injury.

3 Hemodynamically abnormal patients with multiple blunt injuries should be rapidly assessed for intraabdominal bleeding or contamination from the gastrointestinal tract by performing a FAST or DPL.

4 Indications for CT scan in hemodynamically normal patients include an unevaluable abdomen, pain, or tenderness. The decision to operate is based on the specific organ(s) involved and the magnitude of injury.

5 All patients with penetrating wounds in proximity to the abdomen and associated hypotension, peritonitis, or evisceration require emergent laparotomy. Patients with gunshot wounds that obviously traverse the peritoneal cavity or visceral/vascular area of the retroperitoneum on physical examination or routine x-rays also require laparotomy. Asymptomatic patients with anterior abdominal stab wounds that penetrate the fascia or peritoneum on local wound exploration require further evaluation; there are several acceptable alternatives.

6 Asymptomatic patients with flank or back stab wounds that are not obviously superficial are evaluated by serial physical examinations or contrast-enhanced CT. Exploratory laparotomy is an acceptable option with these patients as well.

Chapter Summary (continued)

7 Management of blunt and penetrating trauma to the abdomen and pelvis includes:

▶ Reestablishing vital functions and optimizing oxygenation and tissue perfusion

▶ Prompt recognition of sources of hemorrhage with efforts at hemorrhage control
- Laparotomy
- Pelvic stabilization
- Angiographic embolization

▶ Delineating the injury mechanism

▶ Meticulous initial physical examination, repeated at regular intervals

▶ Selecting special diagnostic maneuvers as needed, performed with a minimal loss of time

▶ Maintaining a high index of suspicion related to occult vascular and retroperitoneal injuries

BIBLIOGRAPHY

1. Agolini SF, Shah K, Jaffe J, et al. Arterial embolization is a rapid and effective technique for controlling pelvic fracture hemorrhage. *J Trauma* 1997;43(3):395-399.

2. Anderson PA, Rivara FP, Maier RV, et al. The epidemiology of seat belt-associated injuries. *J Trauma* 1991;31:60-67.

3. Aquilera PA, Choi T, Durham BH. Ultrasound-aided supra-pubic cystostomy catheter placement in the emergency department. *J Emerg Med* 2004;26(3):319-321.

4. Ballard RB, Rozycki GS, Newman PG, et al. An algorithm to reduce the incidence of false-negative FAST examinations in patients at high risk for occult injury. *J Am Coll Surg* 1999;189(2):145-150.

5. Boyle EM, Maier RV, Salazar JD, et al: Diagnosis of injuries after stab wounds to the back and flank. *J Trauma* 1997;42(2):260-265.

6. Cryer HM, Miller FB, Evers BM, et al. Pelvic fracture classification: correlation with hemorrhage. *J Trauma* 1988;28:973-980.

7. Dalal SA, Burgess AR, Siegel JH, et al. Pelvic fracture in multiple trauma: classification by mechanism is key to pattern of organ injury, resuscitative requirements, and outcome. *J Trauma* 1989;29:981-1002.

8. Demetriades D, Rabinowitz B, Sofianos C, et al. The management of penetrating injuries of the back: a prospective study of 230 patients. *Ann Surg* 1988;207:72-74.

9. Dischinger PC, Cushing BM, Kerns TJ. Injury patterns associated with direction of impact: drivers admitted to trauma centers. *J Trauma* 1993;35:454-459.

10. Fabian TC, Croce MA. Abdominal trauma, including indications for laparotomy. In: Mattox LK, Feliciano DV, Moore EE, eds. *Trauma*. East Norwalk, CT: Appleton & Lange; 2000:583-602.

11. Holmes JF, Harris D, Battistella FD. Performance of abdominal ultrasonography in blunt trauma patients with out-of-hospital or emergency department hypotension. *Ann Emerg Med* 2004;43(3):354-361.

12. Huizinga WK, Baker LW, Mtshali ZW. Selective management of abdominal and thoracic stab wounds with established peritoneal penetration: the eviscerated omentum. *Am J Surg* 1987;153:564-568.

13. Knudson MM, McAninch JW, Gomez R. Hematuria as a predictor of abdominal injury after blunt trauma. *Am J Surg* 1992;164(5):482-486.

14. Koraitim MM. Pelvic fracture urethral injuries: the unresolved controversy. *J Urol* 1999;161(5):1433-1441.

15. Liu M, Lee C, Veng F. Prospective comparison of diagnostic peritoneal lavage, computed tomographic scanning, and ultrasonography for the diagnosis of blunt abdominal trauma. *J Trauma* 1993;35:267-270.

16. McCarthy MC, Lowdermilk GA, Canal DF, et al. Prediction of injury caused by penetrating wounds to the abdomen, flank, and back. *Arch Surg* 1991;26:962-966.

17. Mendez C, Gubler KD, Maier RV. Diagnostic accuracy of peritoneal lavage in patients with pelvic fractures. *Arch Surg* 1994;129(5):477-481.

18. Meyer DM, Thal ER, Weigelt JA, et al. The role of abdominal CT in the evaluation of stab wounds to the back. *J Trauma* 1989;29:1226-1230.

19. Miller KS, McAnnich JW. Radiographic assessment of renal trauma: our 15-year experience. *J Urol* 1995;154(2 Pt 1):352-355.

20. Nordenholz KE, Rubin MA, Gularte GG, et al. Ultrasound in the evaluation and management of blunt abdominal trauma. *Ann Emerg Med* 1997;29(3):357-366.

21. Phillips T, Sclafani SJA, Goldstein A, et al. Use of the contrast-enhanced CT enema in the management of penetrating trauma to the flank and back. *J Trauma* 1986;26:593-601.

22. Reid AB, Letts RM, Black GB. Pediatric Chance fractures: association with intraabdominal injuries and seat belt use. *J Trauma* 1990;30:384-391.

23. Robin AP, Andrews JR, Lange DA, et al. Selective management of anterior abdominal stab wounds. *J Trauma* 1989;29:1684-1689.

24. Routt ML Jr, Simonian PT, Swiontkowski MF. Stabilization of pelvic ring disruptions. *Orthop Clin North Am* 1997;28(3):369-388.

25. Rozycki GS, Ballard RB, Feliciano DV, et al. Surgeon-performed ultrasound for the assessment of truncal injuries: lessons learned from 1540 patients. *Ann Surg* 1998;228(4):557-565.

25. Rozycki GS. Abdominal ultrasonography in trauma. *Surg Clin North Am* 1995;75:175-191.

21. Shackford SR, Rogers FB, Osler TM, et al. Focused abdominal sonography for trauma: the learning curve of non-radiologist clinicians in detecting hemoperitoneum. *J Trauma* 1999;46(4):553-562.

22. Takishima T, Sugimota K, Hirata M, et al. Serum amylase level on admission in the diagnosis of blunt injury to the pancreas: its significance and limitations. *Ann Surg* 1997;226(1):70-76.

24. Udobi KF, Roderiques A, Chiu WC, Scalea TM. Role of ultra-sonography in penetrating abdominal trauma: a prospective clinical study. *J Trauma* 2001;50(3):475-479.

25. Zantut LF, Ivatury RR, Smith RS, et al. Diagnostic and therapeutic laparoscopy for penetrating abdominal trauma: a multicenter experience. *J Trauma* 1997;42(5):825-829.

Focused Assessment Sonography in Trauma (FAST)

▶▶ INTERACTIVE SKILL PROCEDURES

Note: Standard precautions are required whenever caring for trauma patients.

THE FOLLOWING PROCEDURES ARE INCLUDED IN THIS SKILL STATION:

▶▶ **Skill VIII:** Focused Assessment Sonography in Trauma (FAST)

Objectives

Performance at this station will allow participants to become familiar with the technique of focused assessment sonography in trauma (FAST). Accompanying this Skill Station is a series of scenarios for participants to review and use to prepare for this station.

1 List the indications and contraindications of FAST.

2 Describe the views necessary for a complete evaluation using FAST.

3 Identify normal and abnormal FAST images.

▶ SCENARIOS

Note: The following scenarios apply to this Skill Station and Skill Station IX: Diagnostic Peritoneal Lavage (DPL).

SCENARIO VIII-1

A 45-year-old restrained driver is involved in a head-on motor vehicle collision. She is complaining of severe abdominal pain, but does not have any trouble breathing. Her heart rate is 115, blood pressure 85/60, respiratory rate 24, and GCS 15. Intravenous access is obtained, and crystalloid fluid resuscitation is initiated. A chest x-ray shows lower left-sided rib fractures, and a pelvic x-ray is normal.

SCENARIO VIII-2

A 57-year-old construction worker falls from a second story. He complains of back pain and has no sensation or movement in his lower extremities. His heart rate is 100, blood pressure 100/60, respiratory rate 20, and GCS 15. Chest and pelvic x-rays are normal.

SCENARIO VIII-3

A 23-year-old motorcyclist is thrown from his cycle. He is unresponsive, with decreased breath sounds on the right, a heart rate of 130, and blood pressure 70/40. His trachea is midline and he does not have jugular venous distention. As he is being intubated, chest and pelvic radiographs are obtained, along with FAST images.

▶ Skill VIII: Focused Assessment Sonography in Trauma (FAST)

The FAST exam is a tool for the rapid assessment of a trauma patient. In order to develop proficiency with this assessment, more time than is available in the ATLS skill station is required. However, this skill station will provide you with a basic framework for identifying the correct way to perform the FAST exam, and to interpret FAST images in the context of several cases. FAST includes the following views:

- pericardial view
- right upper quadrant (RUQ) view to include diaphragm-liver interface and Morrison's pouch
- left upper quadrant (LUQ) view to include diaphragm-spleen interface and spleen-kidney interface
- suprapubic view

The only equipment necessary to perform a FAST exam is an ultrasound machine and water-based gel (■ FIGURE VIII-1). The FAST exam is performed with a low frequency (3.5 MHz) transducer, which allows the depth of penetration necessary to obtain appropriate images. Either the curved array transducer or the phased array cardiac transducer, with a smaller footprint that fits more easily between the ribs, may be used. Higher frequency transducers may be appropri-

ate for children or extremely thin adults. Even lower frequency transducers may be necessary for the morbidly obese.

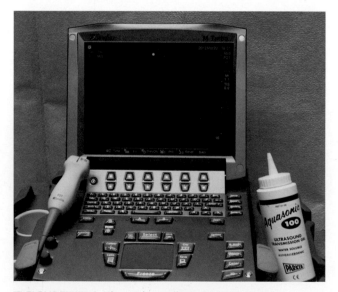

■ FIGURE VIII-1 The only equipment necessary to perform a FAST exam is an ultrasound machine and water-based gel.

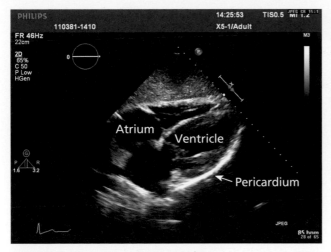

■ **FIGURE VIII-2** The pericardial view.

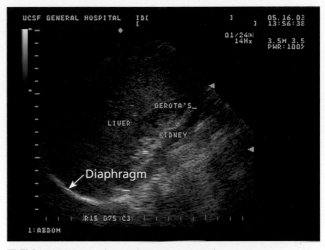

■ **FIGURE VIII-3** The right upper quadrant view.

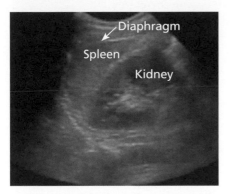

■ **FIGURE VIII-4** The left upper quadrant view.

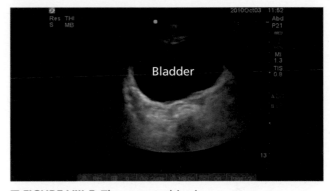

■ **FIGURE VIII-5** The suprapubic view.

STEP 1. Start with the heart to ensure that the gain is set appropriately—fluid within the heart should be black (■ **FIGURE VIII-2**). The heart can be imaged using the subxiphoid or the parasternal view.

STEP 2. The RUQ view is a sagittal view in the midaxillary line, at approximately the 10th or 11th rib space. Structures to visualize include the diaphragm, liver, and kidney (■ **FIGURE VIII-3**). The entire hepatorenal fossa (Morrison's pouch) should be visualized.

STEP 3. The LUQ view is a sagittal view in the midaxillary line, at approximately the 8th or 9th rib space. Structures to visualize include

the diaphragm, spleen, and kidney (■ **FIGURE VIII-4**). The entire splenorenal fossa should be visualized. Air artifacts from the stomach and colon, in addition to the smaller acoustic window, make this the most difficult view to obtain; it may be necessary to move the transducer posteriorly.

STEP 4. The suprapubic view is a transverse view optimally obtained prior to placement of a Foley catheter (■ **FIGURE VIII-5**). Artifacts may be introduced due to posterior enhancement; if areas of fluid disappear with side-to-side movement of the transducer, they are likely artifact.

PITFALLS

■ A negative FAST exam does not rule out intraabdominal injury. It does, however, make an abdominal source less likely as the cause of hemodynamically significant hemorrhage.

■ The pelvic view is best performed prior to insertion of a Foley catheter, as a distended bladder is helpful in seeing free pelvic fluid on FAST.

■ Sound waves do not travel well through air, making FAST more difficult in patients with subcutaneous emphysema.

■ Obesity may make it difficult to obtain interpretable images; adjusting gain and frequency (either on machine or by changing transducers) may improve image quality.

■ As with DPL, an absolute indication for laparotomy is a contraindication for FAST.

■ Pelvic fracture may decrease the accuracy of FAST.

Diagnostic Peritoneal Lavage (Optional)

THE FOLLOWING PROCEDURES ARE INCLUDED IN THIS SKILL STATION:

▸▸ **Skill IX-A:** Diagnostic Peritoneal Lavage—Open Technique

▸▸ **Skill IX-B:** Diagnostic Peritoneal Lavage—Closed Technique

Objectives

Performance at this station will allow participants to practice and demonstrate the technique of diagnostic peritoneal lavage (DPL) on a live, anesthetized animal; a fresh, human cadaver; or an anatomic human body manikin.

1 Identify the indications and contraindications of DPL.

2 Perform the closed procedure and the open procedure for DPL.

3 Describe the complications of DPL.

▶ Skill IX-A: Diagnostic Peritoneal Lavage—Open Technique

STEP 1. Obtain informed consent, if time permits.

STEP 2. Decompress the stomach and urinary bladder by inserting a gastric tube and urinary catheter.

STEP 3. After donning mask, sterile gown, and gloves, surgically prepare the abdomen (costal margin to the pubic area and flank to flank, anteriorly).

STEP 4. Inject local anesthetic midline just below the umbilicus, down to the level of the fascia.

STEP 5. Vertically incise the skin and subcutaneous tissues to the fascia.

STEP 6. Grasp the fascial edges with clamps, and elevate and incise the fascia down to the peritoneum. Make a small nick in the peritoneum, entering the peritoneal cavity.

STEP 7. Insert a peritoneal dialysis catheter into the peritoneal cavity.

STEP 8. Advance the catheter into the pelvis.

STEP 9. Connect the dialysis catheter to a syringe and aspirate.

STEP 10. If gross blood is aspirated, the patient should be taken to laparotomy. If gross blood is not obtained, instill 1 L of warmed isotonic crystalloid solution/normal saline (10 mL/kg in a child) into the peritoneum through the intravenous tubing attached to the dialysis catheter.

STEP 11. Gently agitate the abdomen to distribute the fluid throughout the peritoneal cavity and increase mixing with the blood.

STEP 12. If the patient's condition is stable, allow the fluid to remain a few minutes before placing the crystalloid container on the floor and allowing the peritoneal fluid to drain from the abdomen. Adequate fluid return is >20% of the infused volume.

STEP 13. After the fluid returns, send a sample to the laboratory for Gram stain and erythrocyte and leukocyte counts (unspun). A positive test and thus the need for surgical intervention is indicated by 100,000 red blood cells (RBCs)/mm3 or more, greater than 500 white blood cells (WBCs)/mm3, or a positive Gram stain for food fibers or bacteria. A negative lavage does not exclude retroperitoneal injuries, such as pancreatic and duodenal injuries.

▶▶ COMPLICATIONS OF PERITONEAL LAVAGE

- Hemorrhage, secondary to injection of local anesthetic or incision of the skin or subcutaneous tissues, which produces false positive results
- Peritonitis due to intestinal perforation from the catheter
- Laceration of urinary bladder (if bladder not evacuated prior to procedure)
- Injury to other abdominal and retroperitoneal structures requiring operative care
- Wound infection at the lavage site (late complication)

▶ Skill IX-B: Diagnostic Peritoneal Lavage—Closed Technique

STEP 1. Obtain informed consent, if time permits.

STEP 2. Decompress the stomach and urinary bladder by inserting a gastric tube and urinary catheter.

STEP 3. After donning mask, sterile gown, and gloves, surgically prepare the abdomen (costal margin to the pubic area and flank to flank, anteriorly).

STEP 4. Inject local anesthetic midline just below the umbilicus.

STEP 5. Insert an 18-gauge beveled needle attached to a syringe through the skin and subcutaneous tissue. Resistance is encountered when traversing the skin, fascia, and again when penetrating the peritoneum. Aspirate. If gross blood is not obtained, continue to step 6. If gross blood is aspirated, the patient should be taken to laparotomy.

STEP 6. Pass the flexible end of the guidewire through the 18-gauge needle until resistance is met or 3 cm is still showing outside the needle. Then remove the needle from the abdominal cavity so that only the guidewire remains.

STEP 7. Make a small skin incision at the entrance site of the guidewire and insert the peritoneal lavage catheter over the guidewire into the peritoneal cavity. Remove the guidewire from the abdominal cavity so that only the lavage catheter remains. Reattempt aspiration of the catheter to look for gross blood. If gross blood is aspirated, the patient should be taken to laparotomy.

STEP 8. Instill 1 L of warmed isotonic crystalloid solution (10 mL/kg in a child) into the peritoneum through the intravenous tubing attached to the lavage catheter.

STEP 9. Gently agitate the abdomen to distribute the fluid throughout the peritoneal cavity and increase mixing with the blood.

STEP 10. If the patient's condition is stable, allow the fluid to remain a few minutes before placing the crystalloid container on the floor and allowing the peritoneal fluid to drain from the abdomen. Adequate fluid return is >20% of the infused volume.

STEP 11. After the fluid has returned, send a sample to the laboratory for Gram stain and erythrocyte and leukocyte counts (unspun). A positive test and thus the need for surgical intervention is indicated by 100,000 RBCs/mm3 or more, greater than 500 WBCs/mm3, or a positive Gram stain for food fibers or bacteria. A negative lavage does not exclude retroperitoneal injuries, such as pancreatic and duodenal injuries.

▶▶ COMPLICATIONS OF PERITONEAL LAVAGE

- Hemorrhage, secondary to injection of local anesthetic or incision of the skin or subcutaneous tissues, which produces a false positive result
- Peritonitis due to intestinal perforation from the catheter
- Laceration of urinary bladder (if bladder not evacuated prior to procedure)
- Injury to other abdominal and retroperitoneal structures requiring operative care
- Wound infection at the lavage site (late complication)

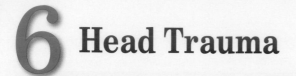

6 Head Trauma

The primary goal of treatment for patients with suspected traumatic brain injury (TBI) is to prevent secondary brain injury.

Scenario A 58-year-old male fell from a second-story roof in a small rural town. He is initially able to say his name, has a heart rate of 115, blood pressure of 100/60, and oxygen saturation of 88%. His initial Glasgow Coma Scale (GCS) score was 12; two hours after transfer to a trauma center, he has sonorous respirations, a heart rate of 120, blood pressure of 100/70, and his GCS score is 6.

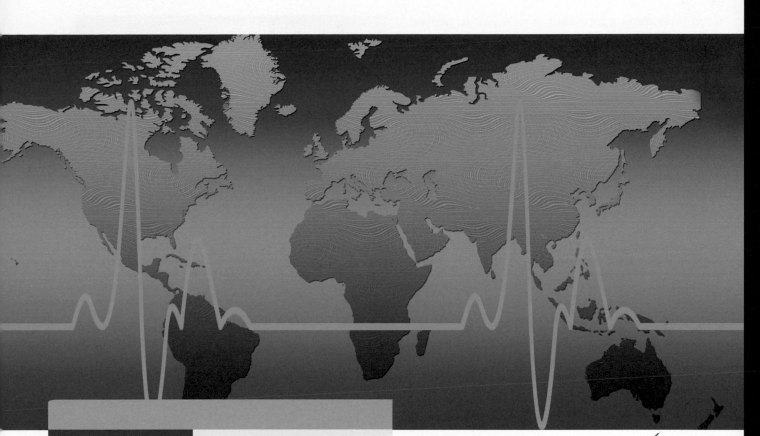

Objectives

1. Describe basic intracranial physiology.

2. Evaluate patients with head and brain injuries.

3. Perform a focused neurologic examination.

4. Explain the importance of adequate resuscitation in limiting secondary brain injury.

5. Given a patient scenario, determine the need for patient transfer, admission, consultation, or discharge.

Head injuries are among the most common types of trauma encountered in emergency departments (EDs). Many patients with severe brain injuries die before reaching a hospital, with almost 90% of prehospital trauma-related deaths involving brain injury. About 75% of patients with brain injuries who receive medical attention can be categorized as having minor injuries, 15% as moderate, and 10% as severe. Most recent United States data estimate 1,700,000 traumatic brain injuries (TBIs) annually, including 275,000 hospitalizations and 52,000 deaths.

Survivors of TBI are often left with neuropsychologic impairments that result in disabilities affecting work and social activity. Every year, an estimated 80,000 to 90,000 people in the United States experience long-term disability from brain injury. In one average European country (Denmark), approximately 300 individuals per million inhabitants suffer moderate to severe head injuries annually, with more than one-third of these individuals requiring brain injury rehabilitation. Given these statistics, it is clear that even a small reduction in the mortality and morbidity resulting from brain injury can have a major impact on public health.

The primary goal of treatment for patients with suspected TBI is to prevent secondary brain injury. Providing adequate oxygenation and maintaining blood pressure at a level that is sufficient to perfuse the brain are the most important ways to limit secondary brain damage and thereby improve the patient's outcome. Subsequent to managing the ABCDEs, identification of a mass lesion that requires surgical evacuation is critical, and this is best achieved by immediately obtaining a computed tomographic (CT) scan of the head. **However, obtaining a CT scan should not delay patient transfer to a trauma center that is capable of immediate and definitive neurosurgical intervention.**

The triage of a patient with brain injury depends on the severity of the injury and the facilities available within a particular community. For facilities without neurosurgical coverage, prearranged transfer agreements with higher-level facilities should be in place. Consultation with a neurosurgeon early in the course of treatment is strongly recommended (Box 6-1).

Anatomy Review

? *What are the unique features of brain anatomy and physiology, and how do they affect patterns of brain injury?*

A review of cranial anatomy includes the scalp, skull, meninges, brain, ventricular system, and intracranial compartments. (■ FIGURE 6-1).

SCALP

Because of the scalp's generous blood supply, scalp lacerations can result in major blood loss, hemorrhagic shock, and even death. This is particularly true in patients with a long transport time.

■ **FIGURE 6-1** Overview of cranial anatomy.

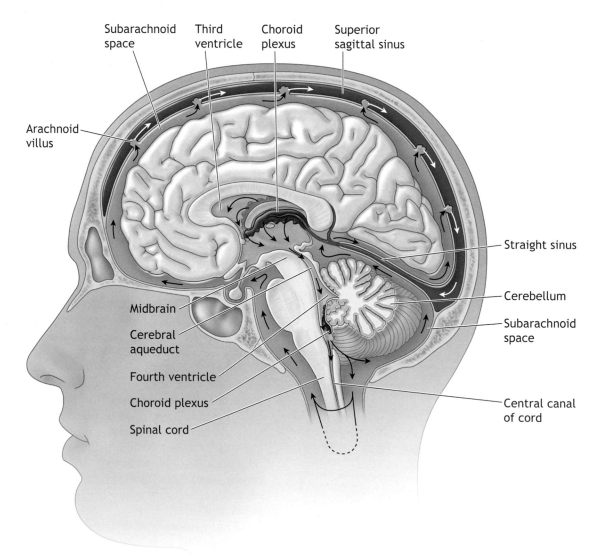

Box 6-1 Neurosurgical Consultation for Patients with TBI

In consulting a neurosurgeon about a patient with TBI, the following information is relayed:

- Age of patient
- Mechanism and time of injury
- Respiratory and cardiovascular status (particularly blood pressure and oxygen saturation)
- Results of the neurologic examination, including the GCS score (with particular emphasis on the motor response), pupil size and reaction to light

- Focal neurological deficits
- Presence and type of associated injuries
- Results of diagnostic studies, particularly CT scan (if available)
- Treatment of hypotension or hypoxia

SKULL

The base of the skull is irregular, which can contribute to injury as the brain moves within the skull during acceleration and deceleration. The anterior fossa houses the frontal lobes, the middle fossa the temporal lobes, and the posterior fossa the lower brainstem and the cerebellum.

MENINGES

The meninges cover the brain and consist of three layers: the dura mater, arachnoid mater, and pia mater (■ FIGURE 6-2). The dura mater is a tough, fibrous membrane that adheres firmly to the internal surface of the skull. At specific sites, the dura splits into two leaves that enclose the large venous sinuses, which provide

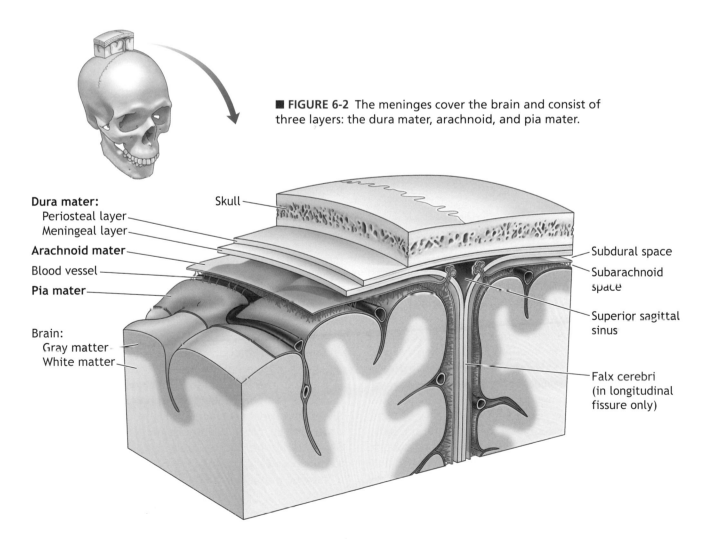

■ **FIGURE 6-2** The meninges cover the brain and consist of three layers: the dura mater, arachnoid, and pia mater.

Dura mater:
Periosteal layer
Meningeal layer
Arachnoid mater
Blood vessel
Pia mater

Skull

Brain:
Gray matter
White matter

Subdural space
Subarachnoid space
Superior sagittal sinus
Falx cerebri (in longitudinal fissure only)

the major venous drainage from the brain. The midline superior sagittal sinus drains into the bilateral transverse and sigmoid sinuses, which are usually larger on the right side. Laceration of these venous sinuses can result in massive hemorrhage.

Meningeal arteries lie between the dura and the internal surface of the skull (the epidural space). Overlying skull fractures can lacerate these arteries and cause an epidural hematoma. The most commonly injured meningeal vessel is the middle meningeal artery, which is located over the temporal fossa. An expanding hematoma from arterial injury in this location may lead to rapid deterioration and death. Epidural hematomas can also result from injury to the dural sinuses and from skull fractures, which tend to expand slowly and put less pressure on the underlying brain. However, most epidural hematomas represent a life-threatening emergency and must be evaluated by a neurosurgeon as soon as possible.

Beneath the dura is a second meningeal layer, the thin, transparent arachnoid mater. Because the dura is not attached to the underlying arachnoid membrane, a potential space between these layers exists (the subdural space), into which hemorrhage can occur. In brain injury, bridging veins that travel from the surface of the brain to the venous sinuses within the dura may tear, leading to the formation of a subdural hematoma.

The third layer, the pia mater, is firmly attached to the surface of the brain. Cerebrospinal fluid (CSF) fills the space between the watertight arachnoid mater and the pia mater (the subarachnoid space), cushioning the brain and spinal cord. Hemorrhage into this fluid-filled space (subarachnoid hemorrhage) is frequently seen in brain contusion or injury to major blood vessels at the base of the brain.

BRAIN

The brain consists of the cerebrum, brainstem, and cerebellum (see Figure 6.1). The cerebrum is composed of the right and left hemispheres, which are separated by the falx cerebri. The left hemisphere contains the language centers in virtually all right-handed people and in more than 85% of left-handed people. The frontal lobe controls executive function, emotions, motor function, and, on the dominant side, expression of speech (motor speech areas). The parietal lobe directs sensory function and spatial orientation. The temporal lobe regulates certain memory functions. The occipital lobe is responsible for vision.

The brainstem is composed of the midbrain, pons, and medulla. The midbrain and upper pons contain the reticular activating system, which is responsible for the state of alertness. Vital cardiorespiratory cen-

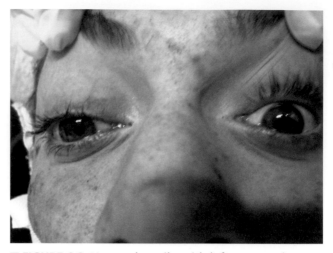

■ **FIGURE 6-3** Unequal pupils, with left greater than right.

ters reside in the medulla, which continues on to form the spinal cord. Even small lesions in the brainstem may be associated with severe neurologic deficits.

The cerebellum, responsible mainly for coordination and balance, projects posteriorly in the posterior fossa and forms connections with the spinal cord, brainstem, and, ultimately, the cerebral hemispheres.

VENTRICULAR SYSTEM

The ventricles are a system of CSF-filled spaces and aqueducts within the brain. CSF is constantly produced within the ventricles and is absorbed over the surface of the brain. The presence of blood in the CSF may impair CSF reabsorption, resulting in increased intracranial pressure. Edema and mass lesions (e.g., hematomas) can cause effacement or shifting of the usually symmetric ventricles that can be easily identified on CT scans of the brain.

INTRACRANIAL COMPARTMENTS

Tough meningeal partitions separate the brain into regions. The tentorium cerebelli divides the intracranial cavity into the supratentorial and infratentorial compartments. The midbrain passes through an opening called the tentorial hiatus or notch. The oculomotor nerve (cranial nerve III) runs along the edge of the tentorium and may become compressed against it during temporal lobe herniation. Parasympathetic fibers that constrict the pupil lie on the surface of the third cranial nerve. Compression of these superficial fibers during herniation causes pupillary dilation due to unopposed sympathetic activity, often referred to as a "blown" pupil (■ **FIGURE 6-3**).

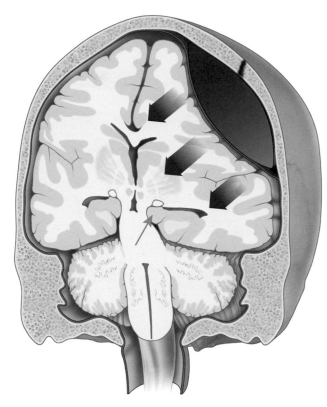

■ FIGURE 6-4 **The Lateral (Uncal) Herniation from a Temporal Epidural Hematoma Caused by a Lesion of the Middle Meningeal Artery from a Fracture in the Temporal Bone.** The uncus compresses the upper brain stem with the reticular system (decreasing GCS), the oculomotor nerve (pupillary changes), and the corticospinal tract in the midbrain (contralateral hemiparesis).

The part of the brain that usually herniates through the tentorial notch is the medial part of the temporal lobe, known as the uncus (■ FIGURE 6-4). Uncal herniation also causes compression of the corticospinal (pyramidal) tract in the midbrain. The motor tract crosses to the opposite side at the foramen magnum, so compression at the level of the midbrain results in weakness of the opposite side of the body (contralateral hemiparesis). **Ipsilateral pupillary dilation associated with contralateral hemiparesis is the classic sign of uncal herniation.** Rarely, the mass lesion may push the opposite side of the midbrain against the tentorial edge, resulting in hemiparesis and a dilated pupil on the same side as the hematoma.

> ## Physiology

Physiologic concepts that relate to head trauma include intracranial pressure, the Monro-Kellie doctrine, and cerebral blood flow (CBF).

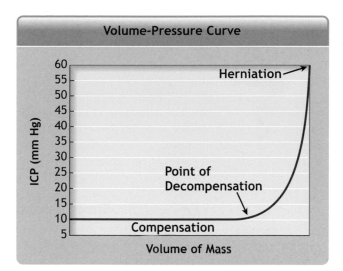

■ FIGURE 6-5 **Volume–Pressure Curve.** The intracranial contents are initially able to compensate for a new intracranial mass, such as a subdural or epidural hematoma. Once the volume of this mass reaches a critical threshold, a rapid increase in intracranial pressure often occurs, which can lead to reduction or cessation of cerebral blood flow.

INTRACRANIAL PRESSURE

Elevation of intracranial pressure (ICP) can reduce cerebral perfusion and cause or exacerbate ischemia. The normal ICP in the resting state is approximately 10 mmHg. Pressures greater than 20 mmHg, particularly if sustained and refractory to treatment, are associated with poor outcomes.

MONRO-KELLIE DOCTRINE

The Monro-Kellie Doctrine is a simple, yet vitally important concept related to the understanding of ICP dynamics. The doctrine states that the total volume of the intracranial contents must remain constant, because the cranium is a rigid, nonexpansile container. Venous blood and cerebrospinal fluid may be compressed out of the container, providing a degree of pressure buffering (■ FIGURE 6-5 and ■ FIGURE 6-6). Thus, very early after injury, a mass such as a blood clot may enlarge while the ICP remains normal. However, once the limit of displacement of CSF and intravascular blood has been reached, ICP rapidly increases.

CEREBRAL BLOOD FLOW

TBI severe enough to cause coma may cause a marked reduction in CBF during the first few hours after injury. It usually increases over the next 2 to 3 days, but for patients who remain comatose, CBF remains below nor-

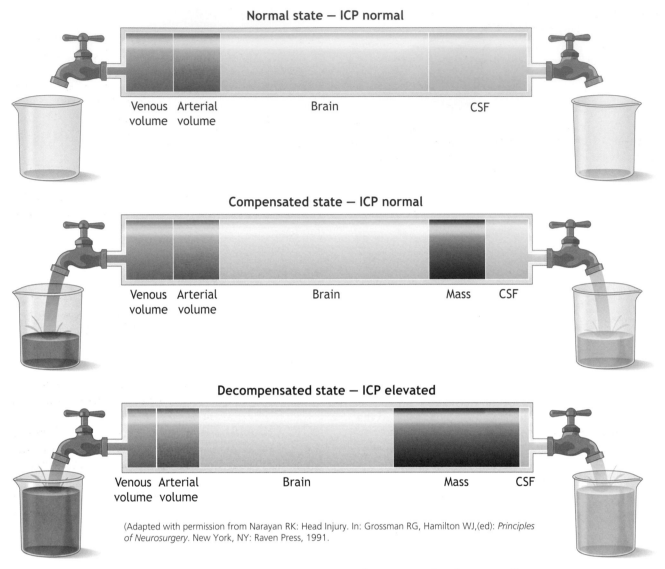

Normal state — ICP normal

Venous volume   Arterial volume   Brain   CSF

Compensated state — ICP normal

Venous volume   Arterial volume   Brain   Mass   CSF

Decompensated state — ICP elevated

Venous volume   Arterial volume   Brain   Mass   CSF

(Adapted with permission from Narayan RK: Head Injury. In: Grossman RG, Hamilton WJ,(ed): *Principles of Neurosurgery*. New York, NY: Raven Press, 1991.

■ **FIGURE 6-6 The Monro-Kellie Doctrine Regarding Intracranial Compensation for Expanding Mass.**
The volume of the intracranial contents remains constant. If the addition of a mass such as a hematoma results in the squeezing out of an equal volume of CSF and venous blood, the ICP remains normal. However, when this compensatory mechanism is exhausted, there is an exponential increase in ICP for even a small additional increase in the volume of the hematoma.

mal for days or weeks after injury. There is increasing evidence that low levels of CBF are inadequate to meet the metabolic demands of the brain early after injury. Regional, even global, cerebral ischemia is common after severe head injury for known and unknown reasons.

The precapillary cerebral vasculature normally has the ability to reflexively constrict or dilate in response to changes in mean arterial blood pressure (MAP). For clinical purposes, cerebral perfusion pressure (CPP) is defined as mean arterial blood pressure minus intracranial pressure (CPP = MAP – ICP). A MAP of 50 to 150 mm Hg is "autoregulated" to maintain a constant CBF (pressure autoregulation). Severe TBI may disrupt pressure autoregulation such that the brain is unable to adequately compensate for changes in CPP. In this setting, if the MAP is too low, ischemia and infarction will result. If the MAP is too high, marked brain swelling will occur with elevated ICP. Cerebral blood vessels also constrict or dilate due to changes in the partial pressure of oxygen (PaO_2) and the partial pressure of carbon dioxide ($PaCO_2$) levels in the blood (chemical regulation).

Therefore, secondary injury may occur due to hypotension, hypoxia, hypercapnia, and iatrogenic hypocapnia. **Every effort should be made to enhance cerebral perfusion and blood flow by reducing elevated ICP, maintaining normal intravascular volume, maintaining a normal mean arterial blood pressure (MAP), and restoring normal oxygenation and normocapnia. Hematomas and other lesions that increase intracranial volume should be evacuated early.** Maintaining a normal cerebral perfusion pressure may help to improve CBF, however, CPP does not equate with or assure adequate CBF. Once compensatory mechanisms are exhausted and there is an exponential increase in ICP, brain perfusion is compromised.

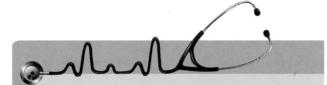

Scenario ■ *continued* The patient is intubated and given a second liter of normal saline. His heart rate improves to 100 bpm, and oxygen saturation improves to 94%. His blood pressure remains 100/70.

Classifications of Head Injuries

Head injuries are classified in several ways. For practical purposes, the severity of injury and morphology are used in this chapter (Table 6.1).

SEVERITY OF INJURY

The GCS score is used as an objective clinical measure of the severity of brain injury (Table 6.2). **A GCS score of 8 or less has become the generally accepted definition of coma or severe brain injury.** Patients with a brain injury who have a GCS score of 9 to 12 are categorized as "moderate," whereas individuals with a GCS score of 13 to 15 are designated as "minor." **In assessing the GCS score, when there is right/left or upper/lower asymmetry, it is important to use the best motor response to calculate the score, because this is the most reliable predictor of outcome.** However, one must record the actual response on both sides of the body, face, arm, and leg.

MORPHOLOGY

Head trauma may include skull fractures and intracranial lesions, such as contusions, hematomas, diffuse injuries, and resultant swelling (edema/hyperemia).

Skull Fractures

Skull fractures may occur in the cranial vault or skull base. They may be linear or stellate, and open or closed. Basilar skull fractures usually require CT scanning with bone-window settings for identification. The clinical signs of a basilar skull fracture include periorbital ecchymosis (raccoon eyes), retroauricular ecchymosis (Battle's sign), CSF leakage from the nose (rhinorrhea) or ear (otorrhea), and seventh- and eighth-nerve dysfunction (facial paralysis and hearing

■ TABLE 6.1 Classifications of Brain Injury				
Severity	• Minor • Moderate • Severe		• GCS Score 13–15 • GCS Score 9–12 • GCS Score 3–8
Morphology	• Skull fractures	• Vault	• Linear vs stellate • Depressed/nondepressed • Open/closed
		• Basilar	• With/without CSF leak • With/without seventh nerve palsy
	• Intracranial lesions	• Focal	• Epidural • Subdural • Intracerebral
		• Diffuse	• Concussion • Multiple contusions • Hypoxic/ischemic injury • Axonal injury

Adapted with permission from Valadka AB, Narayan RK. Emergency room management of the head-injured patient. In Narayan RK, Wilberger JE, Povlishock JT, eds. *Neurotrauma.* New York, NY: McGraw-Hill, 1996: 120.

■ TABLE 6.2 Glasgow Coma Scale (GCS)

ASSESSMENT AREA	SCORE
Eye opening (E)	
Spontaneous	4
To speech	3
To pain	2
None	1
Verbal response (V)	
Oriented	5
Confused conversation	4
Inappropriate words	3
Incomprehensible sounds	2
None	1
Best motor response (M)	
Obeys commands	6
Localizes pain	5
Flexion withdrawal to pain	4
Abnormal flexion (decorticate)	3
Extension (decerebrate)	2
None (flaccid)	1

GCS Score = (E[4] + V[5] + M[6]) = Best possible score 15; Worst possible score 3.

loss), which may occur immediately or a few days after the initial injury. The presence of these signs should increase the index of suspicion and help identify basilar skull fractures. Those fractures that traverse the carotid canals may damage the carotid arteries (dissection, pseudoaneurysm, or thrombosis), and consideration should be given to cerebral arteriography (CT angiography [CT-A] or catheter-based).

Open or compound skull fractures can provide a direct communication between the scalp laceration and the cerebral surface, because the dura may be torn. **The significance of a skull fracture should not be underestimated, since it takes considerable force to fracture the skull.** A linear vault fracture in conscious patients increases the likelihood of an intracranial hematoma by about 400 times.

Intracranial Lesions

Intracranial lesions may be classified as diffuse or focal, although these two forms frequently coexist.

Diffuse Brain Injuries Diffuse brain injuries range from mild concussions, in which the CT scan of the head is normal, to severe hypoxic ischemic injuries. With a concussion, the patient has a transient, nonfocal neurologic disturbance that often includes loss of consciousness. Severe diffuse injuries often result from a hypoxic, ischemic insult to the brain due to prolonged shock or apnea occurring immediately after the trauma. In such cases, the CT scan may initially appear normal, or the brain may appear diffusely swollen, with loss of the normal gray-white distinction. Another diffuse pattern, often seen in high-velocity impact or deceleration injuries, may produce multiple punctate hemorrhages throughout the cerebral hemispheres, which are often seen in the border between the gray matter and white matter. These "shearing injuries," referred to as diffuse axonal injury (DAI), have defined a clinical syndrome of severe brain injury with variable but often poor outcome.

Focal Brain Injuries Focal lesions include epidural hematomas, subdural hematomas, contusions, and intracerebral hematomas (■ FIGURE 6-7).

Epidural Hematomas Epidural hematomas are relatively uncommon, occurring in about 0.5% of patients with brain injuries and in 9% of patients with TBI who are comatose. These hematomas typically become biconvex or lenticular in shape as they push the adherent dura away from the inner table of the skull. They are most often located in the temporal or temporoparietal region and often result from a tear of the middle meningeal artery as the result of a fracture. These clots are classically arterial in origin; however, they also may result from disruption of a major venous sinus or bleeding from a skull fracture. A lucid interval between time of injury and neurologic deterioration is the classic presentation of an epidural hematoma.

Subdural Hematomas Subdural hematomas are more common than epidural hematomas, occurring in approximately 30% of patients with severe brain injuries. They often develop from the shearing of small surface or bridging blood vessels of the cerebral cortex. In contrast to the lenticular shape of an epidural hematoma on a CT scan, subdural hematomas more often appear to conform to the contours of the brain. Brain damage underlying an acute subdural hematoma is typically much more severe than that associated with epidural hematomas due to the presence of concomitant parenchymal injury.

Contusions and Intracerebral Hematomas Cerebral contusions are fairly common (present in approximately 20% to 30% of severe brain injuries). The majority of contusions occur in the frontal and temporal lobes, although they may occur in any part of the brain. Contusions may, in a period of hours or days, evolve to form an intracerebral hematoma or a coalescent contusion with enough mass effect to require immediate surgical evacuation. This occurs in as many as 20% of patients presenting with contusions on initial CT scan of the head. **For this reason, patients with contusions generally undergo repeat CT scanning to evaluate for changes in the pattern of injury within 24 hours of the initial scan.**

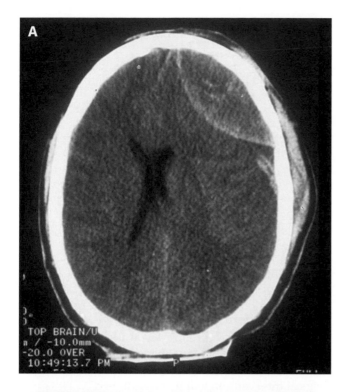

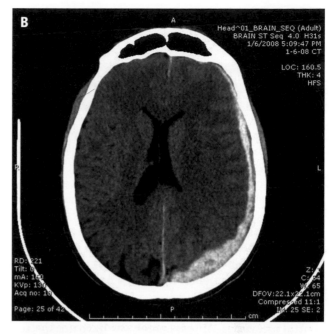

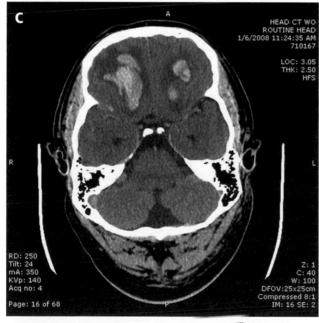

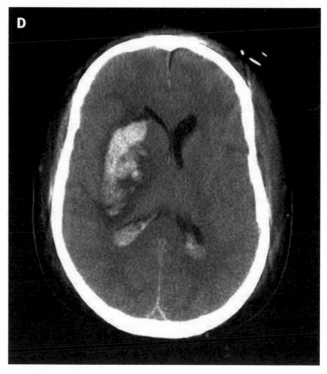

■ **FIGURE 6-7 CT Scans of Intracranial Hematomas.**
(A) Epidural hematoma. **(B)** Subdural hematoma.
(C) Bilateral contusions with hemorrhage. **(D)** Right
intraparenchymal hemorrhage with right to left midline
shift. Associated biventricular hemorrhages.

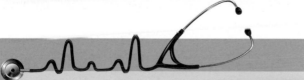

Scenario ■ *continued*   After improvement
in vital signs, the patient undergoes a head and
abdominal CT. The head CT shows a subdural
hematoma with 1 cm of midline shift and two
areas of contusion in the frontal lobes.

? *What is the optimal treatment for patients with brain injuries?*

Management of Minor Brain Injury (GCS Score 13–15)

Minor traumatic brain injury (MTBI) is defined by a history of disorientation, amnesia, or transient loss of consciousness in a patient who is conscious and talking. This correlates with a GCS score between 13 and 15. The history of a brief loss of consciousness can be difficult to confirm, and the picture often is confounded by alcohol or other intoxicants. **However, alterations in mental status must never be ascribed to confounding factors until brain injury can be definitively excluded.** The management of patients with minor brain injury is described in ■ FIGURE 6-8.

Most patients with minor brain injury make uneventful recoveries. Approximately 3% have unexpected deterioration, potentially resulting in severe neurologic dysfunction unless the decline in mental status is detected early.

The secondary survey is particularly important in evaluating patients with MTBI. Note the mechanism of injury, with particular attention to any loss of consciousness, including the length of time the patient was unresponsive, any seizure activity, and the subsequent level of alertness. Determine the duration of amnesia both before (retrograde) and after (antegrade) the traumatic incident. Serial examination and documentation of the GCS score is important in all patients with a GCS score <15. CT scanning is the preferred method of imaging. **A CT scan should be obtained in all patients with suspected brain injury who have a clinically suspected open skull fracture, any sign of basilar skull fracture, more than two episodes of vomiting, or in patients who are older than 65 years (Table 6.3).** CT should also be considered if the patient has had a loss of consciousness for longer than 5 minutes, retrograde amnesia for longer than 30 minutes, a danger-

PITFALL

Patients with minor traumatic brain injuries may appear neurologically normal but continue to be symptomatic for some time. Be sure that these patients avoid any unnecessary risk of a "second impact" during the symptomatic period that could result in devastating brain edema. Emphasize the need for competent follow-up and clearance before resuming normal activities, especially contact sports.

ous mechanism of injury, severe headaches, or a focal neurologic deficit attributable to the brain.

Applying these parameters to patients with a GCS score of 13, approximately 25% will have a CT finding indicative of trauma, and 1.3% will require neurosurgical intervention. Applying this to patients with a GCS score of 15, 10% will have CT findings indicative of trauma, and 0.5% will require neurosurgical intervention. Based on current best evidence, no patient with clinically significant brain injury or requiring neurosurgical intervention will be missed. **Obtaining CT scans should not delay transfer of the patient.**

If abnormalities are observed on the CT scan, or if the patient remains symptomatic or continues to have neurologic abnormalities, he or she should be admitted to the hospital, and a neurosurgeon should be consulted.

If patients are asymptomatic, are fully awake and alert, and have no neurologic abnormalities, they may be observed for several hours, reexamined, and, if still normal, safely discharged. Ideally, the patient is discharged to the care of a companion who can observe the patient continually over the subsequent 24 hours. An instruction sheet directs both the patient and the companion to continue close observation and to return to the ED if the patient develops headaches or experiences a decline in mental status or focal neurologic deficits. In all cases, written discharge instructions should be supplied to and carefully reviewed with the

TABLE 6.3 Indications for CT Scanning MTBI

Head CT is required for patients with minor head injuries (i.e., witnessed loss of consciousness, definite amnesia, or witnessed disorientation in a patient with a GCS score of 13–15) and any one of the following factors:

High risk for neurosurgical intervention	Moderate risk for brain injury on CT
• GCS score less than 15 at 2 hours after injury • Suspected open or depressed skull fracture • Any sign of basilar skull fracture (e.g., hemotympanum, raccoon eyes, CSF otorrhea or rhinorrhea, Battle's sign) • Vomiting (more than two episodes) • Age more than 65 years	• Loss of consciousness (more than 5 minutes) • Amnesia before impact (more than 30 minutes) • Dangerous mechanism (e.g., pedestrian struck by motor vehicle, occupant ejected from motor vehicle, fall from height more than 3 feet or five stairs)

Adapted from Stiell IG, Wells GA, Vandemheen K, et al. The Canadian CT Head Rule for patients with minor head injury. *Lancet* 2001;357;1294.

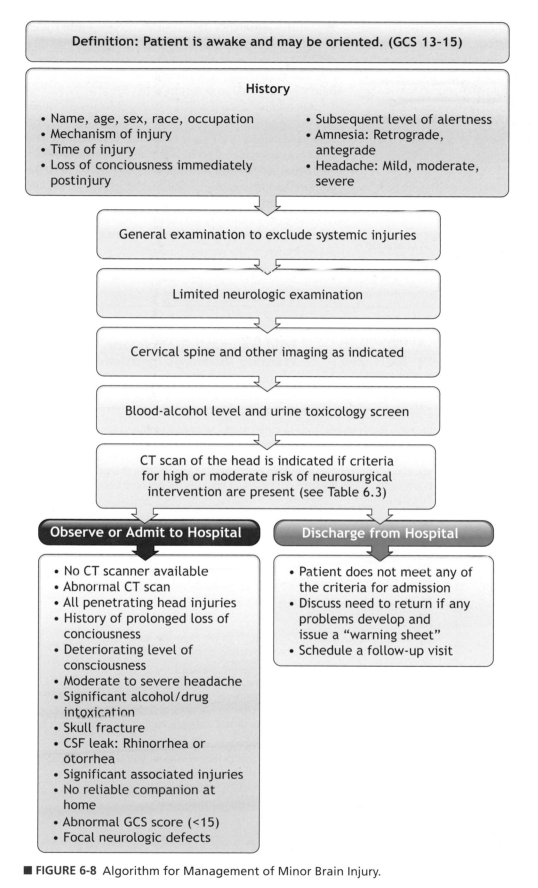

Definition: Patient is awake and may be oriented. (GCS 13-15)

History

- Name, age, sex, race, occupation
- Mechanism of injury
- Time of injury
- Loss of conciousness immediately postinjury

- Subsequent level of alertness
- Amnesia: Retrograde, antegrade
- Headache: Mild, moderate, severe

General examination to exclude systemic injuries

Limited neurologic examination

Cervical spine and other imaging as indicated

Blood-alcohol level and urine toxicology screen

CT scan of the head is indicated if criteria for high or moderate risk of neurosurgical intervention are present (see Table 6.3)

Observe or Admit to Hospital

- No CT scanner available
- Abnormal CT scan
- All penetrating head injuries
- History of prolonged loss of conciousness
- Deteriorating level of consciousness
- Moderate to severe headache
- Significant alcohol/drug intoxication
- Skull fracture
- CSF leak: Rhinorrhea or otorrhea
- Significant associated injuries
- No reliable companion at home
- Abnormal GCS score (<15)
- Focal neurologic defects

Discharge from Hospital

- Patient does not meet any of the criteria for admission
- Discuss need to return if any problems develop and issue a "warning sheet"
- Schedule a follow-up visit

■ **FIGURE 6-8** Algorithm for Management of Minor Brain Injury.

(Adapted with permission from Valadka AB, Narayan RK: Emergency room management of the head-injured patient. In: Narayan RK, Wilberger JE, Povlishock JT, (eds.): *Neurotrauma*. New York, NY: McGraw-Hill, 1996.)

patient and/or companion (■ FIGURE 6-9). If the patient is not alert or oriented enough to clearly understand the written and verbal instructions, the decision for discharge should be reconsidered.

Management of Moderate Brain Injury (GCS Score 9–12)

Approximately 15% of patients with brain injury who are seen in the ED have a moderate injury. They still are able to follow simple commands, but usually are confused or somnolent and can have focal neurologic deficits such as hemiparesis. Approximately 10% to 20% of these patients deteriorate and lapse into coma. For this reason, serial neurologic examinations are critical in the treatment of these patients.

The management of patients with moderate brain injury is described in ■ FIGURE 6-10.

On admission to the ED, a brief history is obtained, and cardiopulmonary stability is ensured before neurologic assessment. A CT scan of the head is obtained, and a neurosurgeon is contacted. All of these patients require admission for observation in an intensive care unit (ICU) or a similar unit capable of close nursing observation and frequent neurologic reassessment for at least the first 12 to 24 hours. A follow-up CT scan within 24 hours is recommended if the initial CT scan is abnormal or if there is deterioration of the patient's neurologic status.

■ FIGURE 6-9 Example of Head Injury Warning Discharge Instructions.

County General Hospital

Mild Traumatic Brain Injury Warning Discharge Instructions

Patient Name: _____

Date: _____

We have found no evidence to indicate that your head injury was serious. However, new symptoms and unexpected complications can develop hours or even days after the injury. The first 24 hours are the most crucial and you should remain with a reliable companion at least during this period. If any of the following signs develop, call your doctor or come back to the hospital.

1 *Drowsiness or increasing difficulty in awakening patient*
2 *Nausea or vomiting*
3 *Convulsions or fits*
4 *Bleeding or watery drainage from the nose or ear*
5 *Severe headaches*
6 *Weakness or loss of feeling in the arm or leg*
7 *Confusion or strange behavior*
8 *One pupil (black part of eye) much larger than the other; peculiar movements of the eyes, double vision, or other visual disturbances*
9 *A very slow or very rapid pulse, or an unusual breathing pattern*

If there is swelling at the site of the injury, apply an ice pack, making sure that there is a cloth or towel between the ice pack and the skin. If swelling increases markedly in spite of the ice pack application, call us or come back to the hospital.

You may eat or drink as usual if you so desire. However, you should NOT drink alcoholic beverages for at least 3 days after your injury.

Do not take any sedatives or any pain relievers stronger than acetaminophen, at least for the first 24 hours. Do not use aspirin-containing medicines.

If you have any further questions, or in case of emergency, we can be reached at: <telephone number>

Physician's Signature _____

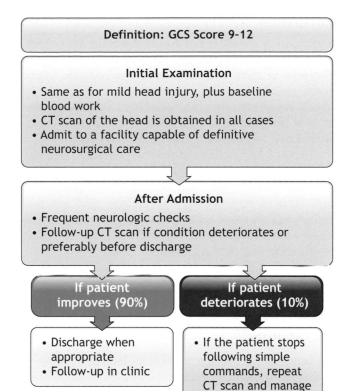

Definition: GCS Score 9-12

Initial Examination
- Same as for mild head injury, plus baseline blood work
- CT scan of the head is obtained in all cases
- Admit to a facility capable of definitive neurosurgical care

After Admission
- Frequent neurologic checks
- Follow-up CT scan if condition deteriorates or preferably before discharge

If patient improves (90%)
- Discharge when appropriate
- Follow-up in clinic

If patient deteriorates (10%)
- If the patient stops following simple commands, repeat CT scan and manage per severe brain injury protocol

■ **FIGURE 6-10 Algorithm for Management of Moderate Brain Injury.**

(Adapted with permission from Valadka AB, Narayan RK: Emergency room management of the head-injured patient. In: Narayan RK, Wilberger JE, Povlishock JT, (eds). *Neurotrauma.* New York, NY: McGraw-Hill, 1996.)

PITFALL

Patients with moderate brain injury can have rapid deterioration with hypoventilation or a subtle loss of their ability to protect their airway from declining mental status. Narcotic analgesics must be used with caution. Avoid hypercapnia with close monitoring of respiratory status and the ability of patients to manage their airway. Urgent intubation may become a necessity under these circumstances.

Management of Severe Brain Injury (GCS Score 3–8)

Approximately 10% of patients with brain injury who are treated in the ED have a severe brain injury. Patients who have sustained a severe brain injury are unable to follow simple commands, even after cardiopulmonary stabilization. Although this definition includes a wide spectrum of brain injury, it identifies the patients who are at greatest risk of suffering significant morbidity and mortality. A "wait and see" approach in such patients can be disastrous, and prompt diagnosis and treatment are extremely important. **Do not delay patient transfer to obtain a CT scan.**

The initial management of severe brain injury is outlined in ■ **FIGURE 6-11.**

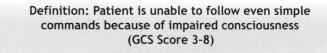

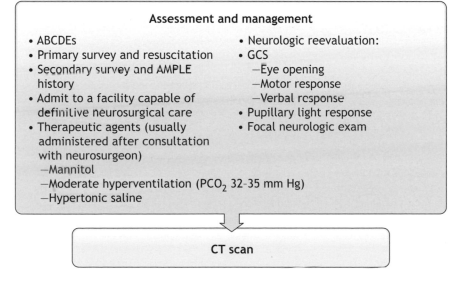

Definition: Patient is unable to follow even simple commands because of impaired consciousness (GCS Score 3-8)

Assessment and management
- ABCDEs
- Primary survey and resuscitation
- Secondary survey and AMPLE history
- Admit to a facility capable of definitive neurosurgical care
- Therapeutic agents (usually administered after consultation with neurosurgeon)
  - Mannitol
  - Moderate hyperventilation (PCO_2 32-35 mm Hg)
  - Hypertonic saline

- Neurologic reevaluation:
- GCS
  - Eye opening
  - Motor response
  - Verbal response
- Pupillary light response
- Focal neurologic exam

CT scan

■ **FIGURE 6-11 Algorithm for Initial Management of Severe Brain Injury.**

(Adapted with permission from Valadka AB, Narayan RK: Emergency room management of the head-injured patient. In: Narayan RK, Wilberger JE, Povlishock JT, (eds). *Neurotrauma.* New York, NY: McGraw-Hill, 1996.)

PRIMARY SURVEY AND RESUSCITATION

Brain injury often is adversely affected by secondary insults. The mortality rate for patients with severe brain injury who have hypotension on admission is more than double that of patients who do not have hypotension. The presence of hypoxia in addition to hypotension is associated with an increase in the relative risk of mortality of 75%. **Therefore, it is imperative that cardiopulmonary stabilization be achieved rapidly in patients with severe brain injury. See Box 6-2 for the priorities of the initial evaluation and triage of patients with severe brain injuries.** See Skill Station X: Head and Neck Trauma: Assessment and Management, Skill X-A: Primary Survey, and Skill X-D: Helmet Removal.

Airway and Breathing

Transient respiratory arrest and hypoxia are common with severe brain injury and may cause secondary brain injury. **Early endotracheal intubation should be performed in comatose patients.**

The patient should be ventilated with 100% oxygen until blood gas measurements are obtained, after which appropriate adjustments to the fraction of inspired oxygen (FIO_2) are made. Pulse oximetry is a useful adjunct, and oxygen saturations of >98% are desirable. Ventilation parameters are set to maintain a PCO_2 of approximately 35 mm Hg. Hyperventilation (PCO_2 <32 mm Hg) should be used cautiously in patients with severe brain injury and only when acute neurologic deterioration has occurred.

Circulation

Hypotension usually is not due to the brain injury itself, except in the terminal stages when medullary failure supervenes or there is a concomitant spinal cord injury. Intracranial hemorrhage cannot cause hemorrhagic shock. Euvolemia should be established as soon as possible if the patient is hypotensive, using blood products, whole blood, or isotonic fluids, as needed.

It must be emphasized that the neurologic examination of patients with hypotension is unreliable. Patients with hypotension who are unresponsive to any form of stimulation may recover and substantially improve soon after normal blood pressure is restored. The primary source of the hypotension must be urgently sought and treated.

Neurologic Examination

? *What is a focused neurological examination?*

As soon as the patient's cardiopulmonary status is managed, a rapid and directed (focused) neurologic examination is performed. It consists primarily of determining the GCS score, pupillary light response, and focal neurological deficit.

It is important to recognize confounding issues in the evaluation of TBI, including the presence of drugs, alcohol, intoxicants, and other injuries. Do not overlook a severe brain injury because the patient is also intoxicated.

Box 6-2 Priorities for the Initial Evaluation and Triage of Patients with Severe Brain Injuries

1. All comatose patients with brain injuries should undergo resuscitation (ABCDEs) on arrival in the ED.

2. As soon as the blood pressure (BP) is normalized, a neurologic exam is performed (GCS score and pupillary reaction). If the BP cannot be normalized, the neurologic examination is still performed, and the hypotension recorded.

3. If the patient's systolic BP cannot be brought up to >100 mm Hg, the priority is to establish the cause of the hypotension, with the neurosurgical evaluation taking second priority. In such cases, the patient undergoes a diagnostic peritoneal lavage (DPL) or ultrasound in the ED and may need to go directly to the operating room (OR) for a laparotomy. CT scans of the head are obtained after the laparotomy. If there is clinical evidence of an intracranial mass, diagnostic burr holes or craniotomy may be undertaken in the OR while the celiotomy is being performed.

4. If the patient's systolic BP is >100 mm Hg after resuscitation and the patient has clinical evidence of a possible intracranial mass (unequal pupils, asymmetric results on motor exam), the first priority is to obtain a CT head scan. A DPL or FAST exam may be performed in the ED, CT area, or OR, but the patient's neurologic evaluation or treatment should not be delayed.

5. In borderline cases—i.e., when the systolic BP can be temporarily corrected but tends to slowly decrease—every effort should be made to get a head CT prior to taking the patient to the OR for a laparotomy or thoracotomy. Such cases call for sound clinical judgment and cooperation between the trauma surgeon and neurosurgeon.

The postictal state after a traumatic seizure will typically worsen the patient's responsiveness for minutes or hours. In a comatose patient, motor responses may be elicited by pinching the trapezius muscle or with nail-bed or supraorbital ridge pressure. **If a patient demonstrates variable responses to stimulation, the best motor response elicited is a more accurate prognostic indicator than the worst response.** Testing for doll's eye movements (oculocephalic), the caloric test with ice water (oculovestibular), and testing of corneal responses are deferred to a neurosurgeon. **Doll's eye testing should never be attempted until a cervical spine injury has been ruled out.**

It is important to obtain the GCS score and to perform a pupillary examination prior to sedating or paralyzing the patient, because knowledge of the patient's clinical condition is important for determining subsequent treatment. Long-acting paralytic and sedating agents should not be used during the primary survey. Sedation should be avoided except when a patient's agitated state could place him or her at risk. The shortest-acting agents available are recommended when pharmacologic paralysis or brief sedation is necessary for safe endotracheal intubation or obtaining good quality diagnostic studies.

SECONDARY SURVEY

Serial examinations (e.g., GCS score, lateralization, and pupillary reaction) should be performed to detect neurologic deterioration as early as possible. A well-known early sign of temporal lobe (uncal) herniation is dilation of the pupil and loss of the pupillary response to light. Direct trauma to the eye also is a potential cause of abnormal pupillary response and may make pupil evaluation difficult. However, in the setting of brain trauma, brain injury should be considered first. See Skill Station X: Head and Neck Trauma: Assessment and Management, Skill X-B: Secondary Survey and Management.

DIAGNOSTIC PROCEDURES

A head CT scan must be obtained as soon as possible after hemodynamic normalization. CT scanning also should be repeated whenever there is a change in the patient's clinical status and routinely within 24 hours after injury for patients with a contusion or hematoma on the initial scan. See Skill Station X: Head and Neck Trauma: Assessment and Management, Skill X-C: Evaluation of CT Scans of the Head.

Findings of significance on the CT images include scalp swelling and subgaleal hematomas at the region of impact. Skull fractures may be seen better with bone windows, but are often apparent even on the soft-tissue windows. The crucial findings on the CT scan are intracranial hematoma, contusions, shift of the midline (mass effect) and obliteration of the basal cisterns (see Figure 6-7). **A shift of 5 mm or greater is often indicative of the need for surgery to evacuate the blood clot or contusion causing the shift.** See Chapter 7: Spine and Spinal Cord Trauma for relevance to spine, and the discussion of basilar skull fracture, above, for relevance to cranial injury.

Caution should be applied in assessing patients with TBI who are anticoagulated or on antiplatelet therapy. The international normalized ratio (INR) should be obtained and a CT should be performed expeditiously in these patients when indicated. Rapid normalization of anticoagulation is the general rule.

Table 6.4 provides an overview of the management of TBI.

PITFALL

Even patients with apparently devastating TBI on presentation may have significant neurologic recovery. Vigorous management and improved understanding of the pathophysiology of severe head injury, especially the role of hypotension, hypoxia, and cerebral perfusion, have made a significant impact on patient outcomes.

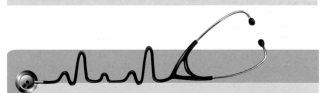

Scenario ▪ *continued* The patient's abdominal CT scan did not show any injury. Due to his intracranial lesion and deterioration in GCS score, he is taken to the operating room for urgent decompression of his subdural hematoma.

Medical Therapies for Brain Injury

The primary aim of intensive care protocols is to prevent secondary damage to an already injured brain. **The basic principle is that if injured neural tissue is provided an optimal milieu in which to recover, it may recover and regain normal function.** Medical therapies for brain injury include intravenous fluids, temporary hyperventilation, mannitol, hypertonic saline, barbiturates, and anticonvulsants.

INTRAVENOUS FLUIDS

Intravenous fluids, blood, and blood products should be administered as required to resuscitate the patient

■ TABLE 6.4 Management Overview of Traumatic Brain Injury

ALL PATIENTS: PERFORM ABCDEs WITH SPECIAL ATTENTION TO HYPOXIA AND HYPOTENSION

GCS CLASSIFICATION	13–15 MILD TRAUMATIC BRAIN INJURY		9–12 MODERATE TRAUMATIC BRAIN INJURY	3–8 SEVERE TRAUMATIC BRAIN INJURY
	May discharge if admission criteria not met	Admit for indications below:	Neurosurgery evaluation required	Urgent neurosurgery consultation required
Initial Management	*AMPLE history and neurological exam:		*Primary survey and resuscitation	*Primary survey and resuscitation
	Determine mechanism, time of injury, initial GCS, confusion, amnestic interval, seizure, headache severity, etc. *Secondary survey including focused neurological exam	No CT available, CT abnormal, skull fracture, CSF leak Focal neurologic deficit GCS does not return to 15 within 2 hours	*Arrange for transfer to definitive neurosurgical evaluation and management *Focused neurological exam *Secondary survey and AMPLE history	*Intubation and ventilation for airway protection *Treat hypotension, hypovolemia and hypoxia *Focused neurological exam *Secondary survey and AMPLE history
Diagnostic	*CT scanning as determined by head CT rules (Table 6.3) *Blood/Urine EtOH and toxicology screens	CT not available, CT abnormal, skull fracture Significant intoxication (admit or observe)	*CT scan in all cases *Evaluate carefully for other injuries *Type and cross, coagulation studies	*CT scan in all cases *Evaluate carefully for other injuries *Type and cross, coagulation studies
Secondary Management	*Serial examinations until GCS is 15 and patient has no perseveration or memory deficit *Rule out indication for CT (Table 6.3)	*Perform serial examinations *Perform follow-up CT scan if first is abnormal or GCS remains less than 15 *Repeat CT if neurological exam deteriorates	*Serial exams *Consider follow-up CT in 12–18 h	*Frequent serial neurological examinations with GCS *PCO$_2$ 35+/-3 *Mannitol, PCO$_2$ 28-32 for deterioration *Avoid PCO$_2$ <28 *Address intracranial lesions appropriately
Disposition	*Home if patient does not meet criteria for admission *Discharge with head injury warning sheet and follow-up arranged	Obtain neurosurgical evaluation if CT or neurological exam is abnormal or patient deteriorates *Arrange for medical follow-up and neuropsychological evaluation as required (may be done as outpatient)	*Repeat CT immediately for deterioration and manage as in severe brain injury (10%) *Discharge with medical and neuropsychological follow-up arranged when stable GCS (90%)	*Transfer as soon as possible to definitive neurosurgical care

*Asterisk denotes action required.

and maintain normovolemia. **Hypovolemia in these patients is harmful.** Care should also be taken not to overload the patient with fluids. Hypotonic fluids should not be used. Furthermore, the use of glucose-containing fluids may result in hyperglycemia, which has been shown to be harmful to the injured brain. Therefore, it is recommended Ringer's lactate solution or normal saline be used for resuscitation. Serum sodium levels need to be very carefully monitored in patients with head injuries. Hyponatremia is associated with brain edema and should be prevented.

HYPERVENTILATION

In most patients, normocarbia is preferred. Hyperventilation acts by reducing PaCO$_2$ and causing cerebral vasoconstriction. Aggressive and prolonged hyperventilation may promote cerebral ischemia in the already injured brain by causing severe cerebral vasoconstriction and thus impaired cerebral perfusion. This is particularly true if the $PaCO_2$ is allowed to fall below 30 mm Hg (4.0 kPa). However, hypercarbia (PCO_2 > 45 mm Hg) will promote vasodilation and increase intracranial pressure, and thus it should be avoided.

Hyperventilation should be used only in moderation and for as limited a period as possible. In general, it is preferable to keep the $PaCO_2$ at approximately 35 mm Hg (4.7 kPa), the low end of the normal range (35 mm Hg to 45 mm Hg). Brief periods of hyperventilation ($PaCO_2$ of 25 to 30 mm Hg [3.3 to 4.7 kPa]) may be necessary for acute neurologic deterioration while other treatments are initiated. Hyperventilation will lower ICP in a deteriorating patient with expanding intracranial hematoma until emergent craniotomy can be performed.

MANNITOL

Mannitol is used to reduce elevated ICP. The preparation most commonly used is a 20% solution (20 g of mannitol per 100 ml solution). Mannitol should not be given to patients with hypotension, because mannitol does not lower ICP in hypovolemia and is a potent osmotic diuretic. This can further exacerbate hypotension and cerebral ischemia. Acute neurologic deterioration, such as the development of a dilated pupil, hemiparesis, or loss of consciousness while the patient is being observed, is a strong indication for administering mannitol in a euvolemic patient. In this setting, a bolus of mannitol (1 g/kg) should be given rapidly (over 5 minutes) and the patient transported immediately to the CT scanner or directly to the operating room if a causative surgical lesion is already identified.

HYPERTONIC SALINE

Hypertonic saline is also used to reduce elevated ICP. Concentrations of 3% to 23.4% are used, and this may be the preferable agent to use in patients with hypotension, as it does not act as a diuretic. However, there is no difference between mannitol and hypertonic saline in lowering ICP, and neither will adequately lower ICP in hypovolemic patients.

BARBITURATES

Barbiturates are effective in reducing ICP refractory to other measures. They should not be used in the presence of hypotension or hypovolemia. Furthermore, hypotension often results from their use. Therefore, barbiturates are not indicated in the acute resuscitative phase. The long half-life of most barbiturates will also prolong the time to brain death determination, a consideration in patients with devastating and likely nonsurvivable injury.

ANTICONVULSANTS

Posttraumatic epilepsy occurs in about 5% of patients admitted to the hospital with closed head injuries and in 15% of individuals with severe head injuries. Three main factors linked to a high incidence of late epilepsy are seizures occurring within the first week, an intracranial hematoma, and a depressed skull fracture. Acute seizures may be controlled with anticonvulsants, but early anticonvulsant use does not change long-term traumatic seizure outcome. **Anticonvulsants may also inhibit brain recovery, so they should be used only when absolutely necessary.** Currently, phenytoin and fosphenytoin are the agents generally used in the acute phase. For adults, the usual loading dose is 1 g of phenytoin given intravenously at a rate no faster than 50 mg/min. The usual maintenance dose is 100 mg/8 hours, with the dose titrated to achieve therapeutic serum levels. Diazepam or lorazepam is frequently used in addition to phenytoin until the seizure stops. Control of continuous seizures may require general anesthesia. It is imperative that acute seizures be controlled as soon as possible, because prolonged seizures (30 to 60 minutes) may cause secondary brain injury.

PITFALLS

- It is important to monitor the ICP if active ICP management is being undertaken. For example, mannitol may have a significant rebound effect on ICP, and additional therapies may be indicated if ongoing management is required.

- It is important to remember that seizures are not controlled with muscle relaxants. Prolonged seizures in a patient whose muscles are relaxed pharmacologically can still be devastating to brain function, and may go undiagnosed and untreated if tonic-clonic muscle contractions are masked by a neuromuscular blocker such as vecuronium or succinylcholine. In a patient with a witnessed seizure, make sure appropriate antiseizure therapy is being initiated and that the seizure is under control before initiating neuromuscular blockade if at all possible.

Surgical Management

Surgical management may be necessary for scalp wounds, depressed skull fractures, intracranial mass lesions, and penetrating brain injuries.

SCALP WOUNDS

It is important to clean and inspect the wound thoroughly before suturing. The most common cause of infected scalp wounds is inadequate cleansing and debridement. Blood loss from scalp wounds may be extensive, especially in children (■ FIGURE 6-12). Scalp hemorrhage usually can be controlled by applying direct pressure and cauterizing or ligating large vessels. Appropriate sutures, clips, or staples may then be applied. Carefully inspect the wound under direct vision for signs of a skull fracture or foreign material. CSF leakage indicates that there is an associated dural tear. A neurosurgeon should be consulted in all cases of open or depressed skull fractures. Not infrequently, a subgaleal collection of blood can feel like a skull fracture. In such cases, the presence of a fracture can be confirmed or excluded by plain x-ray examination of the region and/or a CT scan.

DEPRESSED SKULL FRACTURES

Generally, a depressed skull fracture needs operative elevation if the degree of depression is greater than the thickness of the adjacent skull, or if it is open and grossly contaminated. Less significant depressed fractures can often be managed with closure of the overlying scalp laceration, if present. A CT scan is valuable in identifying the degree of depression, but more importantly in excluding the presence of an intracranial hematoma or contusion.

INTRACRANIAL MASS LESIONS

Intracranial mass lesions are managed by a neurosurgeon. If a neurosurgeon is not available in the facil-

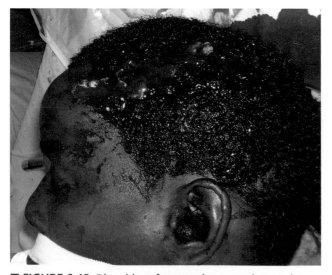

■ **FIGURE 6-12** Blood loss from scalp wounds may be extensive, especially in children.

ity initially receiving the patient with an intracranial mass lesion, early transfer to a hospital with a neurosurgeon is essential. In very exceptional circumstances, a rapidly expanding intracranial hematoma may be imminently life-threatening and may not allow time for transfer if neurosurgical care is some distance away. Although this circumstance is rare in urban settings, it may occur in austere or remote areas. Emergency craniotomy in a rapidly deteriorating patient by a non-neurosurgeon should be considered only in extreme circumstances, and the procedure should be performed by surgeons properly trained in the procedure only after discussion and advice of a neurosurgeon.

The indications for a craniotomy performed by a non-neurosurgeon are few, and its use as a desperation maneuver is neither recommended nor supported by the Committee on Trauma. This procedure is justified only when definitive neurosurgical care is unavailable. The Committee on Trauma strongly recommends that individuals who anticipate the need for this procedure receive proper training from a neurosurgeon.

PENETRATING BRAIN INJURIES

CT scanning of the head is strongly recommended to evaluate patients with penetrating brain injury. Plain radiographs of the head can be helpful in assessing bullet trajectory and fragmentation, and the presence of large foreign bodies and intracranial air. However, when CT is available, plain radiographs are not essential. CT and/or conventional angiography is recommended with any penetrating brain injury, or when a trajectory passes through or near the skull base or a major dural venous sinus. Substantial subarachnoid hemorrhage or delayed hematoma should also prompt consideration of vascular imaging. Patients with a penetrating injury involving the orbitofacial or pterional regions should undergo angiography to identify a traumatic intracranial aneurysm or arteriovenous (AV) fistula. When an aneurysm or AV fistula is identified, surgical or endovascular management is recommended. MRI can play a role in evaluating injuries from penetrating wooden or other nonmagnetic objects. The presence on CT of large contusions, hematomas, or intraventricular hemorrhage is associated with increased mortality, especially when both hemispheres are involved.

Prophylactic broad-spectrum antibiotics are appropriate for patients with penetrating brain injury. Early ICP monitoring is recommended when the clinician is unable to assess the neurologic examination accurately, the need to evacuate a mass lesion is unclear, or imaging studies suggest elevated ICP.

It is appropriate to treat small bullet entrance wounds to the head with local wound care and closure in patients whose scalp is not devitalized and who have no major intracranial pathology.

Objects that penetrate the intracranial compartment or infratemporal fossa and remain partially exteriorized (e.g., arrows, knives, screwdrivers) must be left in place until possible vascular injury has been evaluated and definitive neurosurgical management established. Disturbing or removing penetrating objects prematurely can lead to fatal vascular injury or intracranial hemorrhage.

▼ PITFALLS

Burr hole craniostomy/craniotomy—placing a 10-to-15-mm drill hole in the skull—has been advocated as a method of emergently diagnosing accessible hematomas in patients in austere or remote regions with rapid deterioration when neurosurgeons and imaging are not readily available. Unfortunately, even in very experienced hands, these drill holes are easily placed incorrectly, and they seldom result in draining enough of the hematoma to make a clinical difference. In patients who need an evacuation, bone flap craniotomy (and not a simple burr hole) is the definitive lifesaving procedure to decompress the brain, and every attempt should be made to have a practitioner trained and experienced in doing the procedure perform it in a timely fashion.

▶ Prognosis

All patients should be treated aggressively pending consultation with a neurosurgeon. This is particularly true of children, who have a remarkable ability to recover from seemingly devastating injuries.

▶ Brain Death

? *How do I diagnose brain death?*

The diagnosis of brain death implies that there is no possibility for recovery of brain function. Most experts agree that the following criteria should be satisfied for the diagnosis of brain death:

- Glasgow Coma Scale score = 3
- Nonreactive pupils
- Absent brainstem reflexes (e.g., oculocephalic, corneal, and Doll's eyes, and no gag reflex)
- No spontaneous ventilatory effort on formal apnea testing

Ancillary studies that may be used to confirm the diagnosis of brain death include:

- Electroencephalography: No activity at high gain
- CBF studies: No CBF (e.g., isotope studies, Doppler studies, xenon CBF studies)
- Cerebral angiography

Certain reversible conditions, such as hypothermia or barbiturate coma, may mimic the appearance of brain death; therefore, this diagnosis should be considered only after all physiologic parameters are normalized and central nervous system (CNS) function is not potentially affected by medications. The remarkable ability of children to recover from seemingly devastating brain injuries should be carefully considered prior to diagnosing brain death in children. If any doubt exists, especially in children, multiple serial exams spaced several hours apart are useful in confirming the initial clinical impression. Local organ-procurement agencies should be notified about all patients with the diagnosis or impending diagnosis of brain death prior to discontinuing artificial life support measures.

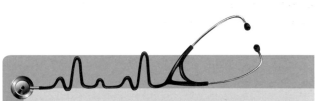

Scenario ■ conclusion The patient underwent successful evacuation of his subdural hematoma and subsequent treatment of a femur fracture found on secondary survey post-evacuation. He was ultimately discharged to a rehabilitation center for ongoing physical, occupational, and speech therapy.

Chapter Summary

1 Understanding basic intracranial anatomy and physiology is key to the management of head injury.

2 Learn to evaluate patients with head and brain injuries efficiently. In a comatose patient, secure and maintain the airway by endotracheal intubation. Perform a neurologic examination after normalizing the blood pressure and before paralyzing the patient. Search for associated injuries.

3 Practice performing a rapid and focused neurologic examination. Become familiar with the Glasgow Coma Scale (GCS) and practice its use. Frequently reassess the patient's neurologic status.

4 Adequate resuscitation is important in limiting secondary brain injury. Prevent hypovolemia and hypoxemia. Treat shock aggressively and look for its cause. Resuscitate with Ringer's lactate solution, normal saline, or similar isotonic solutions without dextrose. Do not use hypotonic solutions. The goal in resuscitating the patient with brain injuries is to prevent secondary brain injury.

5 Determine the need for transfer, admission, consultation, or discharge. Contact a neurosurgeon as early as possible. If a neurosurgeon is not available at the facility, transfer all patients with moderate or severe head injuries.

BIBLIOGRAPHY

1. Amirjamshidi A, Abbassioun K, Rahmat H. Minimal debridement or simple wound closure as the only surgical treatment in war victims with low-velocity penetrating head injuries. Indications and management protocol based upon more than 8 years' follow-up of 99 cases from Iran-Iraq conflict. *Surg Neurol* 2003;60(2):105-110; discussion 110-111.

2. Andrews BT, Chiles BW, Olsen WL, et al. The effect of intra-cerebral hematoma location on the risk of brainstem compression and on clinical outcome. *J Neurosurg* 1988;69:518-522.

3. Atkinson JLD. The neglected prehospital phase of head injury: apnea and catecholamine surge. *Mayo Clin Proc* 2000;75(1):37-47.

4. Aubry M, Cantu R, Dvorak J, et al. Summary and agreement statement of the first International Conference on Concussion in Sport, Vienna 2001. *Phys Sportsmed* 2002;30:57-62 (copublished in *Br J Sports Med* 2002;36:3-7 and *Clin J Sport Med* 2002;12:6-12).

5. Boyle A, Santarius L, Maimaris C. Evaluation of the impact of the Canadian CT head rule on British practice. *Emerg Med J* 2004;21(4):426-428.

6. Brain Trauma Foundation. Early Indicators of Prognosis in Severe Traumatic Brain Injury. http://www2. braintrauma.org/guidelines/downloads/btf_prognosis_ guidelines.pdf?BrainTrauma_Session=1157580cb4d126 eb381748a50424bb99. Accessed May 4, 2012.

7. Brain Trauma Foundation. Guidelines for the Management of Severe Traumatic Brain Injury. http://www2. braintrauma.org/guidelines/downloads/JON_24_Suppl. pdf?BrainTrauma_Session=1157580cb4d126eb381748a 50424bb99. Accessed Accessed May 4, 2012.

8. Chestnut RM, Marshall LF, Klauber MR, et al. The role of secondary brain injury in determining outcome from severe head injury. *J Trauma* 1993;34:216-222.

9. Chibbaro S, Tacconi L. Orbito-cranial injuries caused by penetrating non-missile foreign bodies. Experience with eighteen patients. *Acta Neurochir* (Wien) 2006;148(9), 937-941; discussion 941-942.

10. Clement CM, Stiell IG, Schull MJ, et al. Clinical features of head injury patients presenting with a Glasgow Coma

Scale score of 15 and who require neurosurgical intervention. *Ann Emerg Med* 2006;48(3):245-251.

11. Eisenberg HM, Frankowski RF, Contant CR, et al. High-dose barbiturates control elevated intracranial pressure in patients with severe head injury. *J Neurosurg* 1988;69:15-23.

12. Eelco F.M. Wijdicks, Panayiotis N. Varelas, Gary S. Gronseth and David M. Greer. Evidence-based guideline update: Determining brain death in adults. Report of the Quality Standards Subcommittee of the American Academy of Neurology. *Neurology*. 2010;74:1911-1918.

13. Giri BK, Krishnappa IK, Bryan RMJ, et al. Regional cerebral blood flow after cortical impact injury complicated by a secondary insult in rats. *Stroke* 2000;31:961-967.

14. Gonul E, Erdogan E, Tasar M, et al. Penetrating orbitocranial gunshot injuries. *Surg Neurol* 2005;63(1):24-30; discussion 31.

15. http://www.cdc.gov/traumaticbraininjury/. Accessed May 4, 2012.

16. Johnson U, Nilsson P, Ronne-Engstrom E, et al. Favorable outcome in traumatic brain injury patients with impaired cerebral pressure autoregulation when treated at low cerebral perfusion pressure levels. *Neurosurgery* 2011;68:714-722.

17. Marion DW, Spiegel TP. Changes in the management of severe traumatic brain injury: 1991-1997. *Crit Care Med* 2000;28:16-18.

18. McCrory, P, Johnston, K, Meeuwisse, W, et al. Summary and agreement statement of the 2nd International Conference on Concussion in Sport, Prague 2004. *Br J Sports Med* 2005;39:196-204.

19. Mower WR, et al. Developing a Decision Instrument to Guide Computed Tomographic Imaging of Blunt Head Injury Patients. http://www.ncbi.nlm.nih.gov/pubmed/16374287. *J Trauma* 2005;59:954-9.

20. Muizelaar JP, Marmarou A, Ward JD, et al. Adverse effects of prolonged hyperventilation in patients with severe head injury: a randomized clinical trial. *J Neurosurg* 1991;75:731-739.

21. Part 1: Guidelines for the management of penetrating brain injury. Introduction and methodology. *J Trauma* 2001;51(2 Suppl):S3-S6.

22. Part 2: Prognosis in penetrating brain injury. *J Trauma* 2001;51(2 Suppl):S44-S86. http://journals.lww.com/jtrauma/toc/2001/08001

23. Robertson CS, Valadka AB, Hannay HJ, et al. Prevention of secondary ischemic insults after severe head injury. *Crit Care Med* 1999;27:2086-2095.

24. Rosengart AJ, Huo D, Tolentino J, Novakovic RL, Frank JI, Goldenberg FD, Macdonald RL. Outcome in patients with subarachnoid hemorrhage treated with antiepileptic drugs. *J Neurosurg* 2007;107:253-260.

25. Rosner MJ, Rosner SD, Johnson AH. Cerebral perfusion pressure management protocols and clinical results. *J Neurosurg* 1995;83:949-962.

26. Sakellaridis N, Pavlou E, Karatzas S, Chroni D, Vlachos K, Chatzopoulos K, Dimopoulou E, Kelesis C, Karaouli V. Comparison of mannitol and hypertonic saline in the treatment of severe brain injuries. *J Neurosurg* 2011;114:545-548.

27. Smits M, Dippel DW, de Haan GG, et al. External validation of the Canadian CT Head Rule and the New Orleans Criteria for CT scanning in patients with minor head injury. *JAMA* 2005;294(12):1519-1525.

28. Stiell IG, Clement CM, Rowe BH, et al. Comparison of the Canadian CT Head Rule and the New Orleans Criteria in patients with minor head injury. *JAMA* 2005;294(12):1511-1518.

29. Stiell IG, Lesiuk H, Wells GA, et al. Canadian CT head rule study for patients with minor head injury: methodology for phase II (validation and economic analysis). *Ann Emerg Med* 2001;38(3):317-322.

30. Stiell IG, Lesiuk H, Wells GA, et al. The Canadian CT Head Rule Study for patients with minor head injury: rationale, objectives, and methodology for phase I (derivation). *Ann Emerg Med* 2001;38(2):160-169.

31. Stiell IG, Wells GA, Vandemheen K, et al. The Canadian CT Head Rule for patients with minor head injury. *Lancet* 2001;357(9266):1391-1396.

32. Sultan HY, Boyle A, Pereira M, Antoun N, Maimaris C. Application of the Canadian CT head rules in managing minor head injuries in a UK emergency department: implications for the implementation of the NICE guidelines. *Emerg Med J* 2004;21(4):420-425.

33. Temkin NR, Dikman SS, Wilensky AJ, et al. A randomized, double-blind study of phenytoin for the prevention of post-traumatic seizures. *N Engl J Med* 1990;323:497-502.

34. Valadka AB. Injury to cranium. In Moore, Feliciano, Mattox, eds. *Trauma*, 2008, pp 385-406.

Head and Neck Trauma: Assessment and Management

▶▶ Interactive Skill Procedures

Note: Accompanying some of the skills in this Skill Station is a series of scenarios for you to review and use to prepare for this station. Standard precautions are required whenever caring for trauma patients.

THE FOLLOWING PROCEDURES ARE INCLUDED IN THIS SKILL STATION:

▶▶ **Skill X-A:** Primary Survey

▶▶ **Skill X-B:** Secondary Survey and Management

▶▶ **Skill X-C:** Evaluation of CT Scans of the Head

▶▶ **Skill X-D:** Helmet Removal

Objectives

Performance at this station will allow participants to practice and demonstrate the following activities in a simulated clinical situation:

1 Demonstrate assessment and diagnostic skills in determining the type and extent of injuries, using a head trauma manikin.

2 Describe the significance of clinical signs and symptoms of brain trauma found through assessment.

3 Establish priorities for the initial treatment of patients with brain trauma.

4 Identify diagnostic aids that can be used to determine the area of injury within the brain and the extent of the injury.

5 Demonstrate proper helmet removal while protecting the patient's cervical spine.

6 Perform a complete secondary assessment and determine the patient's Glasgow Coma Scale (GCS) score through the use of scenarios and interactive dialogue with the instructor.

7 Differentiate between normal and abnormal computed tomographic (CT) scans of the head, and identify injury patterns.

▶ SCENARIOS

SCENARIO X-1

A 17-year-old high-school football player, involved in a crushing tackle with a brief loss of consciousness, reports neck pain and paresthesia in his left arm. He is immobilized on a long spine board with his helmet in place and transported to the emergency department (ED). He is not in respiratory distress, talks coherently, and is awake and alert.

SCENARIO X-2

A 25-year-old male is transported to the ED after a car crash while driving home from a tavern. His airway is clear, he is breathing spontaneously without difficulty, and he has no hemodynamic abnormalities. He has a scalp contusion over the left side of his head. There is a strong odor of alcohol on his breath, but he is able to answer questions appropriately. His eyes are open, but he appears confused and pushes away the examiner's hands when examined for response to pain. He is thought to have suffered a concussion and to have alcohol intoxication. He is kept in the ED for observation.

One hour later, the patient is more somnolent, briefly opens his eyes to painful stimuli, and demonstrates an abnormal flexion response to painful stimuli on the right and withdrawal on the left. His left pupil is now 2 mm larger than his right. Both pupils react sluggishly to light. His verbal response consists of incomprehensible sounds.

SCENARIO X-3

A 21-year-old male was thrown from and then kicked in the face by a horse. He was initially unconscious for at least 5 minutes. He now opens his eyes to speech, moves only to painful stimuli by withdrawing his extremities, and utters inappropriate words. His blood pressure is 180/80 mm Hg, and heart rate is 64 beats/min.

SCENARIO X-4

A 40-year-old motorcyclist is brought to the ED with obvious head trauma. The prehospital personnel report that he has unequal pupils and responds only to painful stimuli by abnormally flexing his arms, opening his eyes, and speaking incomprehensibly. When not stimulated, his respirations are very sonorous.

▶ Skill X-A: Primary Survey

STEP 1. ABCDEs.

STEP 2. Immobilize and stabilize the cervical spine.

STEP 3. Perform a brief neurologic examination, looking for:
   A. Pupillary response
   B. GCS score determination
   C. Lateralizing signs

▶ Skill X-B: Secondary Survey and Management

STEP 1. Inspect the entire head, including the face, looking for:
   A. Lacerations
   B. Presence of cerebrospinal fluid (CSF) leakage from the nose and ears

STEP 2. Palpate the entire head, including the face, looking for:
   A. Fractures
   B. Lacerations overlying fractures

STEP 3. Inspect all scalp lacerations, looking for:
   A. Brain tissue
   B. Depressed skull fractures
   C. Debris
   D. CSF leaks

STEP 4. Determine the GCS score and pupillary response, including:
   A. Eye-opening response
   B. Best limb motor response

C. Verbal response
D. Pupillary response

STEP 5. Examine the cervical spine.
   A. Palpate for tenderness/pain and apply a semirigid cervical collar, if needed.
   B. Perform a cross-table lateral cervical spine x-ray examination, if needed

STEP 6. Document the extent of neurologic injury.

STEP 7. Reassess the patient continuously, observing for signs of deterioration.
   A. Frequency
   B. Parameters to be assessed
   C. Serial GCS scores and extremity motor assessment
   D. Remember, reassess ABCDEs

▶ Skill X-C: Evaluation of CT Scans of the Head

The diagnosis of abnormalities seen on CT scans of the head can be very subtle and difficult. Because of the inherent complexity in interpreting these scans, early review by a neurosurgeon or radiologist is important. The steps outlined here for evaluating a CT scan of the head provide one approach to assessing for significant, life-threatening pathology. Remember, obtaining a CT scan of the head should not delay resuscitation or transfer of the patient to a trauma center.

STEP 1. Follow the process for initial review of CT scans of the head.
   A. Confirm that the images being reviewed are of the correct patient.
   B. Ensure that the CT scan of the head was done without an intravenous contrast agent.
   C. Use the patient's clinical findings to focus the review of the CT scan, and use the image findings to enhance further physical evaluation.

STEP 2. Assess the scalp component for contusion or swelling that can indicate a site of external trauma.

STEP 3. Assess for skull fractures. Keep in mind that:
   A. Suture lines (joining of the bones of the cranial vault) may be mistaken for fractures.
   B. Depressed skull fractures (thickness of skull) require neurosurgical consultation.
   C. Open fractures require neurosurgical consultation.
   D. Missile wound tracts may appear as linear areas of low attenuation.

STEP 4. Assess the gyri and sulci for symmetry. If asymmetry exists, consider these diagnoses:

   A. Acute subdural hematomas:
      • Typically are areas of increased density covering and compressing the gyri and sulci over the entire hemisphere
      • Can cause a shift of the underlying ventricles across the midline
      • Occur more commonly than epidural hematomas
      • Can have associated cerebral contusions and intracerebral hematomas
   B. Acute epidural hematomas:
      • Typically are lenticular or biconvex areas of increased density
      • Appear within the skull and compress the underlying gyri and sulci
      • Can cause a shift of the underlying ventricles across the midline
      • Most often are located in the temporal or temporoparietal region

STEP 5. Assess the cerebral and cerebellar hemispheres.
   A. Compare both hemispheres for similar density and symmetry.
   B. Intracerebral hematomas appear as areas of high density.
   C. Cerebral contusions appear as punctate areas of high density.
   D. Diffuse axonal injury can appear normal or have scattered, small areas of cerebral contusion and areas of low density.

STEP 6. Assess the ventricles.
   A. Check size and symmetry.
   B. Significant mass lesions compress and distort the ventricles, especially the lateral ventricles.
   C. Significant intracranial hypertension is often associated with decreased ventricular size.

D. Intraventricular hemorrhage appears as regions of increased density (bright spots) in the ventricles.

STEP 7. Determine the shifts. Midline shifts may be caused by a hematoma or swelling that causes the septum pellucidum, between the two lateral ventricles, to shift away from the midline. The midline is a line extending from the crista galli anteriorly to the tentlike projection posteriorly (inion). After measuring the distance from the midline to the septum pellucidum, the actual shift is determined by correcting against the scale on the CT print. A shift of 5 mm or more is considered indicative of a mass lesion and the need for surgical decompression.

STEP 8. Assess the maxillofacial structures.
A. Assess the facial bones for fractures.
B. Assess the sinuses and mastoid air cells for air-fluid levels.
C. Facial bone fractures, sinus fractures, and sinus or mastoid air-fluid levels may indicate basilar skull or cribriform plate fractures.

STEP 9. Look for the four Cs of increased density:
A. Contrast
B. Clot
C. Cellularity (tumor)
D. Calcification (pineal gland, choroid plexus)

▶ Skill X-D: Helmet Removal

Any patient wearing a helmet should have the head and neck held in a neutral position while the helmet is removed using the two-person procedure. Note: A poster entitled "Techniques of Helmet Removal from Injured Patients" is available from the American College of Surgeons (www.facs.org/trauma/publications/helmet.pdf). This poster provides a pictorial and narrative description of helmet removal. Also see photographs of this procedure in Figure 2-2 of Chapter 2: Airway and Ventilatory Management. Some varieties of helmets have special removal mechanisms that should be used in accordance with the specific helmets.

STEP 1. One person stabilizes the patient's head and neck by placing one hand on either side of the helmet with the fingers on the patient's mandible. This position prevents slippage if the strap is loose.

STEP 2. The second person cuts or loosens the helmet strap at the D-rings.

STEP 3. The second person then places one hand on the mandible at the angle, with the thumb on one side and the fingers on the other. The other hand applies pressure from under the head at the occipital region. This maneuver transfers the responsibility for inline immobilization to the second person.

STEP 4. The first person then expands the helmet laterally to clear the ears and carefully removes the helmet. If the helmet has a face cover, this device must be removed first. If the helmet provides full facial coverage, the patient's nose will impede helmet removal. To clear the nose, the helmet must be tilted backward and raised over the patient's nose.

STEP 5. During this process, the second person must maintain inline immobilization from below to prevent head tilt.

STEP 6. After the helmet is removed, inline manual immobilization is reestablished from above, and the patient's head and neck are secured.

STEP 7. If attempts to remove the helmet result in pain and paresthesia, the helmet should be removed with a cast cutter. The helmet also should be removed with a cast cutter if there is evidence of a cervical spine injury on x-ray film. The head and neck must be stabilized during this procedure, which is accomplished by dividing the helmet in the coronal plane through the ears. The outer, rigid layer is removed easily, and the inside layer is then incised and removed anteriorly. Maintaining neutral alignment of the head and neck, the posterior portions are removed.

7 Spine and Spinal Cord Trauma

Spine injury, with or without neurologic deficits, must always be considered in patients with multiple injuries. Appropriate immobilization is required for all of these patients.

Scenario A 38-year-old male is pulled from a swimming pool. His vitals are: blood pressure: 80/62; heart rate: 58; respiratory rate: 28. He is alert and following commands. Breathing is shallow, and he is not moving his arms or legs.

Outline

Introduction

Anatomy and Physiology
- Spinal Column
- Spinal Cord Anatomy
- Sensory Examination
- Myotomes
- Neurogenic Shock versus Spinal Shock
- Effects on Other Organ Systems

Classifications of Spinal Cord Injuries
- Level
- Severity of Neurologic Deficit
- Spinal Cord Syndromes
- Morphology

Specific Types of Spinal Injuries
- Atlanto-Occipital Dislocation
- Atlas (C1) Fracture
- C1 Rotary Subluxation
- Axis (C2) Fractures
- Fractures and Dislocations (C3 through C7)
- Thoracic Spine Fractures (T1 through T10)
- Thoracolumbar Junction Fractures (T11 through L1)
- Lumbar Fractures
- Penetrating Injuries
- Blunt Carotid and Vertebral Vascular Injuries

X-Ray Evaluation
- Cervical Spine
- Thoracic and Lumbar Spine

General Management
- Immobilization
- Intravenous Fluids
- Medications
- Transfer

Summary

Bibliography

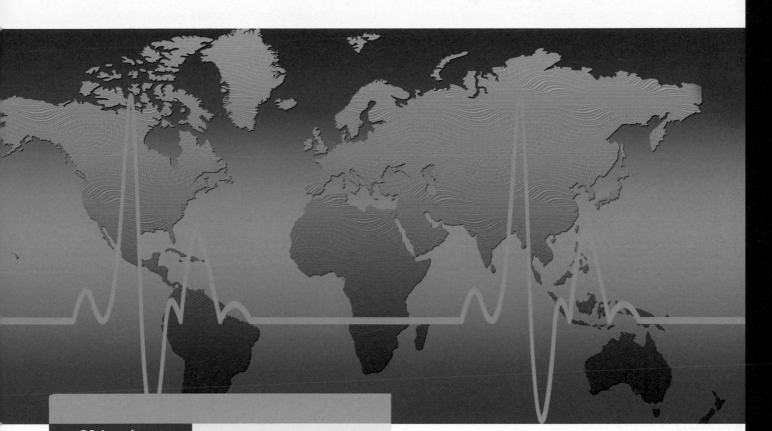

Objectives

1. Describe the basic anatomy and physiology of the spine.

2. Evaluate a patient with suspected spinal injury.

3. Identify the common types of spinal injuries and their x-ray features.

4. Appropriately treat patients with spinal injuries during the first hour after injury.

5. Determine the appropriate disposition of patients with spine trauma.

☆ Suspect Spinal injury!
- *Mechanism*
- *Unconscious pt.*
- *Pain or tenderness of spine.*
- *Neurological Symptoms.*

Spine injury, with or without neurologic deficits, must always be considered in patients with multiple injuries. Approximately 5% of patients with brain injury have an associated spinal injury, whereas 25% of patients with spinal injury have at least a mild brain injury. Approximately 55% of spinal injuries occur in the cervical region, 15% in the thoracic region, 15% at the thoracolumbar junction, and 15% in the lumbosacral area. **Approximately 10% of patients with a cervical spine fracture have a second, noncontiguous vertebral column fracture.**

Doctors and other medical personnel who treat patients with spine injuries must be constantly aware that excessive manipulation and inadequate immobilization of such patients may cause additional neurologic damage and worsen the patient's outcome. At least 5% of patients with spine injury experience the onset of neurologic symptoms or the worsening of preexisting symptoms after reaching the ED. This is usually due to ischemia or progression of spinal cord edema, but it may also result from inadequate immobilization. **As long as the patient's spine is protected, evaluation of the spine and exclusion of spinal injury may be safely deferred, especially in the presence of systemic instability, such as hypotension and respiratory inadequacy.** Cervical spine injury in children is a relatively rare event, occurring in less than 1% of cases. Additionally, anatomical differences, emotional distress, and inability to communicate make evaluation of the spine even more challenging in this population (see Chapter 10: Pediatric Trauma).

In a patient *without* neurological deficit, pain or tenderness along the spine, evidence of intoxication, or distracting injury, excluding the presence of a spinal injury is straightforward. In a neurologically intact patient, the absence of pain or tenderness along the spine virtually excludes the presence of a significant spinal injury. However, in a patient who is comatose or has a depressed level of consciousness, the process is not as simple. In this case, it is incumbent on the clinician to obtain the appropriate x-ray films to exclude a spinal injury. If the x-rays are inconclusive, the patient's spine should remain protected until further testing can be performed.

Although the dangers of inadequate immobilization have been well documented, there also is some danger in prolonged immobilization of patients on a hard surface such as a backboard. In addition to causing severe discomfort in an awake patient, prolonged immobilization may lead to the formation of serious decubitus ulcers in patients with spinal cord injuries. Therefore, the long backboard should be used only as a patient transportation device, and every effort should be made to have the patient evaluated by the appropriate specialists and removed from the spine board as quickly as possible. If this is not feasible within 2 hours, the patient should be removed from the spine board and then logrolled every 2 hours, while maintaining the integrity of the spine, to reduce the risk of the formation of decubitus ulcers.

Anatomy and Physiology

The following review of the anatomy and physiology of the spine and spinal cord includes the spinal column, spinal cord anatomy, sensory examination, myotomes, neurogenic and spinal shock, and effects on other organ systems.

SPINAL COLUMN

The spinal column consists of 7 cervical, 12 thoracic, and 5 lumbar vertebrae, as well as the sacrum and the coccyx (■ FIGURE 7-1). The typical vertebra consists of an anteriorly placed vertebral body, which forms the

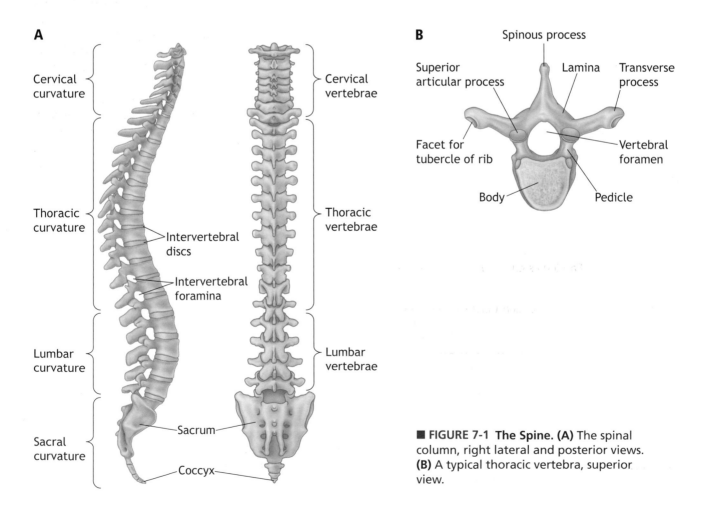

A

Cervical curvature

Thoracic curvature

Intervertebral discs

Intervertebral foramina

Lumbar curvature

Sacral curvature

Sacrum

Coccyx

Cervical vertebrae

Thoracic vertebrae

Lumbar vertebrae

B

Spinous process

Superior articular process

Lamina

Transverse process

Facet for tubercle of rib

Vertebral foramen

Body

Pedicle

■ FIGURE 7-1 The Spine. (A) The spinal column, right lateral and posterior views. (B) A typical thoracic vertebra, superior view.

main weight-bearing column. The vertebral bodies are separated by intervertebral disks, and are held together anteriorly and posteriorly by the anterior and posterior longitudinal ligaments, respectively. Posterolaterally, two pedicles form the pillars on which the roof of the vertebral canal (i.e., the lamina) rests. The facet joints, interspinous ligaments, and paraspinal muscles all contribute to the stability of the spine.

The cervical spine is the most vulnerable to injury, because of its mobility and exposure. The cervical canal is wide in the upper cervical region, or from the foramen magnum to the lower part of C2. The majority of patients with injuries at this level who survive are neurologically intact on arrival at the hospital. However, approximately one-third of patients with upper cervical spine injuries die at the injury scene from apnea caused by loss of central innervation of the phrenic nerves caused by spinal cord injury at C1. Below the level of C3 the diameter of the spinal canal is much smaller relative to the diameter of the spinal cord, and vertebral column injuries are much more likely to cause spinal cord injuries. The cervical spine in children has marked differences from that of adults until approximately 8 years of age. These differences include more flexible joint capsules and interspinous ligaments, as well as flat facet joints and vertebral bodies that are wedged anteriorly and tend to slide forward with flexion. The differences decline steadily until approximately age 12, when the cervical spine is more similar to an adult's (see Chapter 10: Pediatric Trauma).

The mobility of the thoracic spine is much more restricted than that of the cervical spine, and it has additional support from the rib cage. Hence, the incidence of thoracic fractures is much lower. Most thoracic spine fractures are wedge compression fractures that are not associated with spinal cord injury. However, when a fracture-dislocation in the thoracic spine does occur, it almost always results in a complete spinal cord injury (see below) because of the relatively narrow thoracic canal. The thoracolumbar junction is a fulcrum between the inflexible thoracic region and the stronger lumbar levels. This makes it more vulnerable to injury, and 15% of all spinal injuries occur in this region.

SPINAL CORD ANATOMY

The spinal cord originates at the caudal end of the medulla oblongata at the foramen magnum. In adults, it usually ends near the L1 bony level as the conus medullaris. Below this level is the cauda equina, which is somewhat more resilient to injury. Of the many tracts in the spinal cord, only three can be readily assessed clinically: the lateral corticospinal tract, spinothalamic tract, and dorsal columns (■ FIGURE 7-2). Each is a paired tract that can be injured on one or both sides of the cord. The location in the spinal cord, function, and method of testing for each tract are outlined in Table 7.1.

When a patient has no demonstrable sensory or motor function below a certain level, he or she is said to have a *complete spinal cord injury*. During the first weeks after injury, this diagnosis cannot be made with certainty, because of the possibility of spinal shock. An *incomplete spinal cord injury* is one in which any degree of motor or sensory function remains; the prognosis for recovery is significantly better than that for complete spinal cord injury. Sparing of sensation in the perianal region (sacral sparing) may be the only sign of residual function. Sacral sparing can be demonstrated by preservation of some sensory perception in the perianal region and/or voluntary contraction of the rectal sphincter.

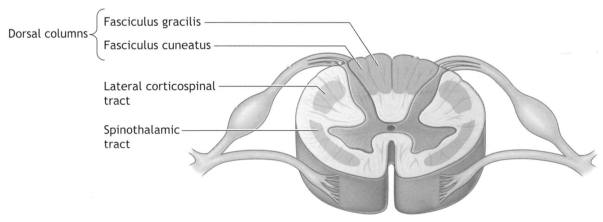

Dorsal columns
{ Fasciculus gracilis
Fasciculus cuneatus

Lateral corticospinal tract

Spinothalamic tract

■ **FIGURE 7-2 Spinal Cord Tracts.** Three of the tracts in the spinal cord can be readily assessed clinically: the lateral corticospinal tract, spinothalamic tract, and dorsal columns. Each is a paired tract that can be injured on one or both sides of the cord.

■ TABLE 7.1 Clinical Assessment of Spinal Cord Tracts

TRACT	LOCATION IN SPINAL CORD	FUNCTION	METHOD OF TESTING
Corticospinal tract	In the posterolateral segment of the cord	Controls motor power on the same side of the body	By voluntary muscle contractions or involuntary response to painful stimuli
Spinothalamic tract	In the anterolateral aspect of the cord	Transmits pain and temperature sensation from the opposite side of the body	By pinprick and light touch
Dorsal columns	In the posteromedial aspect of the cord	Carries position sense (proprioception), vibration sense, and some light-touch sensation from the same side of the body	By position sense in the toes and fingers or vibration sense using a tuning fork

■ TABLE 7.2 Spinal Nerve Segments and Areas of Innervation

SPINAL NERVE SEGMENT	AREA INNERVATED
C5	Area over the deltoid
C6	Thumb
C7	Middle finger
C8	Little finger
T4	Nipple
T8	Xiphisternum
T10	Umbilicus
T12	Symphysis pubis
L4	Medial aspect of the calf
L5	Web space between the first and second toes
S1	Lateral border of the foot
S3	Ischial tuberosity area
S4 and S5	Perianal region

SENSORY EXAMINATION

❓ How do I assess the patient's neurologic status?

A dermatome is the area of skin innervated by the sensory axons within a particular segmental nerve root. Knowledge of the major dermatome levels is invaluable in determining the level of injury and assessing neurologic improvement or deterioration. The sensory level is the lowest dermatome with normal sensory function and can often differ on the two sides of the body. For practical purposes, the upper cervical dermatomes (C1 to C4) are somewhat variable in their cutaneous distribution and are not commonly used for localization. However, it should be remembered that the supraclavicular nerves (C2 through C4) provide sensory innervation to the region overlying the pectoralis muscle (cervical cape). The presence of sensation in this region may confuse the examiner when he or she is trying to determine the sensory level in patients with lower cervical injuries. The key sensory points are outlined in Table 7.2 and illustrated in ■ FIGURE 7-3.

MYOTOMES

Each segmental nerve (root) innervates more than one muscle, and most muscles are innervated by more than one root (usually two). Nevertheless, for the sake of simplicity, certain muscles or muscle groups are identified as representing a single spinal nerve segment. The key myotomes are shown in ■ FIGURE 7-4.

The key muscles should be tested for strength on both sides. Each muscle is graded on a six-point scale from normal strength to paralysis (Table 7.3). Documentation of the strength in key muscle groups helps to assess neurologic improvement or deterioration on subsequent examinations. In addition, the external anal sphincter should be tested for voluntary contraction by digital examination.

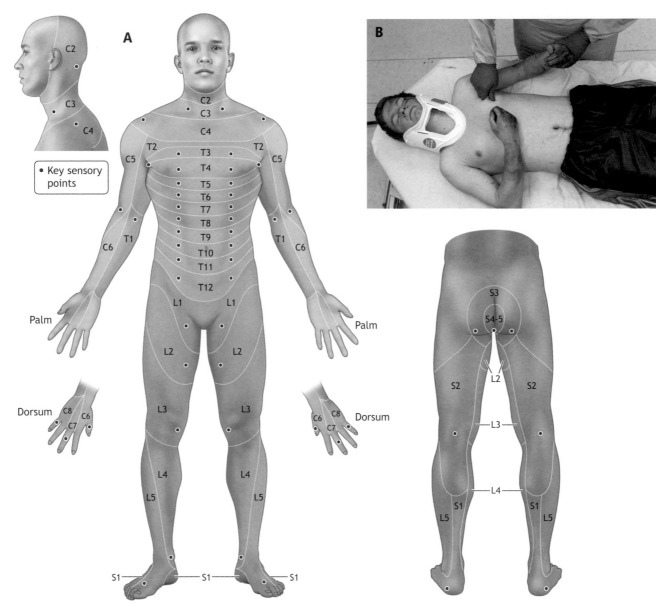

■ **FIGURE 7-3 Spinal Dermatomes. (A)** Key sensory points by spinal dermatomes. **(B)** Assessing sensory response–nipple, T4.

Adapted from the American Spinal Injury Association: *International Standards for Neurological Classification of Spinal Cord Injury,* revised 2002. Chicago, IL: American Spinal Injury Association; 2002.

PITFALLS

- The sensory examination may be confounded by pain.

- Patients sometimes observe the examination itself, which may alter the findings.

- Altered level of consciousness limits the ability to perform a definitive neurologic examination.

NEUROGENIC SHOCK VERSUS SPINAL SHOCK

? *How do I identify and treat neurogenic and spinal shock?*

Neurogenic shock results from impairment of the descending sympathetic pathways in the cervical or upper thoracic spinal cord. This condition results in the loss of vasomotor tone and in sympathetic innervation to the heart. Neurogenic shock is rare in spinal cord injury below the level of T6; if shock is present in these patients, an alternative source should be strongly suspected. Loss of vasomotor tone causes vasodilation of

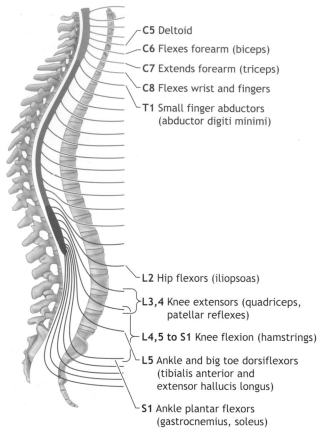

- **C5** Deltoid
- **C6** Flexes forearm (biceps)
- **C7** Extends forearm (triceps)
- **C8** Flexes wrist and fingers
- **T1** Small finger abductors (abductor digiti minimi)
- **L2** Hip flexors (iliopsoas)
- **L3,4** Knee extensors (quadriceps, patellar reflexes)
- **L4,5 to S1** Knee flexion (hamstrings)
- **L5** Ankle and big toe dorsiflexors (tibialis anterior and extensor hallucis longus)
- **S1** Ankle plantar flexors (gastrocnemius, soleus)

■ **FIGURE 7-4 Key Myotomes.**

TABLE 7.3 Muscle Strength Grading	
SCORE	**RESULTS OF EXAMINATION**
0	Total paralysis
1	Palpable or visible contraction
2	Full range of motion with gravity eliminated
3	Full range of motion against gravity
4	Full range of motion, but less than normal strength
5	Normal strength
NT	Not testable

Adapted with permission from Kirshblum SC, Memmo P, Kim N, et al. Comparison of the revised 2000 American Spinal Injury Association classification standards with the 1996 guidelines. *Am J Phys Med Rehabil* 2002;81:502-505.

ments, which innervate the diaphragm via the phrenic nerve. **The inability to perceive pain may mask a potentially serious injury elsewhere in the body, such as the usual signs of an acute abdomen.**

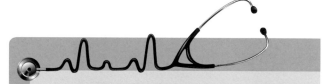

Scenario ■ *continued* The patient is unable to move his legs. He can move his fingers on both hands, can move both wrists, and has weak triceps extension on the left. He is unable to move his elbow on the right. He is able to feel his fingers and thumbs on both hands, but is not able to feel anything above the elbow.

Classifications of Spinal Cord Injuries

❓ *When do I suspect spine injury?*

Spinal cord injuries can be classified according to (1) level, (2) severity of neurologic deficit, (3) spinal cord syndromes, and (4) morphology.

LEVEL

The *neurologic level* is the most caudal segment of the spinal cord that has normal sensory and motor function on both sides of the body. When the term *sensory level* is used, it refers to the most caudal segment of the spinal cord with normal sensory function. The *motor level* is defined similarly with respect to motor func-

---

visceral and lower-extremity blood vessels, pooling of blood, and, consequently, hypotension. Loss of sympathetic innervation to the heart may cause the development of bradycardia or at least a failure of tachycardia in response to hypovolemia. In this condition, the blood pressure may not be restored by fluid infusion alone, and massive fluid resuscitation may result in fluid overload and pulmonary edema. The blood pressure may often be restored by the judicious use of vasopressors after moderate volume replacement. Atropine may be used to counteract hemodynamically significant bradycardia.

Spinal shock refers to the flaccidity (loss of muscle tone) and loss of reflexes seen after spinal cord injury. The "shock" to the injured cord may make it appear completely nonfunctional, although the cord may not necessarily be destroyed. The duration of this state is variable.

EFFECTS ON OTHER ORGAN SYSTEMS

Hypoventilation due to paralysis of the intercostal muscles may result from an injury involving the lower cervical or upper thoracic spinal cord. If the upper or middle cervical cord is injured, the diaphragm also is paralyzed because of involvement of the C3 to C5 seg-

tion as the lowest key muscle that has a grade of at least 3/5 (see Table 7.3). In complete injuries, when some impaired sensory and/or motor function is found just below the lowest normal segment, this is referred to as the zone of partial preservation. As described above, the determination of the level of injury on both sides is important.

A broad distinction may be made between lesions above and below T1. Injuries of the first eight cervical segments of the spinal cord result in quadriplegia, and lesions below the T1 level result in paraplegia. The *bony level of injury* is the vertebra at which the bones are damaged, causing injury to the spinal cord. The *neurologic level of injury* is determined primarily by clinical examination. Frequently, there is a discrepancy between the bony and neurologic levels because the spinal nerves enter the spinal canal through the foramina and ascend or descend inside the spinal canal before actually entering the spinal cord. The further caudal the injury is, the more pronounced this discrepancy becomes. Apart from the initial management to stabilize the bony injury, all subsequent descriptions of the level of injury are based on the neurologic level.

SEVERITY OF NEUROLOGIC DEFICIT

Spinal cord injury may be categorized as:

- Incomplete paraplegia (incomplete thoracic injury)
- Complete paraplegia (complete thoracic injury)
- Incomplete quadriplegia (incomplete cervical injury)
- Complete quadriplegia (complete cervical injury)

It is important to assess for any sign of preservation of function of the long tracts of the spinal cord. Any motor or sensory function below the level of the injury constitutes an incomplete injury. Signs of an incomplete injury include any sensation (including position sense) or voluntary movement in the lower extremities, sacral sparing, voluntary anal sphincter contraction, and voluntary toe flexion. Sacral reflexes, such as the bulbocavernosus reflex or anal wink, do not qualify as sacral sparing.

SPINAL CORD SYNDROMES

Certain characteristic patterns of neurologic injury are frequently encountered in patients with spinal cord injuries, such as central cord syndrome, anterior cord syndrome, and Brown-Séquard syndrome. These patterns should be recognized so they do not confuse the examiner.

Central cord syndrome is characterized by a disproportionately greater loss of motor strength in the upper extremities than in the lower extremities, with varying degrees of sensory loss. Usually this syndrome occurs after a hyperextension injury in a patient with preexisting cervical canal stenosis (often due to degenerative osteoarthritic changes), and the history is commonly that of a forward fall that resulted in a facial impact. Central cord syndrome is thought to be due to vascular compromise of the cord in the distribution of the anterior spinal artery. This artery supplies the central portions of the cord. Because the motor fibers to the cervical segments are topographically arranged toward the center of the cord, the arms and hands are the most severely affected.

Central cord syndrome may occur with or without cervical spine fracture or dislocation. Recovery usually follows a characteristic pattern, with the lower extremities recovering strength first, bladder function next, and the proximal upper extremities and hands last. The prognosis for recovery in central cord injuries is somewhat better than with other incomplete injuries.

Anterior cord syndrome is characterized by paraplegia and a dissociated sensory loss with a loss of pain and temperature sensation. Dorsal column function (position, vibration, and deep pressure sense) is preserved. Usually, anterior cord syndrome is due to infarction of the cord in the territory supplied by the anterior spinal artery. This syndrome has the poorest prognosis of the incomplete injuries.

Brown-Séquard syndrome results from hemisection of the cord, usually as a result of a penetrating trauma. Although this syndrome is rarely seen, variations on the classic picture are not uncommon. In its pure form, the syndrome consists of ipsilateral motor loss (corticospinal tract) and loss of position sense (dorsal column), associated with contralateral loss of pain and temperature sensation beginning one to two levels below the level of injury (spinothalamic tract). Even when the syndrome is caused by a direct penetrating injury to the cord, some recovery is usually seen.

MORPHOLOGY

Spinal injuries can be described as fractures, fracture-dislocations, spinal cord injury without radiographic abnormalities (SCIWORA), and penetrating injuries. Each of these categories may be further described as stable or unstable. However, determining the stability of a particular type of injury is not always simple and, indeed, even experts may disagree. **Therefore, especially in the initial treatment, all patients with radiographic evidence of injury and all those with neurologic deficits should be considered to have an unstable spinal injury.** These patients should be immobilized until after consultation with an appropriately qualified doctor, usually a neurosurgeon or orthopedic surgeon.

Specific Types of Spinal Injuries

Cervical spine injuries can result from one or a combination of the following mechanisms of injury:

- Axial loading

- Flexion

- Extension

- Rotation

- Lateral bending

- Distraction

The injuries identified in this chapter all involve the spinal column. They are listed in anatomic sequence (not in order of frequency), progressing from the cranial to the caudal end of the spine. Of note, upper cervical spine injuries in children (C1–C4) are almost twice as common as lower cervical spine injuries.

ATLANTO-OCCIPITAL DISLOCATION

Craniocervical disruption injuries are uncommon and result from severe traumatic flexion and distraction. Most patients with this injury die of brainstem destruction and apnea or have profound neurologic impairments (e.g., are ventilator-dependent and quadriplegic). Patients may survive if prompt resuscitation is available at the injury scene. Atlanto-occipital dislocation may be identified in up to 19% of patients with fatal cervical spine injuries and is a common cause of death in cases of shaken baby syndrome in which the infant dies immediately after shaking. Spinal immobilization is recommended initially. Aids to the identification of atlanto-occipital dislocation on spine films, including Power's ratio, are included in Skill Station XI: X-Ray Identification of Spine Injuries.

ATLAS (C1) FRACTURE

The atlas is a thin, bony ring with broad articular surfaces. Fractures of the atlas represent approximately 5% of acute cervical spine fractures. Approximately 40% of atlas fractures are associated with fractures of the axis (C2). The most common C1 fracture is a burst fracture (Jefferson fracture). The usual mechanism of injury is axial loading, which occurs when a large load falls vertically on the head or a patient lands on the top of his or her head in a relatively neutral position. The Jefferson fracture involves disruption of both the anterior and posterior rings of C1 with lateral displacement of the lateral masses. The fracture is best seen on an open-mouth view of the C1 to C2 region and axial computed tomography (CT) scans (■ FIGURE 7-5).

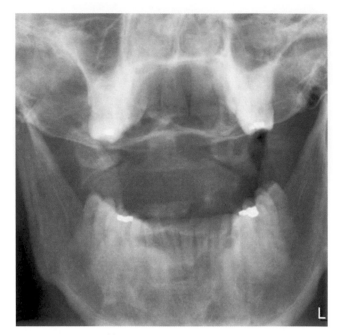

■ FIGURE 7-5 **Jefferson Fracture.** Open-mouth view radiograph showing a Jefferson fracture. This fracture involves disruption of both the anterior and posterior rings of C1 with lateral displacement of the lateral masses.

In patients with an atlas fracture who survive, the fractures usually are not associated with spinal cord injuries. However, they are unstable and should be initially treated with a cervical collar. Unilateral ring or lateral mass fractures are not uncommon and tend to be stable injuries. However, they are treated as unstable until the patient is examined by an appropriately qualified doctor, usually a neurosurgeon or orthopedic surgeon.

C1 ROTARY SUBLUXATION

C1 rotary subluxation injury is most often seen in children (■ FIGURE 7-6). It may occur spontaneously, after major or minor trauma, with an upper respiratory infection, or with rheumatoid arthritis. The patient presents with a persistent rotation of the head (torticollis). This injury is best diagnosed with an open-mouth odontoid view, although the x-ray findings may be confusing. In this injury, the odontoid is not equidistant from the two lateral masses of C1. The patient should not be forced to overcome the rotation, but should be immobilized in the rotated position and referred for further specialized treatment.

AXIS (C2) FRACTURES

The axis is the largest cervical vertebra and is the most unusual in shape. Therefore, it is susceptible to various fractures depending on the force and direction of

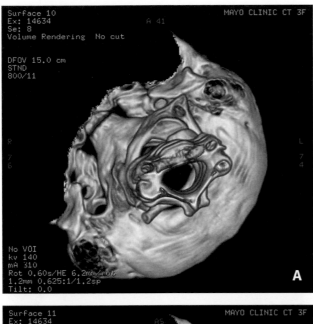

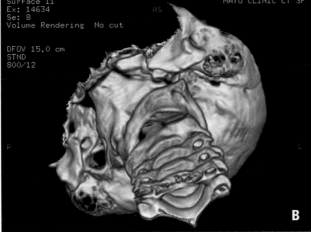

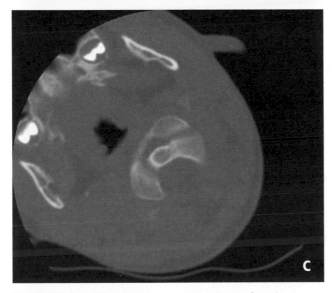

■ **FIGURE 7-6 (A)** 3-D CT reconstructions of patient with C1 rotary subluxation; **(B)** 3-D CT reconstructions of patient with C1 rotary subluxation; **(C)** Axial CT image of patient with C1 rotary subluxation.

the impact. Acute fractures of C2 represent approximately 18% of all cervical spine injuries.

Odontoid Fractures

Approximately 60% of C2 fractures involve the odontoid process, a peg-shaped bony protuberance that projects upward and is normally positioned in contact with the anterior arch of C1. The odontoid process is held in place primarily by the transverse ligament. Odontoid fractures are initially identified by a lateral cervical spine film or open-mouth odontoid views. However, a CT scan usually is required for further delineation. Type I odontoid fractures typically involve the tip of the odontoid and are relatively uncommon. Type II odontoid fractures occur through the base of the dens and are the most common odontoid fracture (■ FIGURE 7-7). In children younger than 6 years of age, the epiphysis may be prominent and may look like a fracture at this level. Type III odontoid fractures occur at the base of the dens and extend obliquely into the body of the axis.

Posterior Element Fractures

A hangman's fracture involves the posterior elements of C2—that is, the pars interarticularis (■ FIGURE 7-8). This type of fracture represents approximately 20% of all axis fractures and usually is caused by an extension-type injury. Patients with this fracture should be maintained in external immobilization until specialized care is available.

Variations of a hangman's fracture include bilateral fractures through the lateral masses or pedicles.

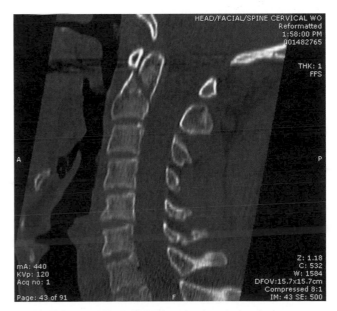

■ **FIGURE 7-7 Odontoid Fracture.** CT view of a Type II odontoid fracture, which occurs through the base of the dens.

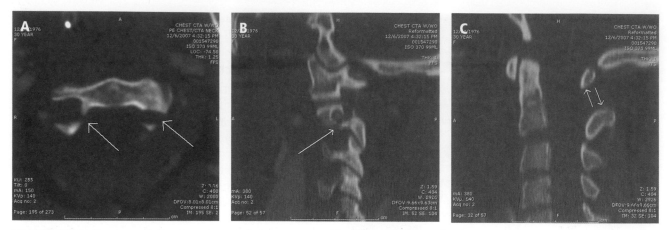

■ **FIGURE 7-8 Hangman's Fracture** (arrows) demonstrated in **(A)** axial; **(B)** sagittal paramedian; and **(C)** sagittal midline CT reconstructions. Note the anterior angulation and excessive distance between the spinous processes of C1 and C2 (double arrows).

Other C2 Fractures

Approximately 20% of all axis fractures are nonodontoid and nonhangman's. These include fractures through the body, pedicle, lateral mass, laminae, and spinous process.

FRACTURES AND DISLOCATIONS (C3 THROUGH C7)

A fracture of C3 is very uncommon, possibly because it is positioned between the more vulnerable axis and the more mobile "relative fulcrum" of the cervical spine—that is, C5 and C6, where the greatest flexion and extension of the cervical spine occur. In adults, the most common level of cervical vertebral fracture is C5, and the most common level of subluxation is C5 on C6. The most common injury patterns identified at these levels are vertebral body fractures with or without subluxation; subluxation of the articular processes (including unilateral or bilateral locked facets); and fractures of the laminae, spinous processes, pedicles, or lateral masses. Rarely, ligamentous disruption occurs without fractures or facet dislocations.

The incidence of neurologic injury increases dramatically with facet dislocations. In the presence of unilateral facet dislocation, 80% of patients have a neurologic injury; approximately 30% have root injuries only, 40% incomplete spinal cord injuries, and 30% complete spinal cord injuries. In the presence of bilateral locked facets, the morbidity is much worse, with 16% incomplete and 84% complete spinal cord injuries.

THORACIC SPINE FRACTURES (T1 THROUGH T10)

Thoracic spine fractures may be classified into four broad categories:

- Anterior wedge compression injuries
- Burst injuries
- Chance fractures
- Fracture-dislocations

Axial loading with flexion produces an *anterior wedge compression injury*. The amount of wedging usually is quite small, and the anterior portion of the vertebral body rarely is more than 25% shorter than the posterior body. Because of the rigidity of the rib cage, most of these fractures are stable.

Burst injury is caused by vertical-axial compression.

Chance fractures are transverse fractures through the vertebral body (■ **FIGURE 7-9**). They are caused by

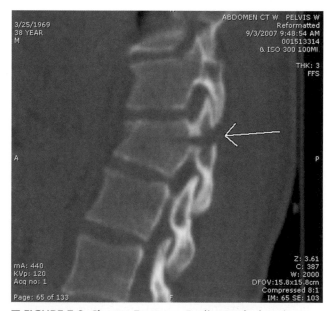

■ **FIGURE 7-9 Chance Fracture.** Radiograph showing a Chance fracture, which is a transverse fracture through the vertebral body.

flexion about an axis anterior to the vertebral column and are most frequently seen following motor vehicle crashes in which the patient was restrained by only a lap belt. Chance fractures may be associated with retroperitoneal and abdominal visceral injuries.

Fracture-dislocations are relatively uncommon in the thoracic and lumbar spine because of the orientation of the facet joints. These injuries almost always are due to extreme flexion or severe blunt trauma to the spine, which causes disruption of the posterior elements (pedicles, facets, and lamina) of the vertebra. The thoracic spinal canal is narrow in relation to the spinal cord, so fracture subluxations in the thoracic spine commonly result in complete neurologic deficits.

Simple compression fractures are usually stable and often treated with a rigid brace. Burst fractures, Chance fractures, and fracture-dislocations are extremely unstable and almost always require internal fixation.

THORACOLUMBAR JUNCTION FRACTURES (T11 THROUGH L1)

Fractures at the level of the thoracolumbar junction are due to the relative immobility of the thoracic spine as compared with the lumbar spine. They most often result from a combination of acute hyperflexion and rotation, and, consequently, they are usually unstable. People who fall from a height and restrained drivers who sustain severe flexion energy transfer are at particular risk for this type of injury.

The spinal cord terminates as the conus medullaris at approximately the level of L1, and injury to this part of the cord commonly results in bladder and bowel dysfunction, as well as in decreased sensation and strength in the lower extremities. **Patients with thoracolumbar fractures are particularly vulnerable to rotational movement. Therefore, logrolling should be performed with extreme care.**

LUMBAR FRACTURES

The radiographic signs associated with a lumbar fracture are similar to those of thoracic and thoracolumbar fractures. However, because only the cauda equina is involved, the probability of a complete neurologic deficit is much less with these injuries.

PENETRATING INJURIES

The most common types of penetrating injuries are those caused by gunshot wounds or stabbings. It is important to determine the path of the bullet or knife. This can be done by analyzing information from the history, clinical examination (entry and exit sites),

plain x-ray films, and CT scans. If the path of injury passes directly through the vertebral canal, a complete neurologic deficit usually results. Complete deficits also may result from energy transfer associated with a high-velocity missile (e.g., bullet) passing close to the spinal cord rather than through it. Penetrating injuries of the spine usually are stable injuries unless the missile destroys a large portion of the vertebra.

BLUNT CAROTID AND VERTEBRAL VASCULAR INJURIES

Blunt trauma to the head and neck is a risk factor for carotid and vertebral arterial injuries. Early recognition and treatment of these injuries may reduce the risk of stroke. Indications for screening are evolving, but suggested criteria for screening include:

- C1–C3 fracture
- Cervical spine fracture with subluxation
- Fractures involving the foramen transversarium

Approximately one-third of these patients will be shown to have blunt carotid and vertebral vascular injury (BCVI) on CT angiography of the neck (■ FIGURE 7-10). The treatment of these injuries is evolving, with either anticoagulation or antiplatelet therapy currently recommended in patients without contraindications.

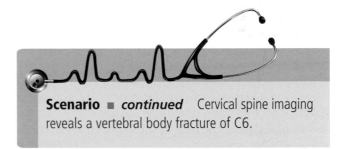

Scenario ■ *continued*   Cervical spine imaging reveals a vertebral body fracture of C6.

X-Ray Evaluation

? *How do I confirm the presence or absence of a significant spine injury?*

Both careful clinical examination and thorough radiographic assessment are critical in identifying significant spine injury. See <u>Skill Station XI: X-Ray Identification of Spine Injuries</u>.

CERVICAL SPINE

Cervical spine radiography is indicated for all trauma patients who have midline neck pain, tenderness on

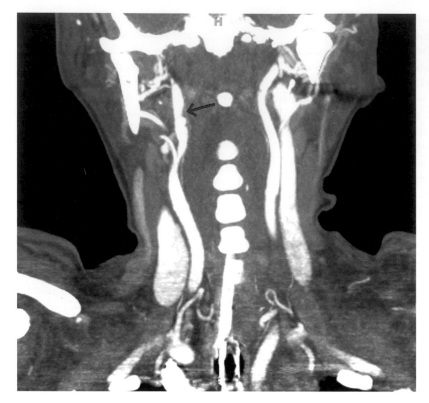

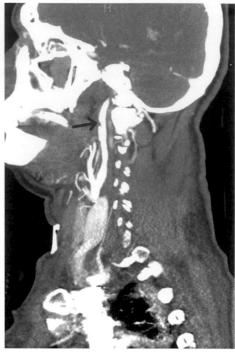

■ **FIGURE 7-10** Neck CT angiogram with a Grade II carotid injury (arrows).

palpation, neurologic deficits referable to the cervical spine, an altered level of consciousness, or a significant mechanism with a distracting injury or in whom intoxication is suspected. Two options for x-ray evaluation exist. In locations with available technology, the primary screening modality is multi-detector axial CT from the occiput to T1 with sagittal and coronal reconstructions. Where this is not available, plain films consisting of lateral, anteroposterior (AP), and open-mouth odontoid views should be obtained.

In plain films, the base of the skull, all seven cervical vertebrae, and the first thoracic vertebra must be visualized on the lateral view. The patient's shoulders may need to be pulled down when obtaining the lateral cervical spine x-ray film to avoid missing fractures or fracture-dislocations in the lower cervical spine. If all seven cervical vertebrae are not visualized on the lateral x-ray film, a swimmer's view of the lower cervical and upper thoracic area should be obtained.

The open-mouth odontoid view should include the entire odontoid process and the right and left C1, C2 articulations. The AP view of the c-spine assists in the identification of a unilateral facet dislocation in cases in which little or no dislocation is identified on the lateral film. Thin-cut axial CT scans should also be obtained through suspicious areas identified on the plain films or through the lower cervical spine if it is not adequately visualized on the plain films. Axial CT images through C1 and C2 may also be more sensi-

tive than plain films for detection of fractures of these vertebrae.

When these films are of good quality and are properly interpreted, unstable cervical spine injuries can be detected with a sensitivity of greater than 97%. **The complete series of cervical spine radiographs must be reviewed by a doctor experienced in the proper interpretation of these films before the spine is considered normal and the cervical collar is removed. CT scans may be used in lieu of plain images to evaluate the cervical spine.**

It is possible for patients to have a purely ligamentous spine injury that results in instability without associated fracture. However, some studies suggest that, if plain three-view cervical spine radiographs or CT films are truly normal (i.e., no anterior soft-tissue swelling and no abnormal angulation), significant instability is unlikely. Patients with neck pain and normal films may be evaluated by magnetic resonance imaging (MRI) or flexion-extension x-ray films, or treated with a semirigid cervical collar for 2–3 weeks with subsequent repeat examination and imaging if necessary. Flexion-extension x-ray films of the cervical spine may detect occult instability or determine the stability of a known fracture, such as a laminar or compression fracture. **Under no circumstances should the patient's neck be forced into a position that elicits pain. All movements must be voluntary. These films should be obtained under the direct supervision and control of a doctor experienced in the interpretation of such films.**

In some patients with significant soft-tissue injury, paraspinal muscle spasm may severely limit the degree of flexion and extension that the patient allows. In such cases, the patient is treated with a semirigid cervical collar for 2 to 3 weeks before another attempt is made to obtain flexion-extension views. MRI appears to be most sensitive for soft tissue injury if done within 72 hours of injury. However, data regarding correlation of cervical spine instability with positive MRI findings are lacking.

Approximately 10% of patients with a cervical spine fracture have a second, noncontiguous vertebral column fracture. This warrants a complete radiographic screening of the entire spine in patients with a cervical spine fracture. Such screening also is advisable in all comatose trauma patients.

In the presence of neurologic deficits, MRI is recommended to detect any soft tissue compressive lesion, such as a spinal epidural hematoma or traumatized herniated disk, that cannot be detected with plain films. MRI may also detect spinal cord contusions or disruption, and paraspinal ligamentous and soft tissue injury. However, MRI is frequently not feasible in patients with hemodynamic instability. When MRI is not available or appropriate, CT myelography may be used to exclude the presence of acute spinal cord compression caused by a traumatic herniated disk or epidural hematoma. These specialized studies usually are performed at the discretion of a spine surgery consultant. Box 7-1 presents guidelines for screening trauma patients with suspected spine injury.

THORACIC AND LUMBAR SPINE

The indications for screening radiography of the thoracic and lumbar spine are the same as those for the cervical spine. Where available, CT scanning of the thoracic and lumbar spine can be used as the initial screening modality. AP and lateral plain radiographs with thin-cut axial CT scans through suspicious areas can detect more than 99% of unstable injuries. On the AP views, the vertical alignment of the pedicles and distance between the pedicles of each thoracic and lumbar vertebra should be observed. Unstable fractures commonly cause widening of the interpedicular distance. The lateral films detect subluxations, compression fractures, and Chance fractures. CT scanning is particularly useful for detecting fractures of the posterior elements (pedicles, lamina, and spinous processes) and determining the degree of canal compromise caused by burst fractures. Sagittal reconstructions of axial CT images or plain tomography may be needed to adequately characterize Chance fractures. **As with the cervical spine, a complete series of good quality radiographs must be properly inter-**preted as normal by an experienced doctor before spine precautions are discontinued. However, due to the possibility of pressure ulcers, removal of the patient from a long board should NOT wait for final radiographic interpretation.

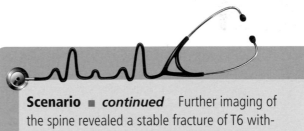

Scenario ■ *continued*   Further imaging of the spine revealed a stable fracture of T6 without other bony injury. Imaging of the abdomen revealed a Grade II splenic injury.

General Management

? *How do I treat patients with spinal cord injury and limit secondary injury?*

General management of spine and spinal cord trauma includes immobilization, intravenous fluids, medications, and transfer, if appropriate. See Skill Station XII: Spinal Cord Injury: Assessment and Management.

IMMOBILIZATION

? *How do I protect the spine during evaluation, management, and transport?*

Prehospital care personnel usually immobilize patients before their transport to the ED. Any patient with a suspected spine injury should be immobilized above and below the suspected injury site until a fracture is excluded by x-ray examination. Remember, spinal protection should be maintained until a cervical spine injury is excluded. Proper immobilization is achieved

Box 7-1 Guidelines for Screening Patients with Suspected Spine Injury

Suspected Cervical Spine Injury

1. **The presence of paraplegia or quadriplegia is presumptive evidence of spinal instability.**

2. *Patients who are awake, alert, sober, and neurologically normal, and have no neck pain or midline tenderness, or a distracting injury:* These patients are extremely unlikely to have an acute c-spine fracture or instability. With the patient in a supine position, remove the c-collar and palpate the spine. If there is no significant tenderness, ask the patient to voluntarily move his or her neck from side to side. **Never force the patient's neck.** When performed voluntarily by the patient, these maneuvers are generally safe. If there is no pain, have the patient voluntarily flex and extend his or her neck. Again, if there is no pain, c-spine films are not necessary.

3. *Patients who are awake and alert, neurologically normal, cooperative, and do not have a distracting injury and are able to concentrate on their spine, but do have neck pain or midline tenderness:* The burden of proof is on the clinician to exclude a spinal injury. Where available, all such patients should undergo multi-detector axial CT from the occiput to T1 with sagittal and coronal reconstructions. Where not available, patients should undergo lateral, AP, and open-mouth odontoid x-ray examinations of the c-spine with axial CT images of suspicious areas or of the lower cervical spine if not adequately visualized on the plain films. Assess the c-spine films for:

   - bony deformity
   - fracture of the vertebral body or processes
   - loss of alignment of the posterior aspect of the vertebral bodies (anterior extent of the vertebral canal)
   - increased distance between the spinous processes at one level
   - narrowing of the vertebral canal
   - increased prevertebral soft tissue space

   If these films are normal, remove the c-collar. Under the care of a knowledgeable clinician, obtain flexion and extension, and lateral cervical spine films with the patient voluntarily flexing and extending his or her neck. If the films show no subluxation, the patient's c-spine can be cleared and the

c-collar removed. However, if any of these films are suspicious or unclear, replace the collar and obtain consultation from a spine specialist.

4. *Patients who have an altered level of consciousness or are too young to describe their symptoms:* Where available, all such patients should undergo multi-detector axial CT from the occiput to T1 with sagittal and coronal reconstructions. Where not available, all such patients should undergo lateral, AP, and open-mouth odontoid films with CT supplementation through suspicious areas (e.g., C1 and C2, and through the lower cervical spine if areas are not adequately visualized on the plain films). In children, CT supplementation is optional. If the entire c-spine can be visualized and is found to be normal, the collar can be removed after appropriate evaluation by a doctor/consultant skilled in the evaluation/management of patients with spine injuries. Clearance of the c-spine is particularly important if pulmonary or other care of the patient is compromised by the inability to mobilize the patient.

5. **When in doubt, leave the collar on.**

6. *Consult:* Doctors who are skilled in the evaluation and management of patients with spine injuries should be consulted in all cases in which a spine injury is detected or suspected.

7. *Backboards:* Patients who have neurologic deficits (e.g., quadriplegia or paraplegia) should be evaluated quickly and removed from the backboard as soon as possible. **A paralyzed patient who is allowed to lie on a hard board for more than 2 hours is at high risk for pressure ulcers.**

8. *Emergency situations:* Trauma patients who require emergency surgery before a complete workup of the spine can be accomplished should be transported carefully, assuming that an unstable spine injury is present. The c-collar should be left on and the patient logrolled when moved to and from the operating table. The patient should not be left on a rigid backboard during surgery. The surgical team should take particular care to protect the neck as much as possible during the operation. The anesthesiologist should be informed of the status of the workup.

(continued)

Box 7-1 (continued)

Suspected Thoracolumbar Spine Injury

1. **The presence of paraplegia or a level of sensory loss on the chest or abdomen is presumptive evidence of spinal instability.**

2. *Patients who are awake, alert, sober, neurologically normal, and have no midline thoracic or lumbar back pain or tenderness:* The entire extent of the spine should be palpated and inspected. If there is no tenderness on palpation or ecchymosis over the spinous processes, an unstable spine fracture is unlikely, and thoracolumbar radiographs may not be necessary.

3. *Patients who have spine pain or tenderness on palpation, neurologic deficits, an altered level of consciousness, or in whom intoxication is suspected:* AP and lateral radiographs of the entire thoracic and lumbar spine should be obtained. Thin-cut axial CT should be obtained through suspicious areas identified on the plain films. **All images must be of good quality and interpreted as normal by an experienced doctor before discontinuing spine precautions.**

4. Consult a doctor skilled in the evaluation and management of spine injuries if a spine injury is detected or suspected.

---

with the patient in the neutral position—that is, supine without rotating or bending the spinal column.

No effort should be made to reduce an obvious deformity. Children may have torticollis, and the elderly may have severe degenerative spine disease that causes them to have a nontraumatic kyphotic or angulation deformity of the spine. Such patients should be immobilized on a backboard in a position of comfort. Supplemental padding is often necessary. **Attempts to align the spine for the purpose of immobilization on the backboard are not recommended if they cause pain.**

Immobilization of the neck with a semirigid collar does not ensure complete stabilization of the cervical spine. Immobilization using a spine board with appropriate bolstering devices is more effective in limiting certain neck motions. The use of long spine boards is recommended. **Cervical spine injury requires continuous immobilization of the entire patient with a semirigid cervical collar, head immobilization, backboard, tape, and straps before and during transfer to a definitive-care facility** (■ FIGURE 7-11). Extension and flexion of the neck should be avoided because these movements are the most dangerous to the spinal cord. The airway is of critical importance in patients with spinal cord injury, and early intubation should be accomplished if there is evidence of respiratory compromise. During intubation, the neck must be maintained in a neutral position.

Of special concern is the maintenance of adequate immobilization of restless, agitated, or violent patients. Such behavior can be due to pain, confusion associated with hypoxia or hypotension, alcohol or drug use, or a personality disorder. The clinician should search for and correct the cause of the behavior, if possible.

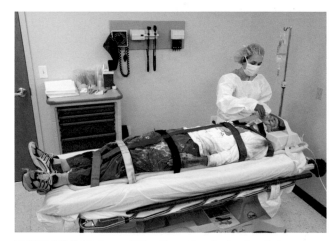

■ **FIGURE 7-11 Immobilization.** Cervical spine injury requires continuous immobilization of the entire patient with a semi-rigid cervical collar, head immobilization, backboard, tape, and straps before and after transfer to a definitive-care facility.

If necessary, a sedative or paralytic agent may be administered, while ensuring adequate airway protection, control, and ventilation. The use of sedatives or paralytic agents in this setting requires considerable clinical judgment, skill, and experience. The use of short-acting, reversible agents is advised.

Once the patient arrives at the ED, every effort should be made to remove the rigid spine board as early as possible to reduce the risk of pressure ulcer formation. Removal of the board is often done as part of the secondary survey when the patient is logrolled for inspection and palpation of the back. It should not be delayed solely for the purpose of obtaining definitive spine radiographs, particularly if radiographic evaluation may not be completed for several hours.

The safe movement, or logrolling, of a patient with an unstable or potentially unstable spine requires planning and the assistance of four or more individuals, depending on the size of the patient (■ FIGURE 7-12). Neutral anatomic alignment of the entire vertebral column must be maintained while rolling and lifting the patient. One person is assigned to maintain in-line immobilization of the head and neck. Other individuals positioned on the same side of the patient's torso manually prevent segmental rotation, flexion, extension, lateral bending, or sagging of the chest or abdomen during transfer of the patient. Another individual is responsible for moving the legs and removing the spine board and examining the patient's back.

PITFALL

Patients being transported to a trauma center may have unrecognized spinal injuries. Such patients should be maintained in complete spinal immobilization.

INTRAVENOUS FLUIDS

In patients in whom spine injury is suspected, intravenous fluids are administered as they would usually be for resuscitation of trauma patients. If active hemorrhage is not detected or suspected, persistent hypotension should raise the suspicion of neurogenic shock. Patients with hypovolemic shock usually have tachycardia, whereas those with neurogenic shock classically have bradycardia. If the blood pressure does

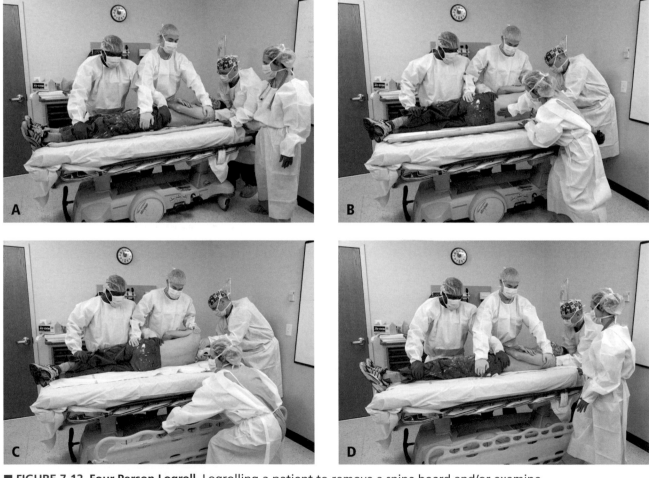

■ FIGURE 7-12 Four-Person Logroll. Logrolling a patient to remove a spine board and/or examine the back should be accomplished using at least four people. **(A)** One person stands at the patient's head to control the head and c-spine, and two are along the patient's sides to control the body and extremities. **(B)** As the patient is rolled, three people maintain alignment of the spine, while **(C)** the fourth person removes the board and examines the back. **(D)** Once the board is removed, the patient is returned to the supine position, while maintaining alignment of the spine.

not improve after a fluid challenge, the judicious use of vasopressors may be indicated. Phenylephrine hydrochloride, dopamine, or norepinephrine is recommended. Overzealous fluid administration may cause pulmonary edema in patients with neurogenic shock. When the fluid status is uncertain, the use of invasive monitoring may be helpful. A urinary catheter is inserted to monitor urinary output and prevent bladder distention.

MEDICATIONS

At present, there is insufficient evidence to support the routine use of steroids in spinal cord injury.

TRANSFER

Patients with spine fractures or neurologic deficit should be transferred to a definitive-care facility. The safest procedure is to transfer the patient after telephone consultation with a spine specialist. Avoid unnecessary delay. Stabilize the patient and apply the necessary splints, backboard, and/or semirigid cervical collar. **Remember, cervical spine injuries above C6 can result in partial or total loss of respiratory function.** If there is any concern about the adequacy of ventilation, the patient should be intubated prior to transfer.

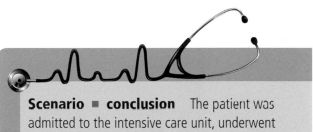

Scenario ▪ conclusion   The patient was admitted to the intensive care unit, underwent fixation of his cervical spine, and was ultimately transferred to a spinal cord rehabilitation center.

Chapter Summary

1 The spinal column consists of cervical, thoracic, and lumbar vertebrae. The spinal cord contains three important tracts: the corticospinal tract, the spinothalamic tract, and the dorsal columns.

2 Obtain images, when indicated, as soon as life-threatening injuries are managed. Document the patient's history and physical examination so as to establish a baseline for any changes in the patient's neurologic status.

3 Spinal cord injuries may be complete or incomplete and may involve any level of the spinal cord.

4 Attend to life-threatening injuries first, minimizing movement of the spinal column. Establish and maintain proper immobilization of the patient until vertebral fractures and spinal cord injuries have been excluded. Obtain early consultation with a neurosurgeon and/or orthopedic surgeon whenever a spinal injury is suspected or detected.

5 Transfer patients with vertebral fractures or spinal cord injuries to a definitive-care facility.

BIBLIOGRAPHY

1. Bach CM, Steingruber IE, Peer S, et al. Radiographic evaluation of cervical spine trauma. Plain radiography and conventional tomography versus computed tomography. *Arch Orthop Trauma Surg* 2001;121(7):385-387.

2. Bachulis BL, Long WI, Hynes GD, et al. Clinical indications for cervical spine radiographs in the traumatized patient. *Am J Surg* 1987;153:473-477.

3. Berne JD, Reuland KS, Villarreal DH, et al. Sixteen-slice multi-detector computed tomographic angiography improves the accuracy of screening for blunt cerebrovascular injury. *J Trauma* 2006;60(6):1204-1209; discussion 1209-1210.

4. Biffl WL, Egglin T, Benedetto B, et al. Sixteen-slice computed tomographic angiography is a reliable noninvasive screening test for clinically significant blunt cerebrovascular injuries. *J Trauma* 2006;60(4):745-751; discussion 751-752.

5. Bracken MB, Shepard MJ, Collins WF, et al. A randomized, controlled trial of methylprednisolone or naloxone in the treatment of spinal cord injury: results of the second National Spinal Cord Injury Study. *N Engl J Med* 1990;322:1405-1411.

6. Bracken MB, Shepard MJ, Holford TR, et al. Methylprednisolone or tirlazad mesylate administration after acute spinal cord injury: 1-year follow up: results of the third national Acute Spinal Cord Injury Randomized Controlled Trial. *J Neurosurg* 1998;89:699-706.

7. Brown CV, Antevil JL, Sise MJ, et al. Spiral computed tomography for the diagnosis of cervical, thoracic, and lumbar spine fractures: its time has come. *J Trauma* 2005;58(5):890-895; discussion 895-896.

8. Coleman WP, Benzel D, Cahill DW, et al. A critical appraisal of the reporting of the National Acute Spinal Cord Injury Studies (II and III) of methylprednisolone in acute spinal cord injury. *J Spinal Disord* 2000;13(3):185-199.

9. Como J, et al. Practice management guidelines for identification of cervical spine injuries following trauma: update from the Eastern Association for the Surgery of Trauma Practice Management Guidelines Committee. *J Trauma* 2009;67:651-659.

10. Cooper C, Dunham CM, Rodriguez A. Falls and major injuries are risk factors for thoracolumbar fractures: cognitive impairment and multiple injuries impede the detection of back pain and tenderness. *J Trauma* 1995;38:692-696.

11. Cothren CC, Biffl WL, Moore EE, et al. Treatment for blunt cerebrovascular injuries: equivalence of anticoagulation and antiplatelet agents. *Arch Surg* 2009;144(7):685-90.

12. Cothren CC, Moore EE, Biffl WL, et al. Anticoagulation is the gold standard therapy for blunt carotid injuries to reduce stroke rate. *Arch Surg* 2004;139(5):540-545; discussion 545-546.

13. Cothren CC, Moore EE, Ray CE, et al. Cervical spine fracture patterns mandating screening to rule out blunt cerebrovascular injury. *Surgery* 2007;141(1):76-82.

14. Daffner RH, Sciulli RL, Rodriguez A, et al. Imaging for evaluation of suspected cervical spine trauma: a 2-year analysis. *Injury* 2006;37(7):652-658.

15. Dziurzynski K, Anderson PA, Bean DB, et al. A blinded assessment of radiographic criteria for atlanto-occipital dislocation. *Spine* 2005;30(12):1427-1432.

16. Eastman AL, Chason DP, Perez CL, et al. Computed tomographic angiography for the diagnosis of blunt cervical vascular injury: is it ready for primetime? *J Trauma* 2006;60(5):925-929; discussion 929.

17. Ghanta MK, Smith LM, Polin RS, et al. An analysis of Eastern Association for the Surgery of Trauma practice guidelines for cervical spine evaluation in a series of patients with multiple imaging techniques. *Am Surg* 2002;68(6):563-567; discussion 567-568.

18. Goodwin RB, Beery PR II, Dorbish RJ, et al. Computed tomographic angiography versus conventional angiography for the diagnosis of blunt cerebrovascular injury in trauma patients. *J Trauma* 2009;67(5):1046-50.

19. Grogan EL, Morris JA, Dittus RS, et al. Cervical spine evaluation in urban trauma centers: lowering institutional costs and complications through helical CT scan. *J Am Coll Surg* 2005;200(2):160-165.

20. Guly HR, Bouamra O, Lecky FE, The incidence of neurogenic shock in patients with isolated spinal cord injury in the emergency department. *Resuscitation* 2008;76:57-62.

21. Harris JH, Carson GC, Wagner LK, et al. Radiologic diagnosis of traumatic occipitovertebral dissociation: 2. Comparison of three methods of detecting occipitovertebral relationships on lateral radiographs of supine subjects. *AJR Am J Roentgenol* 1994;162(4):887-892.

22. Hoffman JR, Mower WR, Wolfson AB, et al. Validity of a set of clinical criteria to rule out injury to the cervical spine in patients with blunt trauma, *N Eng J Med* 2000;343:94-99.

23. Holmes JF, Akkinepalli R. Computed tomography versus plain radiography to screen for cervical spine injury: a meta-analysis. *J Trauma* 2005;58(5):902-905.

24. Hurlbert RJ. Strategies of medical intervention in the management of acute spinal cord injury. *Spine* 2006;31(11 Suppl):S16-S21; discussion S36.

25. Hurlbert RJ. The role of steroids in acute spinal cord injury: an evidence-based analysis. *Spine* 2001;26(24 Suppl):S39-S46.

26. *International Standards for Neurological and Functional Classification of Spinal Cord Injury*. Atlanta, GA: American Spinal Injury Association and International Medical Society of Paraplegia (ASIA/IMSOP);1996.

27. Krassioukov AV, Karlsson AK, Wecht JM, et al. Assessment of autonomic dysfunction following spinal cord injury: rationale for additions to International Standards for Neurological Assessment. *J Rehabil Res Dev* 2007;44:103-112.

28. Marion DW, Pryzybylski G. Injury to the vertebrae and spinal cord. In: Mattox KL, Feliciano DV, Moore EE, eds. *Trauma*. New York, NY: McGraw-Hill; 2000:451-471.

29. McGuire RA, Neville S, Green BA, et al. Spine instability and the log-rolling maneuver. *J Trauma* 1987;27:525-531.

30. Michael DB, Guyot DR, Darmody WR. Coincidence of head and cervical spine injury. *J Neurotrauma* 1989;6:177-189.

31. Mower WR, Hoffman JR, Pollack CV, et al. Use of plain radiography to screen for cervical spine injuries. *Ann Emerg Med* 2001;38(1):1-7.

32. Patel JC, Tepas JJ, Mollitt DL, et al. Pediatric cervical spine injuries: defining the disease. *J Pediatr Surg* 2001;36:373-376.

33. Peretti-Vanmarcke R, et al. Clinical clearance of the cervical spine in blunt trauma patients younger than 3 years: a multi-center study of the American Association for the Surgery of Trauma. *J Trauma* 2009 67:543-550.

34. Sanchez B, Waxman K, Jones T, et al. Cervical spine clearance in blunt trauma: evaluation of a computed tomography-based protocol. *J Trauma* 2005;59(1):179-183.

35. Sayer FT, Kronvall E, Nilsson OG. Methylprednisolone treatment in acute spinal cord injury: the myth challenged through a structured analysis of published literature. *Spine J* 2006;6(3):335-343.

36. Schenarts PJ, Diaz J, Kaiser C, et al. Prospective comparison of admission computed tomographic scan and plain films of the upper cervical spine in trauma patients with altered mental status. *J Trauma* 2001;51(4):663-668; discussion 668-669.

37. Short DJ, El MWS, Jones PW. High dose methylprednisolone in the management of acute spinal cord injury—a systematic review from a clinical perspective. *Spinal Cord* 2000;38(5):273-286.

38. Stein DM, Boswell S, Sliker CW, et al. Blunt cerebrovascular injuries: does treatment always matter? *J Trauma* 2009;66(1):132-42; discussion 143-4.

39. Stiell IG, Clement CM, Grimshaw J, et. al, Implementation of the Canadian C-Spine Rule: prospective 12 centre cluster randomised trial. *BMJ* 2009,339:b4146.

40. Stiell IG, Wells GA, Vandemheen KL, et al. The Canadian C-Spine rule of radiography in alert and stable trauma patients. *JAMA* 2001;286:1841-8.

41. Tator CH, Fehlings MG. Review of the secondary injury theory of acute spinal cord trauma with special emphasis on vascular mechanisms. *J Neurosurg* 1991;75:15-26.

42. Vicellio P, Simon H, Pressman B, et al. A prospective multicenter study of cervical spine injury in children. *Pediatrics* 2001;108(2).

X-Ray Identification of Spine Injuries

▶▶ INTERACTIVE SKILL PROCEDURES

Note: This Skill Station includes a systematic method for evaluating spine x-ray films. A series of x-rays with related scenarios is shown to students for their evaluation and management decisions based on the findings. Standard precautions are required whenever caring for trauma patients.

THE FOLLOWING PROCEDURES ARE INCLUDED IN THIS SKILL STATION:

▶▶ **Skill XI-A:** Cervical Spine X-Ray Assessment

▶▶ **Skill XI-B:** Atlanto-Occipital Joint Assessment

▶▶ **Skill XI-C:** Thoracic and Lumbar X-Ray Assessment

▶▶ **Skill XI-D:** Review Spine X-Rays

Objectives

Performance at this skill station will allow the participant to:

1 Identify various spine injuries by using specific anatomic guidelines for examining a series of spine x-rays.

2 Given a series of spine x-rays and scenarios:
- Define limitations of examination.
- Diagnose fractures.
- Delineate associated injuries.
- Identify other areas of possible injury.

▶ SCENARIOS

PATIENT XI-1

28-year-old male fell while mountain biking. No neurologic deficit.

PATIENT XI-2

54-year-old male hit a tree while driving his car. Symptoms are only slight discomfort of his neck and some numbness in his digit V, left side.

PATIENT XI-3

8-year-old child fell down the stairs and is crying. No neurologic deficit.

PATIENT XI-4

62-year-old male hit an abutment while driving his car. There is no neurologic deficit, the patient is unable to actively move his neck because of pain.

PATIENT XI-5

19-year-old female with head and neck trauma as the result of an assault.

PATIENT XI-6

22-year-old male struck a tree while riding his motorcycle. No neurologic deficit.

PATIENT XI-7

44-year-old male; box fell on head. Painful neck, no neurologic deficit.

PATIENT XI-8

45-year-old female attempted to hang herself. GCS score of 7.

PATIENT XI-9

30-year-old male in motor vehicle crash versus tree. Patient was restrained, but there was no airbag. GCS score of 15; neurologic exam intact; patient reports neck pain.

PATIENT XI-10

36-year-old male fell from a height greater than 3 meters and has back pain.

PATIENT XI-11

30-year-old male involved in motorcycle crash. On examination, he appears to have a sensory and motor deficit involving both legs. Deep-tendon reflexes are absent.

PATIENT XI-12

25-year-old female involved in motor vehicle crash. Patient was wearing a lap belt without shoulder harness. No neurologic deficit.

▶ Skill XI-A: Cervical Spine X-Ray Assessment

STEP 1. Assess adequacy and alignment (■ FIGURE XI-1).

    A. Identify the presence of all 7 cervical vertebrae and the superior aspect of T1.

    B. Identify the:
- Anterior vertebral line
- Anterior spinal line
- Posterior spinal line
- Spinous processes

STEP 2. Assess the bone (■ FIGURE XI-2).

    A. Examine all vertebrae for preservation of height and integrity of the bony cortex.

    B. Examine facets.

    C Examine spinous processes.

STEP 3. Assess the cartilage, including examining the cartilaginous disk spaces for narrowing or widening (see ■ FIGURE XI-2).

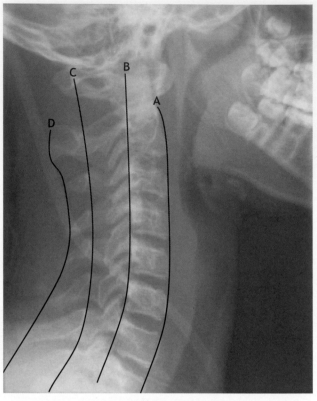

■ **FIGURE XI-1** Assess adequacy and alignment. Line A: Anterior vertebral line; Line B: Anterior spinal line; Line C: Posterior spinal line; Line D: Spinous processes.

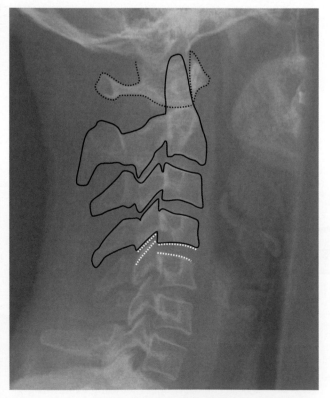

■ **FIGURE XI-2** Assess the bone (black lines), cartilage, and disk space (white dotted lines).

STEP 4. Assess the dens (■ FIGURE XI-3).

    A. Examine the outline of the dens.

    B. Examine the predental space (3 mm).

    C. Examine the clivus; it should point to the dens.

STEP 5. Assess the extraaxial soft tissues.

    A. Examine the extraaxial space and soft tissues
- 7 mm at C3
- 3 cm at C7

    B. Examine the distances between the spinous processes.

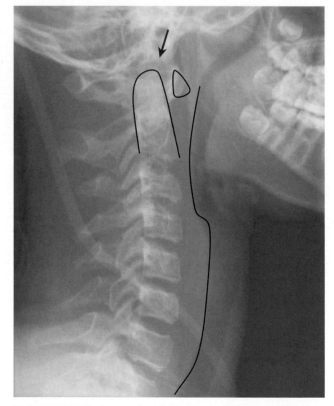

■ **FIGURE XI-3** Assess the dens.

▶ Skill XI-B: Atlanto-Occipital Joint Assessment

Detection of an atlanto-occipital dislocation can be challenging. One useful finding is a Power's ratio >1 (BC/OA, where BC is the distance from the basion [B] to the posterior arch [C] of C1, and OA is the distance from the anterior arch of C1 [A] to the opisthion [O, the posterior margin of the foramen magnum]). Wackenheim's line, drawn along the clivus, does not intersect the dens on a normal lateral cervical spine radiograph. If an atlanto-occipital injury is suspected, spinal immobilization should be preserved, and expert radiologic interpretation should be obtained. ■ FIGURE XI-4A shows a normal Power's ratio, and ■ FIGURE XI-4B shows an abnormal Power's ratio.

NORMAL   **C0-C1 INSTABILITY**

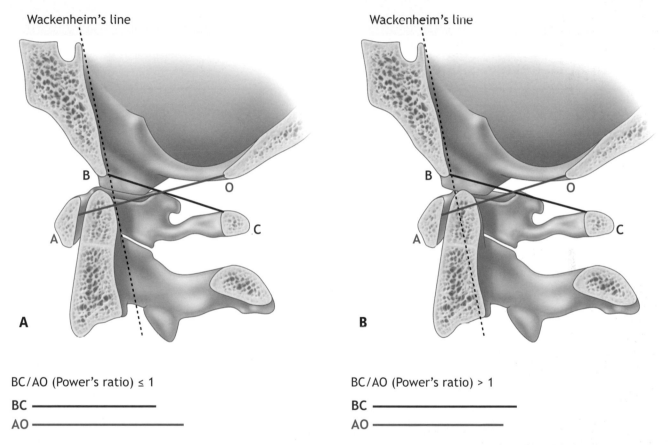

BC/AO (Power's ratio) ≤ 1   BC/AO (Power's ratio) > 1

BC ————————   BC ————————

AO —————————   AO —————————

■ **FIGURE XI-4** Atlanto-occipital joint assessment. **(A)** Normal Power's ratio; **(B)** Abnormal Power's ratio.

▶ Skill XI-C: Thoracic and Lumbar X-Ray Assessment

▶▶ ANTEROPOSTERIOR VIEW

STEP 1.   Assess for:
    A. Alignment
    B. Symmetry of pedicles
    C. Contour of bodies
    D. Height of disk spaces
    E. Central position of spinous processes

▶▶ LATERAL VIEW

STEP 2.   Assess for:
    A. Alignment of bodies/angulation of spine
    B. Contour of bodies
    C. Presence of disk spaces
    D. Encroachment of body on canal

▶ Skill XI-D: Review Spine X-Rays

The instructor will display a series of films to be interpreted and discussed with students.

Spinal Cord Injury Assessment and Management

▶▶ INTERACTIVE SKILL PROCEDURES

Note: Standard precautions are required whenever caring for trauma patients. This Skill Station includes scenarios and related x-rays for use in making evaluation and management decisions based on the findings.

THE FOLLOWING PROCEDURES ARE INCLUDED IN THIS SKILL STATION:

▶▶ **Skill XII-A:** Primary Survey and Resuscitation—Assessing Spine Injuries

▶▶ **Skill XII-B:** Secondary Survey— Neurologic Assessment

▶▶ **Skill XII-C:** Examination for Level of Spinal Cord Injury

▶▶ **Skill XII-D:** Treatment Principles for Patients with Spinal Cord Injuries

▶▶ **Skill XII-E:** Principles of Spine Immobilization and Logrolling

Objectives

Performance at this skill station will allow the participant to:

1 Demonstrate the examination of a patient in whom spine and/or spinal cord injuries are suspected.

2 Explain the principles for immobilizing and logrolling patients with neck and/or spinal injuries, including the indications for removing protective devices.

3 Perform a neurologic examination and determine the level of spinal cord injury.

4 Determine the need for neurosurgical consultation.

5 Determine the need for interhospital or intrahospital transfer, and describe how the patient should be properly immobilized for transfer.

▸ SCENARIOS

SCENARIO XII-1

A 15-year-old male is riding his bicycle through a parking lot. He is distracted and hits a car at low speed when it backs out of a parking space. He is thrown from his bicycle across the trunk of the car and sustains a mild abrasion and an angled deformity of the left wrist. He is brought to the emergency department (ED) immobilized on a long spine board with a semirigid cervical collar in place. He is alert and cooperative and has no hemodynamic abnormalities.

SCENARIO XII-2

A 75-year-old male is walking to the store when he trips and falls forward, striking his chin on a parked car. He is transported to the ED immobilized on a long spine board with a semirigid cervical collar applied. He has an abrasion on his chin and is alert and appropriately responsive. Physical examination reveals paralysis of his hands, with very little finger motion. He has some upper-extremity movement (grade 2/5), but is clearly weak bilaterally. Examination of the lower extremities reveals weakness, but he is able to flex and extend both his legs at the hip and knee. He has various areas of hypesthesia over his body.

SCENARIO XII-3

A 25-year-old male passenger sustains multiple injuries in a car collision. The driver died at the scene. The patient is transported to the ED immobilized on a long spine board with a semirigid cervical collar applied. Oxygen is being administered, and administration of warmed crystalloid fluids with two large-caliber intravenous lines is initiated. His blood pressure is 85/40 mm Hg, his heart rate 130 beats/min, and his respiratory rate 40 breaths/min. His respirations are shallow, and there is a contusion over the chest wall. His eyes are open, and his verbal response is appropriate. He is able to shrug his shoulders, but is unable to raise his elbow to the shoulder level or move his legs.

SCENARIO XII-4

This scenario is essentially the same as Scenario XII-3, but the instructor will make changes in the patient's neurologic status as the student examines the patient. A 25-year-old passenger sustains multiple injuries in a car collision. The driver died at the scene. The passenger is transported to the ED immobilized on a long spine board with a semirigid cervical collar applied. Oxygen is being administered, administration of warmed crystalloid fluids with two large-caliber intravenous lines is initiated.

SCENARIO XII-5

A 6-year-old male fell off his bicycle and hit the back of his head. In the ED, his head and neck are in a flexed position, and he reports pain in his neck. He is immobilized on an unpadded long spine board without a cervical collar.

▶ Skill XII-A: Primary Survey and Resuscitation—Assessing Spine Injuries

Note: The patient should be maintained in a supine, neutral position using proper immobilization techniques.

STEP 1. Airway:
   A. Assess the airway while protecting the cervical spine.
   B. Establish a definitive airway as needed.

STEP 2. Breathing: Assess and provide adequate oxygenation and ventilatory support as needed.

STEP 3. Circulation:
   A. If the patient has hypotension, differentiate hypovolemic shock (decreased blood pressure, increased heart rate, and cool extremities) from neurogenic shock (decreased blood pressure, decreased heart rate, and warm extremities).
   B. Replace fluids for hypovolemia.
   C. If spinal cord injury is present, fluid resuscitation should be guided by monitoring central venous pressure (CVP). (*Note:* Some patients may need inotropic support.)
   D. When performing a rectal examination before inserting the urinary catheter, assess for rectal sphincter tone and sensation.

STEP 4. Disability—Brief Neurologic Examination:
   A. Determine level of consciousness and assess pupils.
   B. Determine Glasgow Coma Scale (GCS) score.
   C. Recognize paralysis/paresis.

▶ Skill XII-B: Secondary Survey—Neurologic Assessment

STEP 1. Obtain AMPLE history.
   A. History and mechanism of injury
   B. Medical history
   C. Identify and record drugs given prior to the patient's arrival and during the assessment and management phases

STEP 2. Reassess level of consciousness and pupils.

STEP 3. Reassess GCS score.

STEP 4. Assess the spine (See Skill XII-C: Examination for Level of Spinal Cord Injury)
   A. Palpate the entire spine posteriorly by carefully logrolling the patient and assessing for:
   • Deformity and/or swelling
   • Crepitus
   • Increased pain with palpation
   • Contusions and lacerations/penetrating wounds
   B. Assess for pain, paralysis, and paresthesia:
   • Presence/absence
   • Location
   • Neurologic level
   C. Test sensation to pinprick in all dermatomes and record the most caudal dermatome that feels the pinprick.
   D. Assess motor function.
   E. Measure deep tendon reflexes (least informative in the emergency setting).
   F. Document and repeat—record the results of the neurologic examination and repeat motor and sensory examinations regularly until consultation is obtained.

STEP 5. Reevaluate—Assess for associated/occult injuries.

▶ Skill XII-C: Examination for Level of Spinal Cord Injury

A patient with a spinal cord injury may have varying levels of neurologic deficit. The level of motor function and sensation must be reassessed frequently and carefully documented, because changes in the level of function can occur.

STEP 1. Best Motor Examination
   A. Determining the level of quadriplegia, nerve root level:
   - Raises elbow to level of shoulder—deltoid, C5
   - Flexes forearm—biceps, C6
   - Extends forearm—triceps, C7
   - Flexes wrist and fingers, C8
   - Spreads fingers, T1
   B. Determining the level of paraplegia, nerve root level
   - Flexes hip—iliopsoas, L2
   - Extends knee—quadriceps, L3-L4
   - Flexes knee—hamstrings, L4-L5 to S1
   - Dorsiflexes big toe—extensor hallucis longus, L5
   - Plantar flexes ankle—gastrocnemius, S1

STEP 2. Sensory Examination: Determining the level of sensation is done primarily by assessing the dermatomes. See Figure 7.3 in Chapter 7: Spine and Spinal Cord Trauma. Remember, the cervical sensory dermatomes of C2 through C4 form a cervical cape or mantle that can extend down as far as the nipples. Because of this unusual pattern, the examiner should not depend on the presence or absence of sensation in the neck and clavicular area, and the level of sensation must be correlated with the motor response level.

▶ Skill XII-D: Treatment Principles for Patients with Spinal Cord Injuries

STEP 1. Patients with suspected spine injury must be protected from further injury. Such protection includes applying a semirigid cervical collar and long back board, performing a modified logroll to ensure neutral alignment of the entire spine, and removing the patient from the long spine board as soon as possible. Paralyzed patients who are immobilized on a long spine board are at particular risk for pressure points and decubitus ulcers. Therefore, paralyzed patients should be removed from the long spine board as soon as possible after a spine injury is diagnosed, i.e., within 2 hours.

STEP 2. Fluid Resuscitation and Monitoring:
   A. CVP monitoring: Intravenous fluids usually are limited to maintenance levels unless specifically needed for the management of shock. A central venous catheter should be inserted to carefully monitor fluid administration.
   B. Urinary catheter: A urinary catheter should be inserted during the primary survey and resuscitation phases to monitor urinary output and prevent bladder distention.
   C. Gastric catheter: A gastric catheter should be inserted in all patients with paraplegia and quadriplegia to prevent gastric distention and aspiration.

▶ Skill XII-E: Principles of Spine Immobilization and Logrolling

▶▶ ADULT PATIENT

Four people are needed to perform the modified log-rolling procedure and to immobilize the patient—for example, on a long spine board:

- one person to maintain manual, inline immobilization of the patient's head and neck
- one for the torso (including the pelvis and hips)
- one for the pelvis and legs
- one to direct the procedure and move the spine board

This procedure maintains the patient's entire body in neutral alignment, thereby minimizing any untoward movement of the spine. This procedure assumes that any extremity suspected of being fractured has already been immobilized.

STEP 1. Place the long spine board with straps next to the patient's side. Position the straps for fastening later across the patient's thorax, just above the iliac crests, across the thighs, and just above the ankles. Straps or tape can be used to secure the patient's head and neck to the long board.

STEP 2. Apply gentle, inline manual immobilization to the patient's head and apply a semirigid cervical collar.

STEP 3. Gently straighten and place the patient's arms (palm in) next to the torso.

STEP 4. Carefully straighten the patient's legs and place them in neutral alignment with the patient's spine. Tie the ankles together with a roller-type dressing or cravat.

STEP 5. While maintaining alignment of the patient's head and neck, another person reaches across and grasps the patient at the shoulder and wrist. A third person reaches across and grasps the patient's hip just distal to the wrist with one hand, and with the other hand firmly grasps the roller bandage or cravat that is securing the ankles together.

STEP 6. At the direction of the person who is maintaining immobilization of the patient's head and neck, cautiously logroll the patient as a unit toward the two assistants at the patient's side, but only to the least degree necessary to position the board under the patient. Maintain neutral alignment of the entire body during this procedure.

STEP 7. Place the spine board beneath the patient and carefully logroll the patient in one smooth movement onto the spine board. The spine board is used only for transferring the patient and should not be left under the patient for any length of time.

STEP 8. Consider padding under the patient's head to avoid hyperextension of the neck and for patient comfort.

STEP 9. Place padding, rolled blankets, or similar bolstering devices on both sides of the patient's head and neck, and firmly secure the patient's head to the board. Tape the cervical collar, further securing the patient's head and neck to the long board.

▶▶ PEDIATRIC PATIENT

A pediatric-sized long spine board is preferable when immobilizing a small child. If only an adult-sized board is available, place blanket rolls along the entire sides of the child to prevent lateral movement. A child's head is proportionately larger than an adult's. Therefore, padding should be placed under the shoulders to elevate the torso so that the large occiput of the child's head does not produce flexion of the cervical spine; this maintains neutral alignment of the child's spine. Such padding extends from the child's lumbar spine to the top of the shoulders and laterally to the edges of the board.

▶▶ COMPLICATIONS

If left immobilized for any length of time (approximately 2 hours or longer) on the long spine board, pressure sores can develop at the occiput, scapulae, sacrum, and heels. Therefore, padding should be applied under these areas as soon as possible, and the patient should be removed from the long spine board as soon as his or her condition permits.

▶▶ REMOVAL FROM A LONG SPINE BOARD

Movement of a patient with an unstable vertebral spine injury can cause or worsen a spinal cord injury. To reduce the risk of spinal cord damage, mechanical protection is necessary for all patients at risk. Such protection should be maintained until an unstable spine injury has been excluded.

STEP 1. As previously described, properly secure the patient to a long spine board, which is the basic technique for splinting the spine. In general, this is done in the prehospital setting, and the patient arrives at the hospital already immobilized. The long spine board provides an effective splint and permits safe transfers of the patient with a minimal number of assistants. However, unpadded spine boards can soon become uncomfortable for conscious patients and pose a significant risk for pressure sores on posterior bony prominences (occiput, scapulae, sacrum, and heels). Therefore, the patient should be transferred from the spine board to a firm, well-padded gurney or equivalent surface as soon as it can be done safely. Before removing the patient from the spine board, c-spine, chest, and pelvis x-ray films should be obtained as indicated, because the patient can be easily lifted and the x-ray plates placed beneath the spine board. While the patient is immobilized on the spine board, it is very important to maintain immobilization of the head and the body continuously. The straps used to immobilize the patient on the board should not be removed from the body while the head remains taped to the upper portion of the spine board.

STEP 2. Remove the patient from the spine board as early as possible. Preplanning is required. A good time to remove the board from under the patient is when the patient is logrolled to evaluate the back.

STEP 3. Safe movement of a patient with an unstable or potentially unstable spine requires continuous maintenance of anatomic alignment of the vertebral column. Rotation, flexion, extension, lateral bending, and shearing-type movements in any direction must be avoided. Manual, in-line immobilization best controls the head and neck. No part of the patient's body should be allowed to sag as the patient is lifted off the sup-

porting surface. The transfer options listed below may be used, depending on available personnel and equipment resources.

STEP 4. Modified Logroll Technique: The modified logroll technique, previously outlined, is reversed to remove the patient from the long spine board. Four assistants are required: one to maintain manual, inline immobilization of the patient's head and neck; one for the torso (including the pelvis and hips); one for the pelvis and legs; and one to direct the procedure and remove the spine board.

STEP 5. Scoop Stretcher: The scoop stretcher is an alternative to using the modified logrolling techniques for patient transfer. The proper use of this device can provide rapid, safe transfer of the patient from the long spine board onto a firm, padded patient gurney. For example, this device can be used to transfer the patient from one transport device to another or to a designated place (e.g., x-ray table).

The patient must remain securely immobilized until a spine injury is excluded. After the patient is transferred from the backboard to the gurney (stretcher) and the scoop stretcher is removed, the patient must again be immobilized securely on the gurney (stretcher). The scoop stretcher is not a device on which the patient is immobilized. In addition, the scoop stretcher is not used to transport the patient, nor should the patient be transferred to the gurney by picking up only the foot and head ends of the scoop stretcher. Without firm support under the stretcher, it can sag in the middle and result in loss of neutral alignment of the spine.

▶▶ IMMOBILIZATION OF THE PATIENT WITH POSSIBLE SPINE INJURY

Patients frequently arrive in the ED with spinal protective devices in place. These devices should cause the examiner to suspect that a c-spine and/or thoracolumbar spine injury may exist, based on mechanism of injury. In patients with multiple injuries with a diminished level of consciousness, protective devices should be left in place until a spine injury is excluded by clinical and x-ray examinations. See Chapter 7: Spine and Spinal Cord Trauma.

If a patient is immobilized on a spine board and is paraplegic, spinal instability should be presumed and all appropriate x-ray films obtained to determine the site of spinal injury. However, if the patient is awake, alert, sober, neurologically normal; is not experiencing neck or back pain; and does not have tenderness to spine palpation, spine x-ray examination and immobilization devices are not needed.

Patients who sustain multiple injuries and are comatose should be kept immobilized on a padded gurney (stretcher) and logrolled to obtain the necessary x-ray films to exclude a fracture. Then, using one of the aforementioned procedures, they can be transferred carefully to a bed.

8 Musculoskeletal Trauma

Injuries to the musculoskeletal system occur in many patients who sustain blunt trauma; they often appear dramatic, but rarely cause an immediate threat to life or limb.

Scenario A wall collapses on a 44-year-old male worker. Vital signs are: blood pressure (BP) 130/75, heart rate (HR) 110, and respiratory rate (RR) 22. Glasgow Coma Scale (GCS) score is 15. He has a painful, bruised, and deformed right leg.

Outline

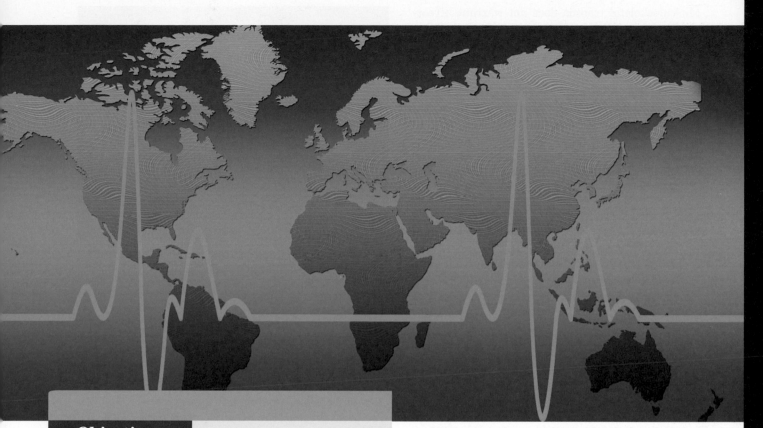

Objectives

Injuries to the musculoskeletal system occur in many patients who sustain blunt trauma; they often appear dramatic, but rarely cause an immediate threat to life or limb. However, musculoskeletal injuries must be assessed and managed properly and appropriately so life and limb are not jeopardized. Clinicians need to recognize the presence of such injuries, be familiar with the anatomy of the injury, protect the patient from further disability, and anticipate and prevent complications.

Major musculoskeletal injuries indicate that significant forces were sustained by the body. For example, a patient with long-bone fractures above and below the diaphragm has an increased likelihood of associated internal torso injuries. Unstable pelvic fractures and open femur fractures may be accompanied by brisk bleeding See Chapter 5: Abdominal and Pelvic Trauma. Severe crush injuries cause the release of myoglobin, which may precipitate in the renal tubules and result in renal failure. Swelling into an intact musculofascial space may cause an acute compartment syndrome that, if not diagnosed and treated, may lead to lasting impairment and loss of use of the extremity. Fat embolism, an uncommon but highly lethal complication of long-bone fractures, may lead to pulmonary failure and impaired cerebral function.

Musculoskeletal trauma does not warrant a reordering of the priorities of resuscitation (ABCDEs). However, the presence of significant musculoskeletal trauma does pose a challenge to clinicians. Musculoskeletal injuries cannot be ignored and treated at a later time. The clinician must treat the whole patient, including musculoskeletal injuries, to ensure an optimal outcome. Despite careful assessment and management of multiple injuries, fractures and soft tissue injuries may not be initially recognized. **Continued reevaluation of the patient is necessary to identify all injuries.**

Primary Survey and Resuscitation

? *What impact do musculoskeletal injuries have on the primary survey?*

During the primary survey, it is imperative to recognize and control hemorrhage from musculoskeletal injuries (■ FIGURE 8-1). Deep soft tissue lacerations may involve major vessels and lead to exsanguinating hemorrhage. Hemorrhage control is best effected by direct pressure.

Hemorrhage from long-bone fractures may be significant, and certain femoral fractures may result in significant blood loss into the thigh. Appropriate splinting of the fracture may significantly decrease bleeding by reducing motion and enhancing a tamponade effect of the muscle. If the fracture is open, application of a sterile pressure dressing usually controls hemorrhage. Appropriate fluid resuscitation is an important supplement to these mechanical measures.

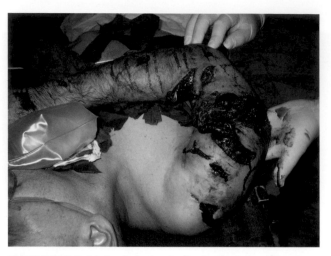

■ FIGURE 8-1 Major injuries indicate that significant forces were sustained by the body, and significant blood loss is possible.

as possible and to prevent excessive fracture-site motion. This is accomplished by the application of in-line traction to realign the extremity and maintained by an immobilization device (■ FIGURE 8-2). The proper application of a splint helps control blood loss, reduce pain, and prevent further soft tissue injury. If an open fracture is present, the clinician need not be concerned about pulling exposed bone back into the wound because open fractures require surgical debridement. See Skill Station XIII: Musculoskeletal Trauma: Assessment and Management, Skill XIII-C: Realigning a Deformed Extremity.

Joint dislocations may require splinting in the position in which they are found. If a closed reduction has successfully relocated the joint, immobilization in an anatomic position may be accomplished in a number of ways: prefabricated splints, pillows, or plaster. These devices will maintain the extremity in its reduced position.

PITFALL

Musculoskeletal injuries are a potential source of blood loss in patients with hemodynamic abnormalities. Sites of hemorrhage include the thigh from femoral fractures and any open fracture with major soft tissue involvement.

Adjuncts to Primary Survey

Adjuncts to the primary survey of patients with musculoskeletal trauma include fracture immobilization and x-ray examination if the fractures are suspected as a cause of shock.

FRACTURE IMMOBILIZATION

The goal of initial fracture immobilization is to realign the injured extremity in as close to anatomic position

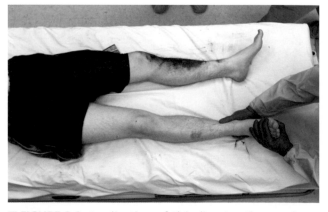

■ FIGURE 8-2 Application of 1) in-line traction, and then 2) rotation of the distal leg to normal anatomic position.

Splints should be applied as soon as possible, as they can control hemorrhage and pain. **However, splint application should not take precedence over resuscitation.**

X-RAY EXAMINATION

X-ray examination of most skeletal injuries occurs as the part of the secondary survey. The decisions regarding which x-ray films to obtain and when to obtain them are determined by the patient's initial and obvious clinical findings, the patient's hemodynamic status, and the mechanism of injury.

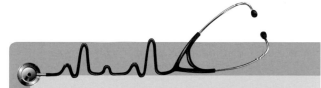

Scenario ■ *continued* The patient has no abnormalities identified on primary survey and continues to complain of pain to his leg. His distal pulses are normal, he is able to move his toes, and he has normal sensation. An x-ray of the lower extremity is obtained along with radiographic evaluation of the cervical spine due to his distracting injury.

Secondary Survey

Elements of the secondary survey of patients with musculoskeletal injuries are the history and physical examination.

HISTORY

Key aspects of the patient history are mechanism of injury, environment, preinjury status and predisposing factors, and prehospital observations and care.

Mechanism of Injury

Information obtained from the transport personnel, the patient, relatives, and bystanders at the scene of the injury should be documented and included as a part of the patient's medical record. It is particularly important to determine the mechanism of injury, which may arouse suspicion of injuries that may not be immediately apparent. See Biomechanics of Injury (electronic version only). The clinician should mentally reconstruct the injury scene, identify other potential injuries that the patient may have sustained, and determine as much of the following information as possible:

1. In a motor vehicle crash, what was the precrash location of the patient in the vehicle—driver or passenger? This fact can indicate the type of fracture—for example, lateral compression fracture of the pelvis resulting from a side impact in a vehicle collision.

2. What was the postcrash location of the patient—inside the vehicle or ejected? Was a seat belt or airbag in use? This information may indicate patterns of injury. If the patient was ejected, determine the distance he or she was thrown and the landing conditions. Ejection generally results in increased injury severity and unpredictable patterns of injury.

3. Was there external damage to the vehicle, such as deformation to the front of the vehicle from a head-on collision? This information raises the suspicion of a hip dislocation.

4. Was there internal damage to the vehicle, such as bent steering wheel, deformation to the dashboard, or damage to the windscreen? These findings indicate a greater likelihood of sternal, clavicular, or spinal fractures or hip dislocation.

5. Was the patient wearing a restraint? If so, what type (lap or three-point safety belt)? Was the restraint applied properly? Faulty application of safety restraints may cause spinal fractures and associated intraabdominal visceral injuries (■ FIGURE 8-3). Was an air bag deployed?

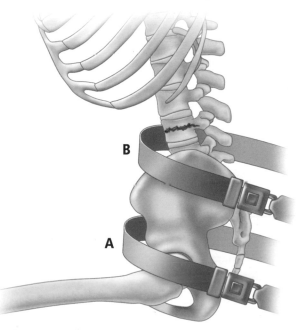

■ **FIGURE 8-3 Safety Restraints.** When worn correctly **(A)**, safety belts can reduce injuries. When worn incorrectly **(B)**, as shown here, burst injuries and organ lacerations can occur. Hyperflexion over an incorrectly applied belt can produce anterior compression fractures of the lumbar spine.

6. Did the patient fall? If so, what was the distance of the fall, and how did the patient land? This information helps identify the spectrum of injuries. Landing on the feet may cause foot and ankle injuries with associated spinal fractures.

7. Was the patient crushed by an object? If so, identify the weight of the crushing object, the site of the injury, and duration of weight applied to the site. Depending on whether a subcutaneous bony surface or a muscular area was crushed, different degrees of soft tissue damage may occur, ranging from a simple contusion to a severe degloving extremity injury with compartment syndrome and tissue loss.

8. Did an explosion occur? If so, what was the magnitude of the blast, and what was the patient's distance from the blast? An individual close to the explosion may sustain primary blast injury from the force of the blast wave. A secondary blast injury may occur from debris and other objects accelerated by the blast effect (e.g., fragments), leading to penetrating wounds, lacerations, and contusions. The patient also may be violently thrown to the ground or against other objects by the blast effect, leading to blunt musculoskeletal and other injuries (tertiary blast effect).

9. Was the patient involved in a vehicle-pedestrian collision? Musculoskeletal injuries may follow predicted patterns (e.g., bumper injury to leg) based on the size and age of the patient.

Environment

Ask prehospital care personnel for information about the environment, including:

- Whether the patient sustained an open fracture in a contaminated environment

- Patient exposure to temperature extremes

- Broken glass fragments (which may also injure the examiner)

- Sources of bacterial contamination (e.g., dirt, animal feces, fresh or salt water)

This information can help the clinician anticipate potential problems and determine the initial antibiotic treatment.

Preinjury Status and Predisposing Factors

It is important to determine the patient's baseline condition prior to injury, because this information may alter the understanding of the patient's condition, treatment regimen, and outcome. The AMPLE history also should include information about the patient's ex-

ercise tolerance and activity level, ingestion of alcohol and/or other drugs, emotional problems or illnesses, and previous musculoskeletal injuries.

Prehospital Observations and Care

Findings at the incident site that may help to identify potential injuries include:

- Position in which the patient was found

- Bleeding or pooling of blood at the scene, including the estimated amount

- Bone or fracture ends that may have been exposed

- Open wounds in proximity to obvious or suspected fractures

- Obvious deformity or dislocation

- Presence or absence of motor and/or sensory function in each extremity

- Delays in extrication procedures or transport

- Changes in limb function, perfusion, or neurologic state, especially after immobilization or during transfer to the hospital

- Reduction of fractures or dislocations during extrication or splinting at the scene

- Dressings and splints applied, with special attention to excessive pressure over bony prominences that may result in peripheral nerve compression injuries, compartment syndromes, or crush syndromes.

The time of the injury also should be noted, especially if there is ongoing bleeding and a delay in reaching the hospital. All prehospital observations and care must be reported and documented.

PHYSICAL EXAMINATION

The patient must be completely undressed for adequate examination. Obvious extremity injuries are often splinted prior to the patient's arrival in the emergency department (ED). There are three goals for the assessment of trauma patients' extremities:

1. Identification of life-threatening injuries (primary survey)

2. Identification of limb-threatening injuries (secondary survey)

3. Systematic review to avoid missing any other musculoskeletal injury (continuous reevaluation)

Assessment of musculoskeletal trauma may be achieved by looking at and talking to the patient, as well as by palpation of the patient's extremities and performance of a logical, systematic review of each extremity. The four components that must be assessed are: skin, which protects the patient from excessive fluid loss and infection; neuromuscular function; circulatory status; and skeletal and ligamentous integrity. Using this evaluation process reduces the risk of missing an injury. See Skill Station XIII: Musculoskeletal Trauma: Assessment and Management, Skill XIII-A: Physical Examination.

Look and Ask

Visually assess the extremities for color and perfusion, wounds, deformity (angulation, shortening), swelling, and discoloration or bruising.

A rapid visual inspection of the entire patient is necessary to identify sites of major external bleeding. A pale or white distal extremity is indicative of a lack of arterial inflow. Extremities that are swollen in the region of major muscle groups may indicate a crush injury with an impending compartment syndrome. Swelling or ecchymosis in or around a joint and/or over the subcutaneous surface of a bone is a sign of a musculoskeletal injury. Extremity deformity is an obvious sign of major extremity injury. Table 8.1 outlines common joint dislocation deformities.

Inspect the patient's entire body for lacerations and abrasions. Open wounds are obvious unless they are located on the dorsum of the body; therefore, patients must be carefully logrolled to assess for an injury or skin laceration. If a bone protrudes or is visualized in the wound, an open fracture exists. Any open wound to a limb with an associated fracture also is considered an open fracture until proven otherwise by a surgeon.

Observe the patient's spontaneous extremity motor function to help identify any neurologic and/or muscular impairment. If the patient is unconscious, absent spontaneous extremity movement may be the only sign of impaired function. With a cooperative patient, active voluntary muscle and peripheral nerve function may be

assessed by asking the patient to contract major muscle groups. The ability to move all major joints through a full range of motion usually indicates that the nerve-muscle unit is intact and the joint is stable.

Feel

Palpate the extremities to determine sensation to the skin (neurologic function) and identify areas of tenderness, which may indicate fracture. Loss of sensation to pain and touch demonstrates the presence of a spinal or peripheral nerve injury. Areas of tenderness or pain over muscles may indicate a muscle contusion or fracture. Pain, tenderness, swelling, and deformity over a subcutaneous bony surface usually confirm the diagnosis of a fracture. If pain or tenderness is associated with painful abnormal motion through the bone, fracture is diagnosed. Attempts to elicit crepitation or demonstrate abnormal motion are not recommended.

At the time of logrolling, palpate the patient's back to identify any lacerations, palpable gaps between the spinous processes, hematomas, or defects in the posterior pelvic region that are indicative of unstable axial skeletal injuries.

Closed soft tissue injuries are more difficult to evaluate. Soft tissue avulsion may shear the skin from the deep fascia, allowing for significant accumulation of blood. Alternatively, the skin may be sheared from its blood supply and undergo necrosis over a few days. This area may have local abrasions or bruised skin, which are clues to a more severe degree of muscle damage and potential compartment or crush syndromes. These soft tissue injuries are best evaluated with knowledge of the mechanism of injury and by palpating the specific component involved.

Joint stability can be determined only by clinical examination. Abnormal motion through a joint segment is indicative of a ligamentous rupture. Palpate the joint to identify any swelling and tenderness of the ligaments as well as intraarticular fluid. Following this, cautious stressing of the specific ligaments can be

■ TABLE 8.1 Common Joint Dislocation Deformities		
JOINT	**DIRECTION**	**DEFORMITY**
Shoulder	Anterior Posterior	Squared off Locked in internal rotation
Elbow	Posterior	Olecranon prominent posteriorly
Hip	Anterior Posterior	Flexed, abducted, externally rotated Flexed, adducted, internally rotated
Knee*	Anteroposterior	Loss of normal contour, extended
Ankle	Lateral is most common	Externally rotated, prominent medial malleolus
Subtalar joint	Lateral is most common	Laterally displaced os calcis

*Knee dislocations can sometimes reduce spontaneously and may not present with any obvious gross external or radiographic anomalies until a physical exam of the joint is performed and instability is detected clinically.

performed. Excessive pain may mask abnormal ligament motion because of guarding of the joint by muscular contraction or spasm; this condition may need to be reassessed later.

Circulatory Evaluation

Palpate the distal pulses in each extremity and assess capillary refill of the digits. If hypotension limits digital examination of the pulse, the use of a Doppler probe may detect blood flow to an extremity. The Doppler signal must have a triphasic quality to ensure no proximal lesion. Loss of sensation in a stocking or glove distribution is an early sign of vascular impairment.

In patients with no hemodynamic abnormalities, pulse discrepancies, coolness, pallor, paresthesia, and even motor function abnormalities can suggest an arterial injury. Open wounds and fractures in proximity to arteries can be clues to an arterial injury. A Doppler ankle/brachial index of less than 0.9 is indicative of an abnormal arterial flow secondary to injury or peripheral vascular disease. The ankle/brachial index is determined by taking the systolic blood pressure value as measured by Doppler at the ankle of the injured leg and dividing it by the Doppler-determined systolic blood pressure of the uninjured arm. Auscultation can reveal a bruit with an associated palpable thrill. Expanding hematomas or pulsatile hemorrhage from an open wound also are indicative of arterial injury.

X-Ray Examination

The clinical examination of patients with musculoskeletal injuries often suggests the need for x-ray examination. Any area over a bone that is tender and deformed likely represents a fracture. In patients who have no hemodynamic abnormalities, an x-ray film should be obtained. Joint effusions, abnormal joint tenderness, or joint deformity represent a joint injury or dislocation that also must be x-rayed. The only reason for electing not to obtain an x-ray film prior to treatment of a dislocation or a fracture is the presence of vascular compromise or impending skin breakdown. This is seen commonly with fracture-dislocations of the ankle.

If there is going to be a delay in obtaining x-rays, immediate reduction or realignment of the extremity should be performed to reestablish the arterial blood supply and reduce the pressure on the skin. Alignment can be maintained by appropriate immobilization techniques.

PITFALL

Not log rolling the patient to look for additional potentially life threatening injuries or failure to perform a thorough secondary survey can result in missing potential life- and limb-threatening injuries.

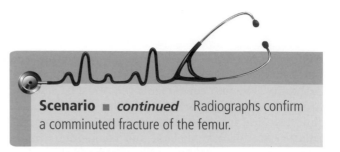

Scenario ■ continued Radiographs confirm a comminuted fracture of the femur.

Potentially Life-Threatening Extremity Injuries

? *What are my priorities and management principles?*

Extremity injuries that are considered potentially life-threatening include major arterial hemorrhage and crush syndrome. (Pelvic disruption is described in Chapter 5: Abdominal and Pelvic Trauma.)

MAJOR ARTERIAL HEMORRHAGE

Injury

Penetrating extremity wounds may result in major arterial vascular injury. Blunt trauma resulting in an extremity fracture or joint dislocation in close proximity to an artery also may disrupt the artery. These injuries may lead to significant hemorrhage through the open wound or into the soft tissues.

Assessment

Assess injured extremities for external bleeding, loss of a previously palpable pulse, and changes in pulse quality, Doppler tone, and ankle/brachial index. A cold, pale, pulseless extremity indicates an interruption in arterial blood supply. A rapidly expanding hematoma suggests a significant vascular injury. See Skill Station XIII: Musculoskeletal Trauma: Assessment and Management, Skill XIII-F: Identification of Arterial Injury.

Management

If a major arterial injury exists or is suspected, immediate consultation with a surgeon is necessary. Management of major arterial hemorrhage includes application of direct pressure to the open wound and appropriate fluid resuscitation.

The judicious use of a tourniquet may be helpful and lifesaving (■ FIGURE 8-4). It is not advisable to apply vascular clamps into bleeding open wounds while the patient is in the ED, unless a superficial vessel is clearly identified. If a fracture is associated with an open hemorrhaging wound, it should be realigned and splinted while direct pressure is applied to the open wound. A joint dislocation should be reduced if possible; if the

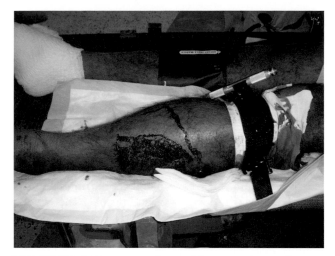

■ **FIGURE 8-4** Trauma patient with manual tourniquet in place.

joint cannot be reduced, emergency orthopedic intervention may be required. The use of arteriography and other investigations is indicated only in resuscitated patients who have no hemodynamic abnormalities; other patients with clear vascular injury require urgent operation. Consultation with a surgeon skilled in vascular and extremity trauma may be necessary.

CRUSH SYNDROME (TRAUMATIC RHABDOMYOLYSIS)

Injury

Crush syndrome refers to the clinical effects of injured muscle that, if left untreated, can lead to acute renal failure. This condition is seen in individuals who have sustained a crush injury of a significant muscle mass, most often a thigh or calf. The muscular insult is a combination of direct muscle injury, muscle ischemia, and cell death with release of myoglobin. Muscular trauma is the most common cause of rhabdomyolysis, which ranges from an asymptomatic illness with elevation of the creatine kinase level to a life-threatening condition associated with acute renal failure and disseminated intravascular coagulation (DIC).

Assessment

The myoglobin produces dark amber urine that tests positive for hemoglobin. The myoglobin assay must be specifically requested to confirm the presence of myoglobin. Rhabdomyolysis may lead to metabolic acidosis, hyperkalemia, hypocalcemia, and DIC.

Management

The initiation of early and aggressive intravenous fluid therapy during the period of resuscitation is critical to protecting the kidneys and preventing renal failure in patients with rhabdomyolysis. Myoglobin-induced renal failure may be prevented by intravascular fluid expansion and osmotic diuresis to maintain a high tubular volume and urine flow. It is recommended to maintain the patient's urinary output at 100 mL/hr until the myoglobinuria is cleared.

Limb-Threatening Injuries

Extremity injuries that are considered potentially limb-threatening include open fractures and joint injuries, vascular injuries, compartment syndrome, and neurologic injury secondary to fracture dislocation.

OPEN FRACTURES AND JOINT INJURIES

Injury

Open fractures represent a communication between the external environment and the bone (■ **FIGURE 8-5**). Muscle and skin must be injured for this to occur. The degree of soft tissue injury is proportional to the energy applied. This damage, along with bacterial contamination, makes open fractures prone to problems with infection, healing, and function.

Assessment

Diagnosis of an open fracture is based on the history of the incident and physical examination of the extremity that demonstrates an open wound on the same limb segment with or without significant muscle damage, contamination, and associated fracture. Management

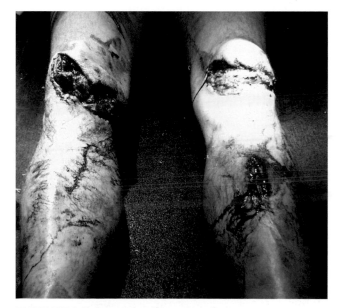

■ **FIGURE 8-5** Example of an open fracture.

decisions should be based on a complete history of the incident and assessment of the injury.

Documentation regarding the open wound begins during the prehospital phase, with the initial description of the injury and any treatment rendered at the scene. At no time should the wound be probed. If a fracture and an open wound exist in the same limb segment, the fracture is considered open until proved otherwise.

If an open wound exists over or near a joint, it should be assumed that this injury connects with or enters the joint, and surgical consultation should be obtained. The insertion of dye, saline, or any other material into the joint to determine whether the joint cavity communicates with the wound is not recommended. The only safe way to determine communication between an open wound and a joint is to surgically explore and debride the wound.

Management

The presence of an open fracture or a joint injury should be promptly determined. Apply appropriate immobilization after an accurate description of the wound is made and associated soft tissue, circulatory, and neurologic involvement is determined. Prompt surgical consultation is necessary. The patient should be adequately resuscitated, with hemodynamic stability achieved if possible. Wounds then may be operatively debrided, fractures stabilized, and distal pulses confirmed. Tetanus prophylaxis should be administered (see Tetanus Immunization [electronic version only]). **All patients with open fractures should be treated with intravenous antibiotics as soon as possible.** Currently first-generation cephalosporins are given to all patients with open fractures and aminoglycosides or other Gram-negative appropriate antibiotics may be given in more severe injuries. Antibiotics are used only after consultation with a surgeon.

VASCULAR INJURIES, INCLUDING TRAUMATIC AMPUTATION

Injury

A vascular injury should be strongly suspected in the presence of vascular insufficiency associated with a history of blunt, crushing, twisting, or penetrating injury to an extremity.

Assessment

The limb may initially appear viable because extremities often have some collateral circulation that provides enough flow. Partial vascular injury results in coolness and prolonged capillary refill in the distal part of an extremity, as well as diminished peripheral pulses and an abnormal ankle/brachial index. Alternatively, the distal extremity may have the complete disruption of flow and be cold, pale, and pulseless.

Management

An acutely avascular extremity must be recognized promptly and treated emergently. The use of a tourniquet may occasionally be lifesaving and/or limb-saving in the presence of ongoing hemorrhage uncontrolled by direct pressure. A properly applied tourniquet, while endangering the limb, may save a life. A tourniquet must occlude arterial inflow, as occluding only the venous system can increase hemorrhage. The risks of tourniquet use increase with time. If a tourniquet must remain in place for a prolonged period to save a life, the clinician must be cognizant of the fact the choice of life over limb has been made.

Muscle does not tolerate a lack of arterial blood flow for longer than 6 hours before necrosis begins. Nerves also are very sensitive to an anoxic environment. Therefore, early operative revascularization is required to restore arterial flow to the impaired distal extremity. If there is an associated fracture deformity, it should be corrected quickly by gently realigning and splinting the injured extremity.

If an arterial injury is associated with a dislocation of a joint, a clinician who is skilled in joint reduction may attempt one gentle reduction maneuver. Otherwise, splinting of the dislocated joint and emergency surgical consultation are necessary. Arteriography must not delay reestablishing arterial blood flow, and is indicated only after consultation with a surgeon. Computed tomography (CT) angiography may be helpful in institutions in which arteriography is not available.

The potential for vascular compromise also exists whenever an injured extremity is splinted or placed in a cast. Vascular compromise can be identified by the loss of or change in the distal pulse, but excessive pain after cast application also must be investigated. The splint, cast, and any other circumferential dressings must be released promptly and the vascular supply reassessed.

Amputation is a traumatic event for the patient, both physically and emotionally. Traumatic amputation, a severe form of open fracture that results in loss of an extremity, may benefit from tourniquet use and requires consultation with and intervention by a surgeon. Certain open fractures with prolonged ischemia, neurologic injury, and muscle damage may require amputation. Amputation of an injured extremity may be lifesaving in patients with hemodynamic abnormalities who are difficult to resuscitate.

Although the potential for replantation should be considered, it must be put into perspective with the patient's other injuries. **A patient with multiple injuries who requires intensive resuscitation and emergency** surgery is not a candidate for replantation. Replantation usually is performed with an injury of an isolated extremity. A patient with clean, sharp amputations of fingers or of a distal extremity, below the knee or elbow, should be transported to an appropriate surgical team skilled in the decision making for and management of replantation procedures.

The amputated part should be thoroughly washed in isotonic solution (e.g., Ringer's lactate) and wrapped in sterile gauze that has been soaked in aqueous penicillin (100,000 units in 50 mL of Ringer's lactate solution). The amputated part is then wrapped in a similarly moistened sterile towel, placed in a plastic bag, and transported with the patient in an insulated cooling chest with crushed ice. Care must be taken not to freeze the amputated part.

COMPARTMENT SYNDROME

Injury

Compartment syndrome develops when the pressure within an osteofascial compartment of muscle causes ischemia and subsequent necrosis. This ischemia may be caused by an increase in compartment size (e.g., swelling secondary to revascularization of an ischemic extremity) or by decreasing the compartment size (e.g., a constrictive dressing). **Compartment syndrome may occur in any site in which muscle is contained within a closed fascial space. (Remember, the skin also may act** as a restricting membrane in certain circumstances.) Common areas for compartment syndrome include the lower leg, forearm, foot, hand, gluteal region, and thigh (■ FIGURE 8-6).

The end results of unchecked compartment syndrome are catastrophic. They include neurologic deficit, muscle necrosis, ischemic contracture, infection, delayed healing of a fracture, and possible amputation.

Assessment

Any injury to an extremity has the potential to cause a compartment syndrome. However, certain injuries or activities are considered high risk, including:

- Tibial and forearm fractures
- Injuries immobilized in tight dressings or casts
- Severe crush injury to muscle
- Localized, prolonged external pressure to an extremity
- Increased capillary permeability secondary to reperfusion of ischemic muscle
- Burns
- Excessive exercise

The signs and symptoms of compartment syndrome are listed in Box 8-1. The key to the successful treatment of acute compartment syndrome is early diagnosis. A high degree of awareness is important,

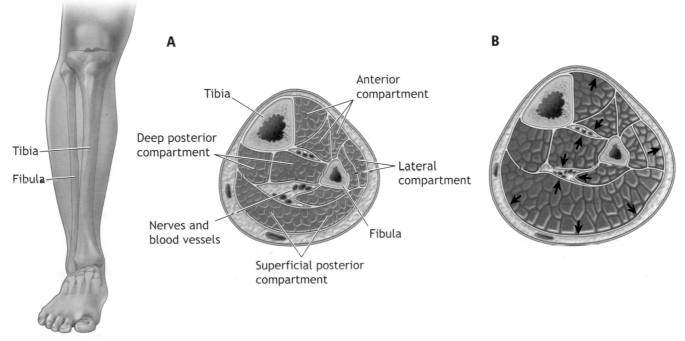

■ **FIGURE 8-6 Compartment Syndrome.** This condition develops when the pressure within an osteofascial compartment of muscle causes ischemia and subsequent necrosis. **(A)** Normal calf. **(B)** Calf with compartment syndrome.

Box 8-1 Signs and Symptoms of Compartment Syndrome

- Increasing pain greater than expected and out of proportion to the stimulus
- Palpable tenseness of the compartment
- Asymmetry of the muscle compartments
- Pain on passive stretch of the affected muscle
- Altered sensation

especially if the patient has an altered mental sensorium and is unable to respond appropriately to pain. See Skill Station XIII: Musculoskeletal Trauma: Assessment and Management, Skill XIII-E: Compartment Syndrome: Assessment and Management.

The absence of a palpable distal pulse usually is an uncommon or late finding in compartment syndrome and should not be relied upon to diagnose compartment syndrome. Weakness or paralysis of the involved muscles and loss of pulses (because the compartment pressure exceeds the systolic pressure) in the affected limb are late signs of compartment syndrome. If pulse abnormalities are present, the possibility of a proximal vascular injury must also be considered.

Remember, changes in distal pulses or capillary refill times are not reliable in diagnosing compartment syndrome. Clinical diagnosis is based on the history of injury and physical signs, coupled with a high index of suspicion.

Intracompartmental pressure measurements may be helpful in diagnosing suspected compartment syndrome. Tissue pressures that are greater than 30 to 45 mm Hg suggest decreased capillary blood flow, which may result in increased muscle and nerve damage caused by anoxia. Many surgeons use the "delta-P" method of calculating tissue pressures. The compartment pressure is subtracted from the diastolic blood pressure, yielding the "delta-P." If this value is 30 mm Hg or less, this suggests that the patient may have a compartment syndrome. Systemic blood pressure is important: the lower the systemic pressure, the lower the compartment pressure that causes a compartment syndrome. Pressure measurement is indicated in all patients who have an altered response to pain.

The physician must realize that compartment syndrome is a clinical diagnosis and is not one that is solely determined by pressure measurements. Compartment measurements are only intended to aid the physician in the diagnosis of compartment syndrome.

Management

All constrictive dressings, casts, and splints applied over the affected extremity must be released. The pa-

tient must be carefully monitored and reassessed clinically for the next 30 to 60 minutes. If no significant changes occur, fasciotomy is required (■ FIGURE 8-7). Compartment syndrome is a time-dependent condition. The higher the compartment pressure and the longer it remains elevated, the greater the degree of resulting neuromuscular damage and functional deficit. A delay in performing a fasciotomy may result in

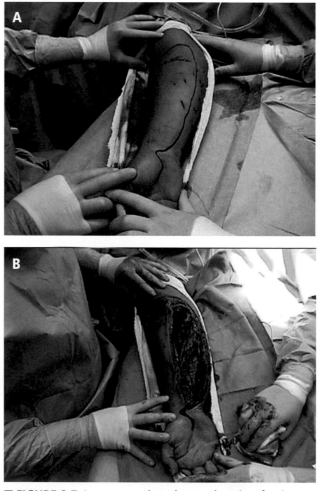

■ FIGURE 8-7 Intraoperative photos showing fasciotomy of upper extremity compartment syndrome secondary to crush injury. **(A)** Planned skin incision for fasciotomy of the forearm. **(B)** Post-surgical decompression of the forearm.

myoglobinuria, which may cause decreased renal function. **Surgical consultation for diagnosed or suspected compartment syndrome must be obtained early.**

◣ PITFALL

Compartment syndrome is limb-threatening. Clinical findings must be recognized and surgical consultation obtained early. Remember that in unconscious patients or those with severe hypovolemia, the classic findings of acute compartment syndrome may be masked.

NEUROLOGIC INJURY SECONDARY TO FRACTURE-DISLOCATION

Injury

Fractures and particularly dislocations may cause significant neurologic injury because of the anatomic relationship and proximity of the nerve to the joint—for example, sciatic nerve compression from posterior hip dislocation or axillary nerve injury from anterior shoulder dislocation. Optimal functional outcome is jeopardized unless this injury is recognized and treated early.

Assessment

A thorough examination of the neurologic system is essential in patients with musculoskeletal injury. Determination of neurologic impairment is important, and progressive changes must be documented.

Assessment usually demonstrates a deformity of the extremity. Assessment of nerve function usually requires a cooperative patient. For each significant peripheral nerve, voluntary motor function and sensation must be confirmed systematically. Table 8.2 and Table 8.3 outline peripheral nerve assessment of the upper extremities and lower extremities, respectively. Muscle testing must include palpation of the contracting muscle.

In most patients with multiple injuries, it is difficult to initially assess nerve function. However, assessment must be continually repeated, especially after the patient is stabilized. Progression of neurologic findings is indicative of continued nerve compression. The

■ TABLE 8.2 Peripheral Nerve Assessment of Upper Extremities

NERVE	MOTOR	SENSATION	INJURY
Ulnar	Index and little finger abduction	Little finger	Elbow injury
Median distal	Thenar contraction with opposition	Index finger	Wrist fracture or dislocation
Median, anterior interosseous	Index tip flexion	None	Supracondylar fracture of humerus (children)
Musculocutaneous	Elbow flexion	Radial forearm	Anterior shoulder dislocation
Radial	Thumb, finger metacarpophalangeal extension	First dorsal web space	Distal humeral shaft, anterior shoulder dislocation
Axillary	Deltoid	Lateral shoulder	Anterior shoulder dislocation, proximal humerus fracture

■ TABLE 8.3 Peripheral Nerve Assessment of Lower Extremities

NERVE	MOTOR	SENSATION	INJURY
Femoral	Knee extension	Anterior knee	Pubic rami fractures
Obturator	Hip adduction	Medial thigh	Obturator ring fractures
Posterior tibial	Toe flexion	Sole of foot	Knee dislocation
Superficial peroneal	Ankle eversion	Lateral dorsum of foot	Fibular neck fracture, knee dislocation
Deep peroneal	Ankle/toe dorsiflexion	Dorsal first to second web space	Fibular neck fracture, compartment syndrome
Sciatic nerve	Plantar dorsiflexion	Foot	Posterior hip dislocation
Superior gluteal	Hip abduction	Upper buttocks	Acetabular fracture
Inferior gluteal	Gluteus maximus hip extension	Lower buttocks	Acetabular fracture

most important aspect of any neurologic assessment is the documentation of progression of neurologic findings. It also is an important aspect of surgical decision making.

Management

The injured extremity should be immobilized in the dislocated position, and surgical consultation obtained immediately. If indicated and if the treating clinician is knowledgeable, a careful reduction of the dislocation may be attempted. After reducing a dislocation, neurologic function should be reevaluated and the limb splinted. If the clinician is able to reduce the dislocation, the subsequent treating physician must be notified that the joint was dislocated and successfully reduced.

Other Extremity Injuries

Other significant extremity injuries include contusions and lacerations, joint injuries, and fractures.

CONTUSIONS AND LACERATIONS

Simple contusions and/or lacerations should be assessed to rule out vascular and/or neurologic injury. In general, lacerations require debridement and closure. If a laceration extends below the fascial level, it requires operative intervention to more completely debride the wound and assess for damage to underlying structures.

Contusions usually are recognized by pain in the area and decreased function of the extremity. Palpation confirms localized swelling and tenderness. The patient usually cannot use the muscle or experiences decreased function because of pain in the affected extremity. If the patient is seen early, contusions are treated by limiting function of the injured part and applying cold packs.

Small wounds, especially those resulting from crush injuries, may be significant. When a very strong force is applied very slowly over an extremity, significant devascularization and crushing of muscle may occur with only a small skin wound. Crush and degloving injuries can be very subtle and must be suspected based on the mechanism of injury.

The risk of tetanus is increased with wounds that are more than 6 hours old, are contused and/or abraded, are more than 1 cm in depth, result from high-velocity missiles, are due to burns or cold, and have significant contamination (especially burn wounds and wounds with denervated or ischemic tissue). See Tetanus Immunization (electronic version only).

JOINT INJURIES

Injury

Joint injuries that are not dislocated (i.e., the joint is within its normal anatomic configuration but has sustained significant ligamentous injury) usually are not limb-threatening. However, such joint injuries may decrease the function of the limb.

Assessment

With joint injuries, the patient usually reports some form of abnormal stress to the joint, for example, impact to the anterior tibia that subluxates the knee posteriorly, impact to the lateral aspect of the leg that resulted in a valgus strain to the knee, or a fall onto an outstretched arm that caused a hyperextension injury to the elbow.

Physical examination reveals tenderness throughout the affected ligament. A hemarthrosis usually is present unless the joint capsule is disrupted and the bleeding diffuses into the soft tissues. Passive ligamentous testing of the affected joint reveals instability. X-ray examination usually reveals no significant injury. However, some small avulsion fractures from ligamentous insertions or origins may be present radiographically.

Management

Joint injuries should be immobilized. The vascular and neurologic status of the limb distal to the injury should be reassessed. Surgical consultation usually is warranted.

FRACTURES

Injury

Fractures are defined as a break in the continuity of the bone cortex. They may be associated with abnormal motion, some form of soft tissue injury, bony crepitus, and pain. A fracture can be open or closed.

Assessment

Examination of the extremity demonstrates pain, swelling, deformity, tenderness, crepitation, and abnormal motion at the fracture site. The evaluation for crepitation and abnormal motion at the fracture site may occasionally be necessary to make the diagnosis, but this is painful and may potentially increase soft tissue damage. These diagnostic tests must not be done routinely or repetitively. Usually the swelling, tenderness, and deformity are sufficient to confirm a fracture. It is important to periodically reassess the neurovascular status of a limb, especially if a splint is in place.

X-ray films taken at right angles to one another confirm the history and physical examinations (■ FIGURE 8-8). Depending on the hemodynamic status of the patient, x-ray examination may need to be delayed until the patient is stabilized. X-ray films through the joint above and below the suspected fracture site must be included to exclude occult dislocation and concomitant injury.

Management

Immobilization must include the joint above and below the fracture. After splinting, the neurologic and vascular status of the extremity must be reassessed. Surgical consultation is required for further treatment.

Principles of Immobilization

Splinting of extremity injuries, unless associated with life-threatening injuries, usually can be accomplished during the secondary survey. However, all such injuries must be splinted before a patient is transported. Assess the limb's neurovascular status after applying splints or realigning a fracture.

Specific types of splints can be applied for specific fracture needs.

A long spine board provides a total body splint for patients with multiple injuries who have possible or confirmed unstable spine injuries. However, its hard, unpadded surface may cause pressure sores on the patient's occiput, scapulae, sacrum, and heels. Therefore, as soon as possible, the patient should be moved carefully to an equally supportive padded surface, using a scoop-style stretcher or an appropriate logrolling maneuver to facilitate the transfer. The patient should be fully immobilized, and an adequate number of personnel should be available during this transfer. See Skill Station XII: Spinal Cord Injury: Assessment and Management, Skill XII-E: Principles of Spine Immobilization and Logrolling, and Skill Station XIII: Musculoskeletal Trauma: Assessment and Management, Skill XIII-B: Principles of Extremity Immobilization.

FEMORAL FRACTURES

Femoral fractures are immobilized temporarily with traction splints (■ FIGURE 8-9). The traction splint's force is applied distally at the ankle or through the skin. Proximally, the splint is pushed into the thigh and hip areas by a ring that applies pressure to the buttocks, perineum, and groin. Excessive traction can cause skin damage to the foot, ankle, or perineum. Neurovascular compromise can result from stretching

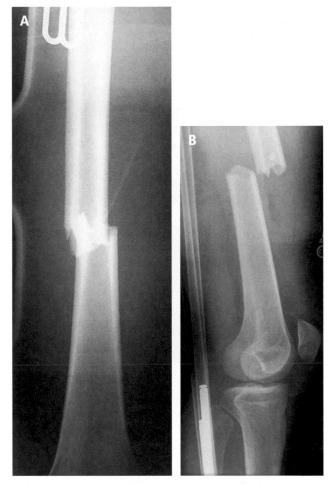

■ FIGURE 8-8 X-ray films taken at right angles to one another confirm the history and physical examinations. **(A)** AP view of the distal femur. **(B)** Lateral view of the distal femur. Satisfactory x-rays of an injured long bone should include two orthogonal views, but the entire bone should be visualized. Thus the above images alone would be inadequate.

the peripheral nerves. Hip fractures can be similarly immobilized with a traction splint, but are more suitably immobilized with skin traction or a foam boot traction with the knee in slight flexion. A simple method of splinting is to bind the injured leg to the opposite leg. See Skill Station XIII: Musculoskeletal Trauma: Assessment and Management, Skill XIII-D: Application of a Traction Splint.

KNEE INJURIES

The use of commercially available knee immobilizers or the application of a long-leg plaster splint is very helpful in maintaining comfort and stability. The knee should not be immobilized in complete extension, but should be immobilized with about 10 degrees of flexion to reduce tension on the neurovascular structures.

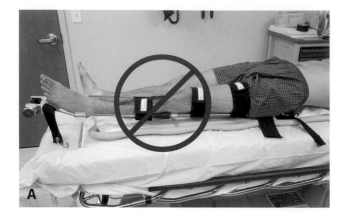

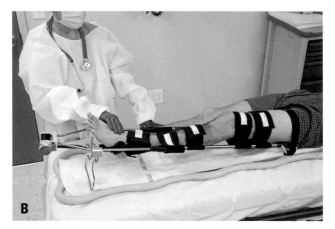

■ **FIGURE 8-9 Traction Splinting.** Proper application of a traction splint includes proper position against the crease of the buttock and sufficient length to apply traction. The straps should be positioned above and below the knee, with the stand extended to suspend the leg. Distal pulses should be evaluated before and after application of the splint. **(A)** It is improper to use the splint without properly placing the straps and securing traction to the device. **(B)** Proper immobilization.

PITFALL

Traction splint of a femur fracture should be avoided if there is a concomitant ipsilateral lower leg fracture.

TIBIA FRACTURES

Tibia fractures are best immobilized with a well-padded cardboard or metal gutter long-leg splint. If readily available, plaster splints immobilizing the lower thigh, the knee, and the ankle may be used.

ANKLE FRACTURES

Ankle fractures may be immobilized with a pillow splint or padded cardboard splint, thereby avoiding pressure over bony prominences.

UPPER-EXTREMITY AND HAND INJURIES

The hand may be temporarily splinted in an anatomic, functional position, with the wrist slightly dorsiflexed and the fingers gently flexed 45 degrees at the metacarpophalangeal joints. This position usually can be achieved by gently immobilizing the hand over a large roll of gauze and using a short-arm splint.

The forearm and wrist are immobilized flat on padded or pillow splints. The elbow usually is immobilized in a flexed position, either by using padded splints or by direct immobilization with respect to the body using a sling and swath device. The upper arm usually is immobilized by splinting it to the body or applying a sling or swath, which can be augmented by a thoracobrachial bandage. Shoulder injuries are managed by a sling-and-swath device or a Velcro-type of dressing.

Pain Control

Analgesics are indicated for joint injuries and fractures. The appropriate use of splints significantly decreases the patient's discomfort by controlling the amount of motion that occurs at the injured site.

Patients who do not appear to have significant pain and discomfort from a major fracture may have other associated injuries—for example, intracranial lesions or hypoxia—or may be under the influence of alcohol and/or other drugs.

Effective pain relief usually requires the administration of narcotics, which should be given in small doses intravenously and repeated as needed. Muscle relaxants and sedatives should be administered cautiously in patients with isolated extremity injuries—for example, reduction of a dislocation. Regional nerve blocks have a role in pain relief and the reduction of appropriate fractures. It is essential to assess and document any peripheral nerve injury before administering a nerve block.

Whenever analgesics, muscle relaxants, or sedatives are administered to an injured patient, the potential exists for respiratory arrest. Consequently, appropriate resuscitative equipment must be immediately available.

Associated Injuries

Certain musculoskeletal injuries, because of their common mechanism of injury, are often associated with other injuries that are not immediately apparent or

■ TABLE 8.4 Injuries Associated with Musculoskeletal Injuries	
INJURY	**MISSED/ASSOCIATED INJURY**
Clavicular fracture Scapular fracture Fracture and/or dislocation of shoulder	Major thoracic injury, especially pulmonary contusion and rib fractures
Displaced thoracic spine fracture	Thoracic aortic rupture
Spine fracture	Intraabdominal injury
Fracture/dislocation of elbow	Brachial artery injury Median, ulnar, and radial nerve injury
Femur fracture	Femoral neck fracture Posterior hip dislocation
Posterior knee dislocation	Femoral fracture Posterior hip dislocation
Knee dislocation or displaced tibial plateau fracture	Popliteal artery and nerve injuries
Calcaneal fracture	Spine injury or fracture Fracture-dislocation of hind foot Tibial plateau fracture
Open fracture	70% incidence of associated nonskeletal injury

may be missed (Table 8.4). Steps to ensure recognition and management of these injuries include:

1. Review the injury history, especially the mechanism of injury, to determine whether another injury is present.

2. Thoroughly reexamine all extremities, placing special emphasis on the hands, wrists, feet, and the joint above and below a fracture or dislocation.

3. Visually examine the patient's dorsum, including the spine and pelvis. Open injuries and closed soft tissue injuries that may be indicative of an unstable injury must be documented.

4. Review the x-rays obtained in the secondary survey to identify subtle injuries that may be associated with more obvious trauma.

Occult Skeletal Injuries

Remember, not all injuries can be diagnosed during the initial assessment and management of injury. Joints or bones that are covered or well padded within muscular areas may contain occult injuries. It can be difficult to identify nondisplaced fractures or joint ligamentous injuries, especially if the patient is unresponsive or there are other severe injuries. It is important to recognize that injuries are commonly discovered days after the injury incident—for example, when the patient is being mobilized. Therefore, is it important to reassess the patient routinely and to relate this possibility to other members of the trauma team and the patient's family.

PITFALL

Despite a thorough examination, occult associated injuries may not be identified during the initial evaluation. It is imperative to repeatedly reevaluate the patient to assess for these injuries.

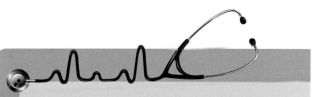

Scenario ■ conclusion   A traction splint is applied to the patient's extremity. He is given intravenous pain medication and transferred to the nearest trauma center with an orthopedic surgeon for early fixation of his femoral fracture.

Chapter Summary

1 Musculoskeletal injuries, although generally not life-threatening, may pose delayed threats to life and limb.

2 The goal of the initial assessment of musculoskeletal trauma is to identify injuries that pose a threat to life and/or limb. Although uncommon, life-threatening musculoskeletal injuries must be properly assessed and managed. Most extremity injuries are appropriately diagnosed and managed during the secondary survey.

3 It is essential to recognize and manage in a timely manner arterial injuries, compartment syndrome, open fractures, crush injuries, and fracture-dislocations. Knowledge of the mechanism of injury and history of the injury-producing event enables the clinician to be aware of what associated conditions potentially exist with the injured extremity.

4 Early splinting of fractures and dislocations may prevent serious complications and late sequelae.

BIBLIOGRAPHY

1. Beekley AC, Starnes BW, Sebesta JA. Lessons learned from modern military surgery. *Surg Clin North Am* 2007;87(1):157-84,vii.

2. Brown CV, Rhee P, Chan L, Evans K, Demetriades D, Velmahos GC. Preventing renal failure in patients with rhabdomyolysis: do bicarbonate and mannitol make a difference? *J Trauma* 2004;56:1191.

3. Clifford CC. Treating traumatic bleeding in a combat setting. *Mil Med* 2004;169(12Suppl):8-10, 14.

5. Elliot GB, Johnstone AJ. Diagnosing acute compartment syndrome. *J Bone Joint Surg Br* 2003;85:625-630.

6. Gustilo RB, Mendoza RM, Williams DN. Problems in the management of type III (severe) open fractures: a new classification of type III open fractures. *J Trauma* 1985;24:742.

9. King RB, Filips D, Blitz S, Logsetty S. Evaluation of possible tourniquet systems for use in the Canadian Forces. *J Trauma* 2006;60(5):1061-1071.

10. Kostler W, Strohm PC, Sudkamp NP. Acute compartment syndrome of the limb. *Injury* 2004;35(12):1221-1227.

12. Lakstein D, Blumenfeld A, Sokolov T, et al. Tourniquets for hemorrhage control on the battlefield: a 4-year accumulated experience. *J Trauma* 2003;54(5 Suppl):S221-S225.

13. Mabry RL. Tourniquet use on the battlefield. *Mil Med* 2006;171(5):352-356.

14. Ododeh M. The role of reperfusion-induced injury in the pathogenesis of the crush syndrome. *N Engl J Med* 1991;324:1417-1421.

15. Okike K, Bhattacharyya T. Trends in the management of open fractures. A critical analysis. *J Bone Joint Surg Am* 2006;88:2739-2748.

16. Olson SA, Glasgow RR. Acute compartment syndrome in lower extremity musculoskeletal trauma. *J Am Acad Orthop Surg* 2005;13(7):436-444.

17. Ulmer T. The clinical diagnosis of compartment syndrome of the lower leg: are clinical findings predictive of the disorder? *J Orthop Trauma* 2002;16(8):572-577.

18. Walters TJ, Mabry RL. Issues related to the use of tourniquets on the battlefield. *Mil Med* 2005;170(9):770-775.

19. Walters TJ, Wenke JC, Kauvar DS, McManus JG, Holcomb JB, Baer DG. Effectiveness of self-applied tourniquets in human volunteers. *Prehosp Emerg Care* 2005;9(4):416-422.

20. Welling DR, Burris DG, Hutton JE, Minken SL, Rich NM. A balanced approach to tourniquet use: lessons learned and relearned. *J Am Coll Surg* 2006;203(1):106-115.

Musculoskeletal Trauma: Assessment and Management

▶▶ INTERACTIVE SKILL PROCEDURES

Note: Standard precautions are required when caring for trauma patients. A series of x-rays with related scenarios is provided for use during this Skill Station in making evaluation and management decisions based on the radiographic findings.

The goal of splinting is to prevent further soft tissue injury and control bleeding and pain. Consider the immobilization of fractured extremities with the use of splints as "secondary resuscitation devices" that aid in the control of bleeding.

THE FOLLOWING PROCEDURES ARE INCLUDED IN THIS SKILL STATION:

> ▶▶ **Skill XIII-A:** Physical Examination

> ▶▶ **Skill XIII-B:** Principles of Extremity Immobilization

> ▶▶ **Skill XIII-C:** Realigning a Deformed Extremity

> ▶▶ **Skill XIII-D:** Application of a Traction Splint

> ▶▶ **Skill XIII-E:** Compartment Syndrome: Assessment and Management

> ▶▶ **Skill XIII-F:** Identification of Arterial Injury

Objectives

Performance at this skill station will allow the participant to:

1 Perform a rapid assessment of the essential components of the musculoskeletal system.

2 Identify life-threatening and limb-threatening injuries of the musculoskeletal system, and institute appropriate initial management of these injuries.

3 Identify patients who are at risk for compartment syndrome.

4 Explain the indications for and the value of appropriate splinting of musculoskeletal injuries.

5 Apply standard splints to the extremities, including a traction splint.

6 List the complications associated with the use of splints.

▶ SCENARIOS

SCENARIO XIII-1

A 28-year-old male is involved in a head-on motorcycle collision with a car. At the scene, he was combative, his systolic blood pressure was 80 mm Hg, his heart rate 120 beats/min, and his respiratory rate was 20 breaths/min. In the emergency department (ED), his vital signs have returned to normal, and the patient reports pain in his right upper extremity and both lower extremities. His right thigh and left lower extremity are deformed. Prehospital personnel report a large laceration to the left leg, to which they applied a dressing.

SCENARIO XIII-2

Scenario A: A 20-year-old female is found trapped in her automobile. Several hours are required to extricate her because her left leg was trapped and twisted beneath the dashboard. In the hospital, she has no hemodynamic abnormalities and is alert. She reports severe pain in her left leg, which is splinted.

Scenario B: A 34-year-old male is shot in the right leg while cleaning his handgun. He is unable to walk because of knee pain and states that his lower extremity is painful, weak, and numb.

SCENARIO XIII-3

A 16-year-old male is thrown approximately 100 feet (33 meters) from the back of a pickup truck. In the ED his skin is cool, and he is lethargic and unresponsive. His systolic blood pressure is 75 mm Hg, his heart rate is 145 beats/min, and his respirations are rapid and shallow. Breath sounds are equal and clear on auscultation. Two large-caliber IV catheters are initiated, and 1500 mL of warmed crystalloid solution is infused. However, the patient's hemodynamic status does not improve significantly. His blood pressure now is 84/58 mm Hg, and his heart rate is 135 beats/min.

▶ Skill XIII-A: Physical Examination

▶▶ LOOK, GENERAL OVERVIEW

External hemorrhage is identified by obvious external bleeding from an extremity, pooling of blood on the stretcher or floor, blood-soaked dressings, and bleeding that occurs during transport to the hospital. The examiner should ask about characteristics of the injury incident and prehospital care. Remember, open wounds may not bleed, but may be indicative of an open fracture.

STEP 1. Splint deformed extremities, which are indicative of a fracture or joint injury, before patient transport or as soon as is safely possible.

STEP 2. Assess the color of the extremity. The presence of bruising indicates muscle injury or significant soft tissue injury over bones or joints. These changes may be associated with swelling or hematoma. Vascular impairment may be first identified by a pale distal extremity.

STEP 3. Note the position of the extremity, which can be helpful in determining specific injury patterns. Certain nerve deficits lead to specific positions of the extremity. For example, injury to the radial nerve results in wrist drop, and injury to the peroneal nerve results in foot drop.

STEP 4. Observe spontaneous activity to help determine the severity of injury. **Observing whether the patient spontaneously moves an extremity may suggest to the examiner other obvious or occult injuries.** An example is a patient with a brain injury who does not follow commands and has no spontaneous lower-extremity movement; this patient could have a thoracic or lumbar fracture.

STEP 5. Note gender and age, which are important clues to potential injuries. Children may sustain growth plate injuries and fractures that may not manifest themselves (e.g., buckle fracture).

▶▶ FEEL

Life- and limb-threatening injuries are excluded first.

STEP 1. Palpate pulses in all extremities and document the findings. Any perceived abnormality or difference must be explained. Normal capillary refill (<2 seconds) of the pulp space or nail bed provides a good indication of satisfactory blood flow to the distal parts of the extremity. Loss or diminishment of pulses with normal capillary refill indicates a viable extremity; however, surgical consultation is required. **If an extremity has no pulses and no capillary refill, a surgical emergency exists.** A Doppler device is useful to assess pulses and determine the ankle/arm systolic pressure ratio. Blood pressure is measured at the ankle and on an uninjured arm. The normal ratio exceeds 0.9. If the ratio is below 0.9, a potential injury exists and surgical consultation is required.

STEP 2. Palpate the muscle compartments of all the extremities for compartment syndromes and fractures. This is done by gentle palpation of the muscle and bone. If a fracture is present, the patient reports pain. A compartment syndrome should be considered if the muscle compartment is very firm or tender. Compartment syndromes may be associated with fractures.

STEP 3. Assess joint stability by asking the cooperative patient to move the joint through a range of motion. This should not be done if there is an obvious fracture or deformity, or if the patient cannot cooperate. Palpate each joint for tenderness, swelling, and intraarticular fluid. Assess joint stability by applying lateral, medial, and anterior-posterior stress. Any deformed or dislocated joint should be splinted and x-rayed before testing for stability.

STEP 4. Perform a rapid, thorough neurologic examination of the extremities and document the findings. Repeat and record testing as indicated by the patient's clinical condition. Test sensation by light touch and pinprick in each of the extremities. Progression of the neurologic findings indicates a potential problem.

A. C5—Lateral aspect of the upper arm (also axillary nerve)
B. C6—Palmar aspect of the thumb and index finger (median nerve)
C. C7—Palmar aspect of the long finger
D. C8—Palmar aspect of the little finger (ulnar nerve)
E. T1—Medial aspect of the forearm
F. L3—Medial aspect of the thigh
G. L4—Medial aspect of the lower leg, especially over the medial malleolus
H. L5—Dorsum of the foot between the first and second toes (common peroneal)
I. S1—Lateral aspect of the foot

STEP 5. Perform motor examination of the extremities.

A. Shoulder abduction—Axillary nerve, C5
B. Elbow flexion—Musculocutaneous nerve, C5 and C6
C. Elbow extension—Radial nerve, C6, C7, and C8
D. Hand and wrist—Power grip tests dorsiflexion of the wrist (radial nerve, C6) and flexion of the fingers (median and ulnar nerves, C7 and C8)
E. Finger add/abduction—Ulnar nerve, C8 and T1
F. Lower extremity—Dorsiflexion of the great toe and ankle tests the deep peroneal nerve, L5, and plantar dorsiflexion tests the posterior tibial nerve, S1
G. Muscle power is graded in the standard form. The motor examination is specific to a variety of voluntary movements of each extremity. See Chapter 7: Spine and Spinal Cord Trauma.

STEP 6. Assess the deep tendon reflexes.

STEP 7. Assess the patient's back.

▶ Skill XIII-B: Principles of Extremity Immobilization

STEP 1. Assess the ABCDEs, and treat life-threatening situations first.

STEP 2. Remove all clothing and completely expose the patient, including the extremities. Remove watches, rings, bracelets, and other potentially constricting devices. Remember to prevent the development of hypothermia.

STEP 3. Assess the neurovascular status of the extremity before applying the splint. Assess for pulses and external hemorrhage, which must be controlled, and perform a motor and sensory examination of the extremity.

STEP 4. Cover any open wounds with sterile dressings.

STEP 5. Select the appropriate size and type of splint for the injured extremity. The device should immobilize the joint above and the joint below the injury site.

STEP 6. Apply padding over bony prominences that will be covered by the splint.

STEP 7. Place the extremity in a splint if normally aligned. If malaligned, the extremity needs to be realigned and then splinted. Do not force realignment of a deformed extremity with a normal pulse. Careful rotation and realignment may be required if circulation is compromised; this is best done by an experienced provider.

STEP 8. Obtain orthopedic consultation.

STEP 9. Document the neurovascular status of the extremity before and after every manipulation or splint application.

STEP 10. Administer appropriate tetanus prophylaxis. See Tetanus Immunization (electronic version only).

▶ Skill XIII-C: Realigning a Deformed Extremity

Physical examination determines whether a deformity is from a fracture or a dislocation. The principle of realigning an extremity fracture is to restore length by applying gentle longitudinal traction to correct the residual angulation and then rotational deformities. While maintaining realignment with manual traction, a splint is applied and secured to the extremity by an assistant.

▶▶ HUMERUS

STEP 1. Grasp the elbow and manually apply distal traction.

STEP 2. After alignment is obtained, apply a splint and secure the arm to the chest wall with a sling and swath.

▶▶ FOREARM

STEP 1. Manually apply distal traction through the wrist while holding the elbow and applying countertraction.

STEP 2. Secure a splint to the forearm and elevate the injured extremity.

▶▶ FEMUR

STEP 1. Realign the femur by manually applying traction through the ankle if the tibia and fibula are not fractured.

STEP 2. As the muscle spasm is overcome, the leg will straighten and the rotational deformity can be corrected. This maneuver may take several minutes, depending on the size of the patient.

▶▶ TIBIA

STEP 1. Manually apply distal traction at the ankle and countertraction just above the knee, provided that the femur is intact.

▶▶ VASCULAR AND NEUROLOGIC DEFICITS

Fractures associated with neurovascular deficits require prompt realignment. Immediate consultation with a surgeon is necessary. If the vascular or neurologic status worsens after realignment and splinting, the splint should be removed and the extremity returned to the position in which blood flow and neurologic status are maximized. The extremity is then immobilized in that position.

▶ Skill XIII-D: Application of a Traction Splint

Note: Application of this device requires two people—one person to handle the injured extremity, and the second to apply the splint.

STEP 1. Remove all clothing, including footwear, to expose the extremity.

STEP 2. Apply sterile dressings to open wounds.

STEP 3. Assess the neurovascular status of the extremity.

STEP 4. Cleanse any exposed bone and muscle of dirt and debris before applying traction. Document that the exposed bone fragments were reduced into the soft tissues.

STEP 5. Determine the length of the splint by measuring the uninjured leg. The upper cushioned ring should be placed under the buttocks and adjacent to the ischial tuberosity. The distal end of the splint should extend beyond the ankle by approximately 6 inches (15 cm). The straps on the splint should be positioned to support the thigh and calf.

STEP 6. Align the femur by manually applying traction through the ankle. After realignment is achieved, gently elevate the leg to allow the assistant to slide the splint under the extremity so that the padded portion of the splint rests against the ischial tuberosity.

STEP 7. Reassess the neurovascular status of the distal injured extremity after applying traction.

STEP 8. Position the ankle hitch around the patient's ankle and foot while the assistant maintains manual traction on the leg. The bottom strap should be slightly shorter than, or at least the same length as, the two upper crossing straps.

STEP 9. Attach the ankle hitch to the traction hook while the assistant maintains manual traction and support. Apply traction in increments using the windlass knob until the extremity appears stable, or until pain and muscular spasm are relieved.

STEP 10. Reassess the neurovascular status of the injured extremity. If perfusion of the extremity distal to the injury appears worse after applying traction, gradually release the traction.

STEP 11. Secure the remaining straps.

STEP 12. Frequently reevaluate the neurovascular status of the extremity. Document the neurovascular status after every manipulation of the extremity.

STEP 13. Administer tetanus prophylaxis, as indicated. See Tetanus Immunization (electronic version only).

▶ Skill XIII-E: Compartment Syndrome: Assessment and Management

STEP 1. Consider the following important facts:
- Compartment syndrome can develop insidiously.
- Compartment syndrome can develop in an extremity as the result of compression or crushing forces and without obvious external injury or fracture.
- Frequent reevaluation of the injured extremity is essential.
- The patient who has had hypotension or is unconscious is at increased risk for compartment syndrome.
- Pain is the earliest symptom that heralds the onset of compartment ischemia, especially pain on passive stretch of the involved muscles of the extremity.
- Unconscious or intubated patients cannot communicate the early signs of extremity ischemia.
- Loss of pulses and other classic findings of ischemia occur late, after irreversible damage has occurred.

STEP 2. Palpate the muscular compartments of the extremities, comparing the compartment tension in the injured extremity with that in the noninjured extremity.

   A. Asymmetry may be a significant finding.

   B. Frequent examination for tense muscular compartments is essential.

   C. Measurement of compartment pressures may be helpful.

STEP 3. Obtain orthopedic or general surgical consultation early.

▶ Skill XIII-F: Identification of Arterial Injury

STEP 1. Recognize that ischemia is a limb-threatening and potentially life-threatening condition.

STEP 2. Palpate peripheral pulses bilaterally (dorsalis pedis, anterior tibial, femoral, radial, and brachial) for quality and symmetry.

STEP 3. Document and evaluate any evidence of asymmetry in peripheral pulses.

STEP 4. Reevaluate peripheral pulses frequently, especially if asymmetry is identified. Use Doppler and measurement of ankle/brachial index to assess the presence and quality of distal pulses.

STEP 5. Obtain early surgical consultation.

9 Thermal Injuries

All thermal injuries require the identification and management of associated mechanical injuries and the maintenance of hemodynamic normality with volume resuscitation.

Scenario A 54-year-old male is rescued from a smoke-filled room in a burning house. He is conscious, agitated, and coughing carbonaceous sputum. The patient's head and upper body appear to be extensively burned.

Outline

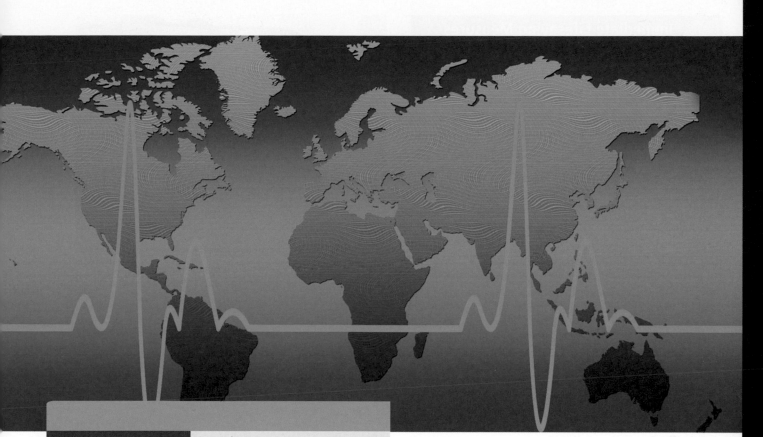

Objectives

1 Given a patient with burn injury, estimate the burn size and determine the presence of associated injuries.

2 Demonstrate the initial assessment and treatment of patients with thermal injuries.

3 Identify the unique problems that can be encountered in the treatment of patients with thermal injuries, and explain how to resolve them.

4 List the criteria for transferring patients with burn injuries to burn centers.

Thermal injuries are major causes of morbidity and mortality. Attention to the basic principles of initial trauma resuscitation and the timely application of simple emergency measures can help to minimize the morbidity and mortality of these injuries. These principles include a high index of suspicion for the presence of airway compromise following smoke inhalation, identification and management of associated mechanical injuries, and maintenance of hemodynamic normality with volume resuscitation. Clinicians also must take measures to prevent and treat the potential complications of thermal injuries, such as rhabdomyolysis and cardiac dysrhythmias, which can be seen in electrical burns. Temperature control and removal from the injury-provoking environment also are major principles of thermal injury management.

Note: Heat injuries, including heat exhaustion and heat stroke, are explained in Appendix B: Hypothermia and Heat Injuries.

Immediate Lifesaving Measures for Burn Injuries

? *What is my first priority?*

Lifesaving measures for patients with burn injuries include establishing airway control, stopping the burning process, and gaining intravenous access.

AIRWAY

Because burns can result in massive edema, the upper airway is at risk for obstruction. Signs of obstruction may initially be subtle until the patient is in crisis; therefore, early evaluation of the need for endotracheal intubation is essential. Factors that increase the risk for upper airway obstruction are increasing burn size and depth, burns to the head and face, inhalation injury, and burns inside the mouth (■ **FIGURE 9-1**). Burns localized to the face and mouth cause more localized edema and pose a greater risk for airway compromise. Because their airways are smaller, children are at higher risk for airway problems.

? *How do I identify inhalation injury?*

Although the larynx protects the subglottic airway from direct thermal injury, the airway is extremely susceptible to obstruction as a consequence of exposure to heat. Clinical indications of inhalation injury include:

- Face and/or neck burns

- Singeing of the eyebrows and nasal vibrissae

- Carbon deposits in the mouth and/or nose and carbonaceous sputum

- Acute inflammatory changes in the oropharynx, including erythema

- Hoarseness

- History of impaired mentation and/or confinement in a burning environment

- Explosion with burns to head and torso

- Carboxyhemoglobin level greater than 10% in a patient who was involved in a fire

Any of the above findings suggests an inhalation injury and the need for intubation. **Transfer to a burn center is indicated if there is inhalation injury, but if the transport time is prolonged, intubation should be performed prior to transport. Stridor occurs late and is an indication for immediate endotracheal intubation. Circumferen-**

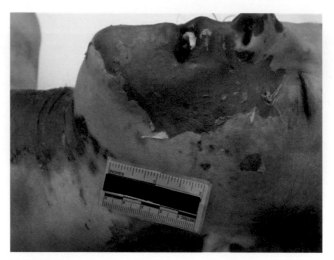

■ FIGURE 9-1 Factors that increase the risk for upper airway obstruction are increasing burn size and depth, burns to the head and face, inhalation injury, associated trauma, and burns inside the mouth.

tial burns of the neck can lead to swelling of the tissues around the airway; therefore, early intubation is also indicated for these injuries.

STOP THE BURNING PROCESS

All clothing should be removed to stop the burning process (■ **FIGURE 9-2**); however, do not peel off adherent clothing. Synthetic fabrics can ignite, burn rapidly at high temperatures, and melt into hot residue that continues to burn the patient. Any clothing that was burned by chemicals should be removed carefully. Dry chemical powders should be brushed from the wound, with the individual caring for the patient avoiding direct contact with the chemical. Then the involved body-surface areas should be rinsed with copious amounts of warm tap water. The patient then should be covered with warm, clean, dry linens to prevent hypothermia.

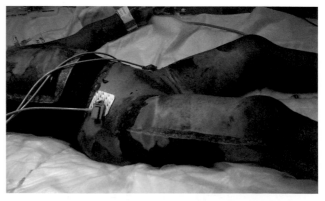

■ FIGURE 9-2 All clothing and jewelry should be removed from the patient to stop the burning process and to prevent constriction from edema.

INTRAVENOUS ACCESS

Any patient with burns over more than 20% of the body surface requires fluid resuscitation. After establishing airway patency and identifying and treating immediately life-threatening injuries, intravenous access must be established. Large-caliber (at least 16-gauge) intravenous lines should be introduced immediately in a peripheral vein. If the extent of the burn precludes placement of the catheter through unburned skin, the IV should be placed through the burned skin into an accessible vein. The upper extremities are preferable to the lower extremities as a site for venous access because of the increased risk of phlebitis and septic phlebitis when the saphenous veins are used for venous access. Begin infusion with an isotonic crystalloid solution, preferably lactated Ringer's solution. Guidelines for establishing the flow rate are outlined later in this chapter.

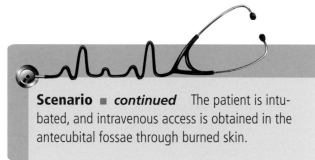

Scenario ■ *continued* The patient is intubated, and intravenous access is obtained in the antecubital fossae through burned skin.

![Assessment of Patients with Burns]

The assessment of patients with burn injuries begins with the patient history and is followed by estimation of the body-surface area burned and the depth of the burn injury.

HISTORY

The injury history is extremely valuable in the treatment of patients with burns. Associated injuries can be sustained while the victim attempts to escape the fire, and injury from explosions can result in internal injuries or fractures (e.g., central nervous system, myocardial, pulmonary, and abdominal injuries). It is essential that the time of the burn injury be established. Burns sustained within an enclosed space suggest the potential for inhalation injury and anoxic brain injury if there is an associated loss of consciousness.

The history, from the patient or a relative, should include a brief survey of preexisting illnesses (e.g., diabetes, hypertension, cardiac, pulmonary, and/or renal disease) and drug therapy, as well as any allergies and/or drug sensitivities. Some patients attempt suicide through self-immolation, so the clinician should be aware of this possibility. In addition, the patient history should be matched with the burn pattern. If the "story" is suspicious, the clinician should be concerned about the possibility of maltreatment. The patient's tetanus immunization status also should be ascertained.

BODY-SURFACE AREA

How do I estimate burn size and depth?

The Rule of Nines is a useful and practical guide for determining the extent of a burn (■ FIGURE 9-3). The adult body configuration is divided into anatomic regions that represent 9%, or multiples of 9%, of the total body surface. Body-surface area (BSA) differs considerably for children. The infant's or young child's head represents a larger proportion of the surface area, and the lower extremities represent a smaller proportion than an adult's. The percentage of total body surface of an infant's head is twice that of the normal adult. **The palmar surface (including the fingers) of the patient's hand represents approximately 1% of the patient's body surface.** The Rule of Nines guideline helps estimate the extent of burns with irregular outlines or distribution and is considered the preferred tool for calculating and documenting the extent of a burn injury.

DEPTH OF BURN

The depth of burn is important in evaluating the severity of a burn, planning for wound care, and predicting functional and cosmetic results.

First-degree burns (e.g., sunburn) are characterized by erythema, pain, and the absence of blisters. They are not life-threatening and generally do not require intravenous fluid replacement because the epidermis remains intact. This type of burn is not discussed further in this chapter and is not included in the assessment of burn size.

Partial-thickness burns are characterized by a red or mottled appearance with associated swelling and blister formation (■ FIGURE 9-4 A and B). The surface can have a weeping, wet appearance and is painfully hypersensitive, even to air current.

Full-thickness burns usually appear dark and leathery (■ FIGURE 9-4 C and D). The skin also may appear translucent or waxy white. The surface is painless and generally dry; it may be red, but does not blanch with pressure. There is little swelling of the full-thickness burned tissue, although the surrounding tissue may swell a significant amount.

Pediatric

Adult

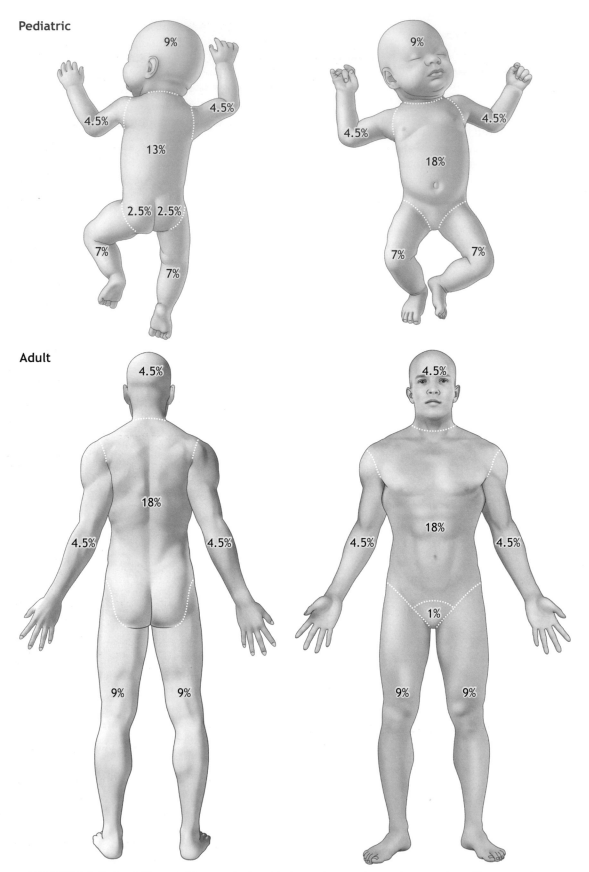

■ **FIGURE 9-3 Rule of Nines.** This practical guide is used to evaluate the severity of burns and determine fluid management. The adult body is generally divided into surface areas of 9% each and/or fractions or multiples of 9%.

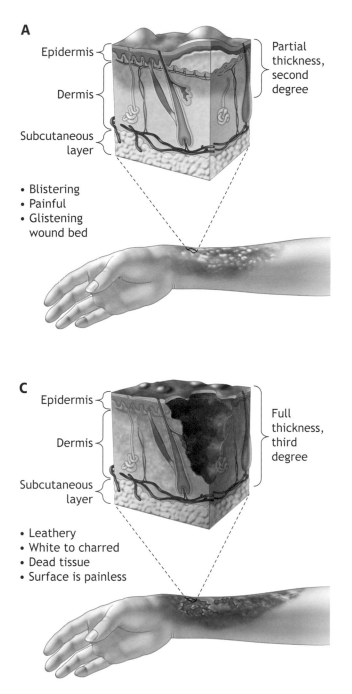

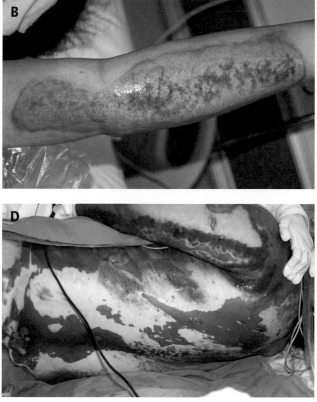

■ **FIGURE 9-4 Depth of Burns. (A)** Shallow partial-thickness burn injury. **(B)** Partial-thickness burn. **(C)** Deep partial, full-thickness burn injury. **(D)** Full-thickness burn injury on a patient's upper arm and back.

Primary Survey and Resuscitation of Patients with Burns

The primary survey and resuscitation of patients with burn injuries focuses on airway, breathing, and circulation.

AIRWAY

A history of confinement in a burning environment or early signs of airway injury on arrival in the emergency department (ED) necessitates evaluation of the airway with definitive management. Pharyngeal thermal injuries can produce marked upper airway edema, and early protection of the airway is important. The clinical manifestations of inhalation injury may be subtle and frequently do not appear in the first 24 hours. If the provider waits for x-ray evidence of pulmonary injury or change in blood gas determinations, airway edema can preclude intubation, and a surgical airway may be required.

BREATHING

Direct thermal injury to the lower airway is very rare and essentially only occurs after exposure to super-heated steam or ignition of inhaled flammable gases. Breathing concerns arise from three general areas: hypoxia, carbon monoxide poisoning, and smoke inhalation injury.

Hypoxia may be related to inhalation injury, inadequate ventilation due to circumferential chest burns, or traumatic thoracic injury unrelated to the thermal injury. Supplemental oxygen with or without intubation should be administered.

Always assume carbon monoxide (CO) exposure in patients who were burned in enclosed areas. The diagnosis of CO poisoning is made primarily from a history of exposure and direct measurement of carboxyhemoglobin (HbCO). Patients with CO levels of less than 20% usually have no physical symptoms. Higher CO levels can result in:

- headache and nausea (20%–30%)
- confusion (30%–40%)
- coma (40%–60%)
- death (>60%)

Cherry-red skin color is rare, and may only be seen in the moribund patient. Because of the increased affinity of CO for hemoglobin, 240 times that of oxygen, it displaces oxygen from the hemoglobin molecule and shifts the oxyhemoglobin dissociation curve to the left. CO dissociates very slowly, and its half-life is 250 minutes (4 hours) when the patient is breathing room air, compared with 40 minutes when breathing 100% oxygen. Therefore, any patient in whom CO exposure could have occurred should receive high-flow oxygen via a non-rebreathing mask.

Early management of inhalation injury may require endotracheal intubation and mechanical ventilation. Prior to intubation, the patient should be preoxygenated with continuous administration of oxygen. Intubation should be performed early in patients with suspected airway injury. Because there is a high probability of the need for bronchoscopy in burn patients with airway injury, an endotracheal tube of sufficient size should be chosen for a definitive airway. Arterial blood gas determinations should be obtained as a baseline for the evaluation of the patient's pulmonary status. However, measurements of arterial PaO_2 do not reliably predict CO poisoning, because a CO partial pressure of only 1 mm Hg results in an HbCO level of 40% or greater. Therefore, baseline HbCO levels should be obtained, and 100% oxygen should be administered.

Inhalation of products of combustion, including carbon particles and toxic fumes, is important to diagnose, because it doubles the mortality of burn patients when compared with patients of a similar age and burn size who do not have inhalation injury. The pathophysiology involves smoke particles settling into the distal bronchioles, leading to damage and death of the mucosal cells. Damage to the airways then leads to an increased inflammatory response that, in turn, leads to an increase in capillary leakage, which results in an oxygen diffusion defect. The necrotic cells tend to slough and obstruct the airways. This plugging of the airways and an impaired ability to fight infection lead to an increased risk of pneumonia.

The American Burn Association has defined two requirements for the diagnosis of smoke inhalation injury: (1) exposure to a combustible agent, and (2) signs of exposure to smoke in the lower airway, below the vocal cords, by bronchoscopy. The possibility of smoke inhalation injury is much higher if the injury occurred within an enclosed place. Prolonged exposure also increases the likelihood for smoke inhalation injury.

An initial chest x-ray and arterial blood gas determination should be obtained as a baseline for evaluating the patient's pulmonary status. Although the initial x-ray and blood gas may be normal, they may deteriorate over time. The treatment of smoke inhalation injury is supportive. A patient with a high likelihood of smoke inhalation injury associated with a significant burn should be intubated. If the patient's hemodynamic condition permits and spinal injury has been excluded, elevation of the head and chest by 30 degrees helps to reduce neck and chest wall edema. If a full-thickness burn of the anterior and lateral chest wall leads to severe restriction of chest wall motion, even in the absence of a circumferential burn, chest wall escharotomy may be required.

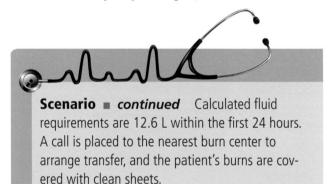

Scenario ■ *continued* Calculated fluid requirements are 12.6 L within the first 24 hours. A call is placed to the nearest burn center to arrange transfer, and the patient's burns are covered with clean sheets.

Circulation—Burn Shock Resuscitation

? *What is the rate and type of fluid administered to patients with burns?*

Evaluation of circulating blood volume is often difficult in severely burned patients. In addition, these patients may have accompanying injuries that contribute to the hypovolemic shock. Shock should be treated according to the resuscitation principles as outlined in Chapter 3: Shock. Burn resuscitation fluids also should be provided (■ FIGURE 9-5). Blood pressure measurements can be difficult to obtain and may be unreliable in patients with severe burn injuries, but monitoring of hourly urinary output can reliably assess circulating blood volume in the absence of osmotic diuresis (e.g., glycosuria). Therefore, an indwelling urinary catheter should be inserted.

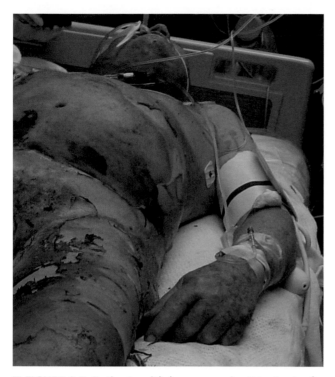

■ **FIGURE 9-5** Patients with burns require 2 to 4 mL of Ringer's lactate solution per kilogram of body weight per percentage BSA of deep partial-thickness and full-thickness burns during the first 24 hours to maintain an adequate circulating blood volume and provide adequate renal perfusion.

The initial fluid rate for burn patients is based on several well-known formulas: Patients with burns require 2 to 4 mL of Ringer's lactate solution per kilogram of body weight per percentage BSA of deep partial-thickness and full-thickness burns during the first 24 hours to maintain an adequate circulating blood volume and provide adequate renal perfusion. The calculated fluid volume is initiated in the following manner: one-half of the total fluid is provided in the first 8 hours after the burn injury. (For example, a 100 kg man with 80% total BSA burns requires 2 to 4 × 80 × 100 = 16,000 to 32,000 mL in 24 hours. One half of that volume, 8,000 to 16,000 mL should be provided in the first 8 hours, so the patient should be started at a rate of 1,000–2,000 mL/hr.) The remaining one-half of the total fluid is administered during the subsequent 16 hours.

It is important to understand that formulas are only for providing a starting target rate. After starting at this target rate, the amount of fluids provided should be adjusted based on the urine output target of 0.5 mL/kg/hr for adults and 1 mL/kg/hr for children <30 kg.

The actual fluid rate that a patient requires depends on the severity of injury. If the target urine output is not reached with the initial resuscitation rate, the fluid rate should be increased until the urine output is appropriate. If the patient has a less severe burn, a lower starting rate can be initiated. Likewise, if the urine output is at or above the 0.5 mL/kg/hr target, the IV rate should be decreased. The IV rate should *not* be decreased by one-half at 8 hours; reduction in IV fluid rate should be based on urine output.

Similarly, fluid rates should *not* be based on the time of the actual injury. Rather, start the fluids based on the initial calculation and adjust based on urine output irrespective of the time from injury. In very small children (i.e., <10 kg), it may be necessary to add glucose to their IV fluids to avoid hypoglycemia.

Cardiac dysrhythmias may be the first sign of hypoxia and electrolyte or acid-base abnormalities. Electrocardiography (ECG) should be performed for cardiac rhythm disturbances. Persistent acidemia may be caused by cyanide poisoning. Consultation with a burn center or poison control center should occur if this diagnosis is suspected. Cyanide is a naturally occurring toxin that may be inhaled in a confined-space fire.

PITFALLS

- Failure to recognize the increased fluid requirement for patients with inhalation injury and those with concomitant blunt or crush trauma, and for pediatric burn patients.

- Failure to adjust the fluid administration rate based on a patient's physiologic response.

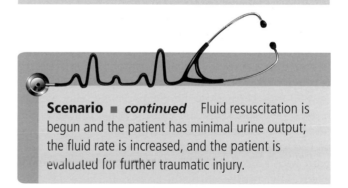

Scenario ■ *continued*   Fluid resuscitation is begun and the patient has minimal urine output; the fluid rate is increased, and the patient is evaluated for further traumatic injury.

Secondary Survey and Related Adjuncts

Key aspects of the secondary survey and its related adjuncts include physical examination, documentation, baseline blood levels and x-rays, maintenance of peripheral circulation in circumferential extremity burns, gastric tube insertion, narcotic analgesics and sedatives, wound care, and tetanus immunization.

PHYSICAL EXAMINATION

In order to plan and direct patient treatment, the provider must estimate the extent and depth of the burn, assess for associated injuries, and weigh the patient.

DOCUMENTATION

A flow sheet or other report that outlines the patient's treatment should be initiated when the patient is admitted to the ED. This flow sheet should accompany the patient when transferred to the burn unit.

BASELINE DETERMINATIONS FOR PATIENTS WITH MAJOR BURNS

Obtain samples for a complete blood count (CBC), type and crossmatch/screen, an arterial blood gas with HbCO, serum glucose, electrolytes, and pregnancy test in all females of childbearing age. A chest x-ray should be obtained for those patients who are intubated or have a suspected smoke inhalation injury, with repeat films as necessary. Other x-rays may be indicated for appraisal of associated injuries.

PERIPHERAL CIRCULATION IN CIRCUMFERENTIAL EXTREMITY BURNS

The goal for assessing peripheral circulation in a patient with burns is to rule out *compartment syndrome*. Compartment syndrome results from an increase in the pressure inside a compartment that interferes with perfusion to the structures within that compartment. For an extremity, perfusion to the muscle within the compartment is the main concern. Although a compartment pressure greater than systolic blood pressure is required to lose a pulse distal to the burn, a pressure of >30 mm Hg within the compartment may lead to muscle necrosis. Once the pulse is gone, it may be too late to save the muscle. Thus, clinicians must be aware of the signs of a compartment syndrome: increased pain with passive motion, tightness, numbness, and, eventually, decreased distal pulses. If there are concerns about a compartment syndrome, the compartment pressure is easily measured by inserting a needle connected to pressure tubing (arterial or central pressure monitor) into the compartment. If the pressure is >30 mm Hg, escharotomy is indicated.

Compartment syndromes may also present with circumferential chest and abdominal burns, leading to increased peak inspiratory pressures. Chest and abdominal escharotomies performed down the anterior axillary lines with a cross-incision at the junction of the thorax and abdomen usually relieve the problem (■ FIGURE 9-6). With aggressive fluid resuscitation,

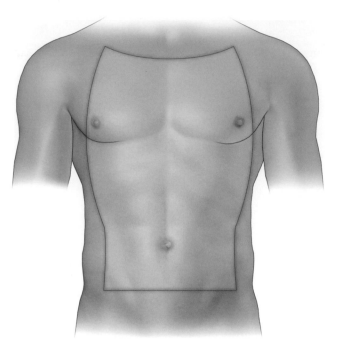

■ **FIGURE 9-6 Escharotomy.** Compartment syndromes may present with circumferential chest and abdominal burns, leading to increased peak inspiratory pressures. Chest and abdominal escharotomies performed down the anterior axillary lines with a cross-incision at the junction of the thorax and abdomen usually relieve the problem.

abdominal compartment syndrome may occur, so the clinicians should watch for this potential problem.

In order to maintain peripheral circulation in patients with circumferential extremity burns, the clinician should:

■ Remove all jewelry on the patient's extremities.

■ Assess the status of distal circulation, checking for cyanosis, impaired capillary refill, and progressive neurologic signs, such as paresthesia and deep-tissue pain. Assessment of peripheral pulses in patients with burns is best performed with a Doppler ultrasonic flow meter.

■ Relieve circulatory compromise in a circumferentially burned limb by escharotomy, always with surgical consultation. Escharotomies usually are not needed within the first 6 hours after a burn injury.

■ Although fasciotomy is seldom required, it may be necessary to restore circulation for patients with associated skeletal trauma, crush injury, high-voltage electrical injury, and burns involving tissue beneath the investing fascia.

GASTRIC TUBE INSERTION

Insert a gastric tube and attach it to a suction setup if the patient experiences nausea, vomiting, or abdominal distention, or if burns involve more than 20% total BSA. Prior to transfer, it is essential that a gastric tube be inserted and functioning in patients with these symptoms in order to avoid vomiting and possible aspiration.

NARCOTICS, ANALGESICS, AND SEDATIVES

Severely burned patients may be restless and anxious from hypoxemia or hypovolemia rather than pain. Consequently, hypoxemia and inadequate fluid resuscitation should be managed before administration of narcotic analgesics or sedatives, which can mask the signs of hypoxemia and hypovolemia. Narcotic analgesics and sedatives should be administered in small, frequent doses by the intravenous route only. Remember that simply covering the wound will improve the pain.

WOUND CARE

Partial-thickness burns are painful when air currents pass over the burned surface. Gently covering the burn with clean sheets relieves the pain and deflects air currents. Do not break blisters or apply an antiseptic agent. Any applied medication must be removed before appropriate antibacterial topical agents can be applied. Application of cold compresses can cause hypothermia. Do not apply cold water to a patient with extensive burns (>10% total BSA).

ANTIBIOTICS

There is NO indication for prophylactic antibiotics in the early post-burn period. Antibiotics should be reserved for the treatment of infection.

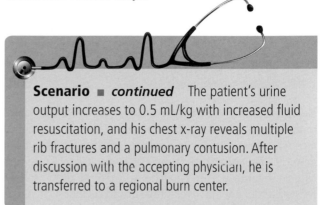

PITFALLS

- Failure to recognize development of compartment syndrome.
- Failure to adequately perform escharotomy.
- Lack of recognition that fasciotomies are seldom necessary.
- Failure to treat carbon monoxide toxicity.
- Failure to provide adequate pain relief.

TETANUS

Determination of the patient's tetanus immunization status is very important. See Tetanus Immunization (electronic version only).

Scenario ■ *continued* The patient's urine output increases to 0.5 mL/kg with increased fluid resuscitation, and his chest x-ray reveals multiple rib fractures and a pulmonary contusion. After discussion with the accepting physician, he is transferred to a regional burn center.

Chemical Burns

Chemical injury can result from exposure to acids, alkalies, and petroleum products. Alkali burns are generally more serious than acid burns, because the alkalies penetrate more deeply. Rapid removal of the chemical and immediate attention to wound care is essential. Chemical burns are influenced by the duration of contact, concentration of the chemical, and amount of the agent. If dry powder is still present on the skin, brush it away before irrigating with water. Otherwise, immediately flush away the chemical with large amounts of water, for at least 20 to 30 minutes, using a shower or hose (■ **FIGURE 9-7**). Alkali burns require longer irrigation. Neutralizing agents offer no advantage over water lavage, because reaction with the neutralizing agent can itself produce heat and cause further

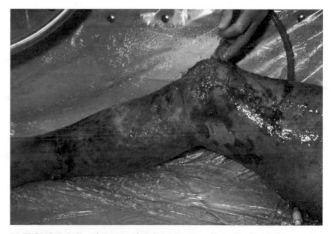

■ **FIGURE 9-7 Chemical Burn.** Immediately flush away the chemical with large amounts of water, for at least 20 to 30 minutes.

tissue damage. Alkali burns to the eye require continuous irrigation during the first 8 hours after the burn. A small-caliber cannula can be fixed in the palpebral sulcus for irrigation. There are specific chemical burns (such as hydrofluoric acid burns) that require specialized burn unit consultation.

Electrical Burns

Electrical burns result when a source of electrical power makes contact with a patient's body. The body can serve as a volume conductor of electrical energy, and the heat generated results in thermal injury to tissue. Different rates of heat loss from superficial and deep tissues allow for relatively normal overlying skin to coexist with deep-muscle necrosis. As such, electrical burns frequently are more serious than they appear on the body surface, and extremities, especially digits, are particularly prone to injury. In addition, the current travels inside blood vessels and nerves and thus may cause local thrombosis and nerve injury. Patients with electrical injuries frequently need fasciotomies and should be transferred to burn centers early in their course of treatment.

Immediate treatment of a patient with a significant electrical burn includes attention to the airway and breathing, establishment of an intravenous line in an uninvolved extremity, ECG monitoring, and placement of an indwelling bladder catheter. Electricity may cause cardiac arrhythmias that may require chest compressions. If there are no arrhythmias within the first few hours of injury, prolonged monitoring is not necessary.

Since electricity causes forced contraction of muscles, clinicians need to examine the patient for associated skeletal and muscular damage, including the possibility of spinal injuries. Rhabdomyolysis results in myoglobin release, which can cause acute renal failure. Do not wait for laboratory confirmation before instituting therapy for myoglobinuria. If the patient's urine is dark, assume that hemochromogens are in the urine. Fluid administration should be increased to ensure a urinary output of 100 mL/hr in adults or 2 mL/kg/hr in children <30 kg. Metabolic acidosis should be corrected by maintaining adequate perfusion.

Patient Transfer

? *Who do I transfer to a burn center?*

The criteria for transfer must be met and procedures must be followed in the transfer of patients to burn centers.

CRITERIA FOR TRANSFER

The American Burn Association has identified the following types of burn injuries that typically require referral to a burn center:

1. Partial-thickness and full-thickness burns on greater than 10% of the BSA in any patient

2. Partial-thickness and full-thickness burns involving the face, eyes, ears, hands, feet, genitalia, and perineum, as well as those that involve skin overlying major joints

3. Full-thickness burns of any size in any age group

4. Significant electrical burns, including lightning injury (significant volumes of tissue beneath the surface can be injured and result in acute renal failure and other complications)

5. Significant chemical burns

6. Inhalation injury

7. Burn injury in patients with preexisting illness that could complicate treatment, prolong recovery, or affect mortality

8. Any patient with a burn injury who has concomitant trauma poses an increased risk of morbidity or mortality, and may be treated initially in a trauma center until stable before being transferred to a burn center

9. Children with burn injuries who are seen in hospitals without qualified personnel or equipment to manage their care should be transferred to a burn center with these capabilities

10. Burn injury in patients who will require special social and emotional or long-term rehabilitative support, including cases involving suspected child maltreatment and neglect

TRANSFER PROCEDURES

Transfer of any patient must be coordinated with the burn center staff. All pertinent information regarding test results, temperature, heart rate, fluids administered, and urinary output should be documented on the burn/trauma flow sheet and sent with the patient. Any other information deemed important by the referring or receiving doctor also is sent with the patient.

PITFALLS

- Failure to secure the patient's airway.
- Failure to provide adequate documentation of treatment to the receiving facility.

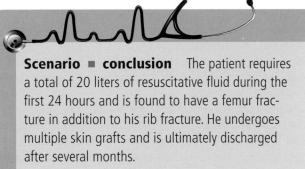

Scenario ■ conclusion The patient requires a total of 20 liters of resuscitative fluid during the first 24 hours and is found to have a femur fracture in addition to his rib fracture. He undergoes multiple skin grafts and is ultimately discharged after several months.

Cold Injury: Local Tissue Effects

❓ *How does cold affect my patient?*

The severity of cold injury depends on temperature, duration of exposure, environmental conditions, amount of protective clothing, and the patient's general state of health. Lower temperatures, immobilization, prolonged exposure, moisture, the presence of peripheral vascular disease, and open wounds all increase the severity of the injury.

TYPES OF COLD INJURY

❓ *How do I recognize a cold injury?*

Three types of cold injury are seen in trauma patients: frostnip, frostbite, and nonfreezing injury.

Frostnip

Frostnip is the mildest form of cold injury. It is characterized by initial pain, pallor, and numbness of the affected body part. It is reversible with rewarming and does not result in tissue loss, unless the injury is repeated over many years, which causes fat pad loss or atrophy.

Frostbite

Frostbite is due to freezing of tissue with intracellular ice crystal formation, microvascular occlusion, and subsequent tissue anoxia (■ FIGURE 9-8). Some of the tissue damage also can result from reperfusion injury that occurs on rewarming. Frostbite is classified into first-degree, second-degree, third-degree, and fourth-degree according to depth of involvement.

1. First-degree frostbite: Hyperemia and edema without skin necrosis

2. Second-degree frostbite: Large, clear vesicle formation accompanies the hyperemia and edema with partial-thickness skin necrosis

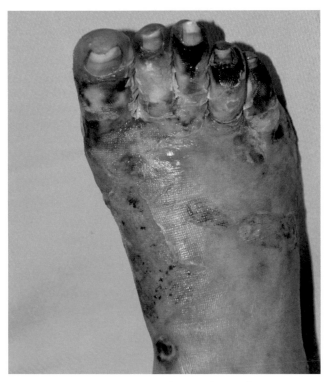

■ **FIGURE 9-8 Frostbite.** Frostbite is due to freezing of tissue with intracellular ice crystal formation, microvascular occlusion, and subsequent tissue anoxia. Some of the tissue damage also can result from reperfusion injury that occurs on rewarming.

3. Third-degree frostbite: Full-thickness and subcutaneous tissue necrosis occurs, commonly with hemorrhage vesicle formation

4. Fourth-degree frostbite: Full-thickness skin necrosis, including muscle and bone with gangrene

Although the affected body part is typically initially hard, cold, white, and numb, the appearance of the lesion changes frequently during the course of treatment. In addition, the initial treatment regimen is applicable for all degrees of insult, and the initial classification is often not prognostically accurate. Hence, some authorities simply classify frostbite as superficial or deep.

Nonfreezing Injury

Nonfreezing injury is due to microvascular endothelial damage, stasis, and vascular occlusion. Trench foot or cold immersion foot (or hand) describes a nonfreezing injury of the hands or feet, typically in soldiers, sailors, and fishermen, resulting from long-term exposure to wet conditions and temperatures just above freezing (1.6°C to 10°C, or 35°F to 50°F). Although the entire foot can appear black, deep-tissue destruction may not be present. Alternating arterial vasospasm and vasodilation occur, with the affected tissue first cold and numb, then progressing to hyperemia in 24 to 48 hours. With hyperemia comes intense, painful burning and dysesthesia, as well as tissue damage characterized by edema, blistering, redness, ecchymosis, and ulcerations. Complications of local infection, cellulitis, lymphangitis, and gangrene can occur. Proper attention to foot hygiene can prevent the occurrence of most such injuries.

MANAGEMENT OF FROSTBITE AND NONFREEZING COLD INJURIES

? *How do I treat local cold injuries?*

Treatment should be immediate to decrease the duration of tissue freezing, although rewarming should not be undertaken if there is the risk of refreezing. Constricting, damp clothing should be replaced by warm blankets, and the patient should be given hot fluids by mouth, if he or she is able to drink. Place the injured part in circulating water at a constant 40°C (104°F) until pink color and perfusion return (usually within 20 to 30 minutes). This is best accomplished in an inpatient setting in a large tank, such as a whirlpool tank. Avoid dry heat, and do not rub or massage the area. Rewarming can be extremely painful, and adequate analgesics (intravenous narcotics) are essential. Cardiac monitoring during rewarming is advised.

Local Wound Care of Frostbite

The goal of wound care for frostbite is to preserve damaged tissue by preventing infection, avoiding opening uninfected vesicles, and elevating the injured area, which is left open to air. The affected tissue should be protected by a tent or cradle, and pressure spots should be avoided.

Only rarely is fluid loss massive enough to require resuscitation with intravenous fluids, although patients may be dehydrated. Tetanus prophylaxis depends on the patient's tetanus immunization status. Systemic antibiotics are not indicated empirically, but are reserved for identified infections. The wounds should be kept clean, and uninfected blebs left intact for 7 to 10 days to provide a sterile biologic dressing to protect underlying epithelialization. Tobacco,

nicotine, and other vasoconstrictive agents must be withheld. Weight bearing is prohibited until edema is resolved. Numerous adjuvants have been attempted in an effort to restore blood supply to cold-injured tissue. Unfortunately, most are ineffective. Sympathetic blockade (sympathectomy, drugs) and vasodilating agents have generally not proven helpful in altering the natural history of the acute cold injury. Heparin and hyperbaric oxygen also have failed to demonstrate substantial treatment benefit. Low-molecular weight dextran has shown some benefit during the rewarming phase in animal models. Thrombolytic agents have also shown some promise.

With all cold injuries, estimations of depth of injury and extent of tissue damage are not usually accurate until demarcation is evident. This often requires several weeks or months of observation. Earlier surgical debridement or amputation is seldom necessary, unless infection with sepsis occurs.

PITFALLS

- Failure to rapidly rewarm the affected area.
- Overzealous debridement of tissue of questionable viability.

Cold Injury: Systemic Hypothermia

Trauma patients also are susceptible to hypothermia, and any degree of hypothermia in trauma patients can be detrimental. In trauma patients, hypothermia should be considered to be any core temperature below 36°C (96.8°F), and severe hypothermia is any core temperature below 32°C (89.6°F). Hypothermia is common in the severely injured, but further loss of core temperature can be limited with the administration of only warmed intravenous fluids and blood, judicious exposure of the patient, and maintenance of a warm environment. **Avoiding iatrogenic hypothermia during exposure and fluid administration is important, as hypothermia may worsen coagulopathy.**

The signs of hypothermia and its treatment are explained in more detail in Appendix B: Hypothermia and Heat Injuries.

Chapter Summary

1 The Rule of Nines is a useful and practical guide to determine the extent of the burn. Body surface area differs considerably for children. The infant's or young child's head represents a larger proportion of the surface area, and the lower extremities represent a smaller proportion than an adult's.

2 Associated injuries can be sustained while the victim attempts to escape the fire, and injury from explosions can result in internal injuries or fractures (e.g., central nervous system, myocardial, pulmonary, and abdominal injuries).

3 Immediate lifesaving measures for patients with burn injury include the recognition of inhalation injury and subsequent endotracheal intubation, and the rapid institution of intravenous fluid therapy. Early management of cold-injured patients includes adhering to the ABCDEs of resuscitation; identifying the type and extent of cold injury; measuring the patient's core temperature; initiating a patient-care flow sheet; and initiating rapid rewarming techniques.

4 Attention must be paid to special problems unique to thermal injuries. Carbon monoxide poisoning should be suspected and identified. Circumferential burns may require escharotomy. Chemical burns require immediate removal of clothing to prevent further injury, as well as copious irrigation. Electrical burns may be associated with extensive occult myonecrosis. Patients sustaining thermal injury are at risk for hypothermia. Judicious analgesia should not be overlooked.

5 The American Burn Association has identified types of burn injuries that typically require referral to a burn center: Transfer principles are similar to non-burned patients but include an accurate assessment of the patient's burn size and depth.

▶ BIBLIOGRAPHY

1. Cioffi WG, Graves TA, McManus WF, et al. High frequency percussive ventilation in patients with inhalation injury. *J Trauma* 1989;29:350-354.

2. Danzl D, Pozos R, Auerbach P, et al. Multicenter hypothermia survey. *Ann Emerg Med* 1987;16:1042-1055.

3. Demling HR. Burn care in the immediate resuscitation period. Section III, Thermal injury. In: Wilmor DW, ed. *Scientific American Surgery.* New York: Scientific American; 1998.

4. Edlich R, Change D, Birk K, et al. Cold injuries. *Compr Ther* 1989;15(9):13-21.

5. Gentilello LM, Cobean RA, Offner PJ, et al. Continuous arteriovenous rewarming: rapid reversal of hypothermia in critically ill patients. *J Trauma* 1992;32(3):316-327.

6. Gentilello LM, Jurkovich GJ, Moujaes S. Hypothermia and injury: thermodynamic principles of prevention and treatment. In: Levine B, ed. *Perspectives in Surgery.* St. Louis: Quality Medical; 1991.

7. Graves TA, Cioffi WG, McManus WF, et al. Fluid resuscitation of infants and children with massive thermal injury. *J Trauma* 1988;28:1656-1659.

8. Gunning K, ed. *Burns Trauma Handbook.* 5th ed. Liverpool, UK: Liverpool Hospital Department of Trauma Services; 1994.

9. Halebian P, Robinson N, Barie P, et al. Whole body oxygen utilization during carbon monoxide poisoning and isocapneic nitrogen hypoxia. *J Trauma* 1986;26:110-117.

10. Haponik EF, Munster AM, eds. *Respiratory Injury: Smoke Inhalation and Burns.* New York: McGraw-Hill; 1990.

11. Herndon D. ed. *Total Burn Care.* 3rd ed. Philadelphia, PA: Saunders; 2007.

12. Jacob J, Weisman M, Rosenblatt S, et al. Chronic pernio: a historical perspective of cold-induced vascular disease. *Arch Intern Med* 1986;146:1589-1592.

13. Jurkovich GJ. Hypothermia in the trauma patient. In: Maull KI, Cleveland HC, Strauch GO, et al., eds. *Advances in Trauma.* Vol. 4. Chicago: Yearbook; 1989:11-140.

14. Jurkovich GJ, Greiser W, Luterman A, et al. Hypothermia in trauma victims: an ominous predictor of survival. *J Trauma* 1987;27:1019-1024.

15. Lund T, Goodwin CW, McManus WF, et al. Upper airway sequelae in burn patients requiring endotracheal intubation or tracheostomy. *Ann Surg* 1985;201:374-382.

16. Mills WJ Jr. Summary of treatment of the cold injured patient: frostbite [1983 classic article]. *Ala Med* 1993;35(1):61-66.

17. Moss J. Accidental severe hypothermia. *Surg Gynecol Obstet* 1986;162:501-513.

18. Mozingo DW, Smith AA, McManus WF, et al. Chemical burns. *J Trauma* 1988;28:642-647.

19. O'Malley J, Mills W, Kappes B, et al. Frostbite: general and specific treatment, the Alaskan method. *Ala Med* 1993;27(1):pullout.

20. Perry RJ, Moore CA, et al. Determining the approximate area of burn: an inconsistency investigated and reevaluated. *BMJ* 1996;312:1338.

21. Pruitt BA Jr. The burn patient: I. Initial care. *Curr Probl Surg* 1979;16(4):1-55.

22. Pruitt BA Jr. The burn patient: II. Later care and complications of thermal injury. *Curr Probl Surg* 1979;16(5):1-95.

23. Reed R, Bracey A, Hudson J, et al. Hypothermia and blood coagulation: dissociation between enzyme activity and clotting factor levels. *Circ Shock* 1990;32:141-152.

24. Saffle JR, Crandall A, Warden GD. Cataracts: a long-term complication of electrical injury. *J Trauma* 1985;25:17-21.

25. Schaller M, Fischer A, Perret C. Hyperkalemia: a prognostic factor during acute severe hypothermia. *JAMA* 1990;264:1842-1845.

26. Sheehy TW, Navari RM. Hypothermia. *Ala J Med Sci* 1984;21(4):374-381.

27. Stratta RJ, Saffle JR, Kravitz M, et al. Management of tar and asphalt injuries. *Am J Surg* 1983;146:766-769.

10 Pediatric Trauma

Injury continues to be the most common cause of death and disability in childhood. Injury morbidity and mortality surpass all major diseases in children and young adults, making injury the most serious public health and health care problem in this population.

Outline

Scenario A 7-year-old boy is struck by a moving car while riding his bicycle. He was not wearing a helmet. He is unresponsive on arrival, breathing rapidly, and pale with mottled extremities. Vital signs on admission: heart rate: 144; respiratory rate 38; blood pressure 80/57; Glasgow Coma Scale score 5 (E = 1, V = 2, M = 2).

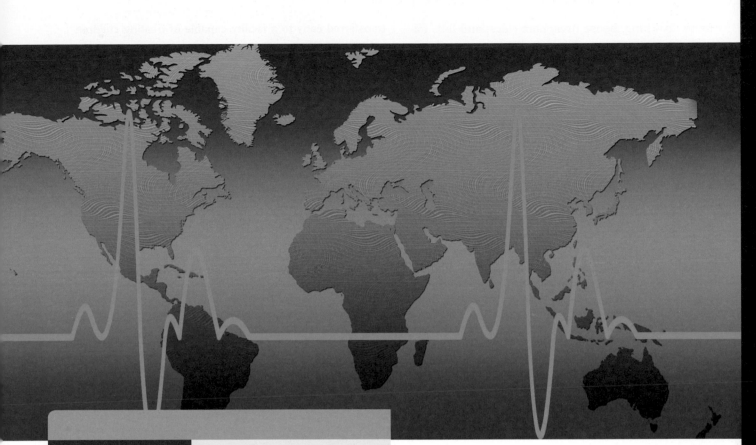

Objectives

1 Identify the unique characteristics of the child as a trauma patient, including common types of injuries, patterns of injury, anatomic and physiologic differences in children as compared with adults, and the long-term effects of injury.

2 Describe the primary management of the following critical injuries in children, to include related issues unique to pediatric patients, emphasizing the anatomic and physiologic differences as compared with adults and their impact on resuscitation:

- Airway with cervical spine control
- Breathing with recognition and management of immediately life-threatening chest injuries
- Circulation with bleeding control and shock recognition and management
- Disability with recognition and initial management of altered mental status and intracranial mass lesions
- Exposure with maintenance of body heat
- Central nervous system and cervical spine injuries
- Chest, abdomen and pelvic injuries
- Musculoskeletal injuries
- Fluid and medication dosages
- Psychological and family support

3 Identify the injury patterns associated with child maltreatment, and describe the elements that lead to the suspicion of child maltreatment.

4 List the ABCDEs of injury prevention.

Injury continues to be the most common cause of death and disability in childhood. Each year, more than 10 million children in the United States require emergency department care for the treatment of injuries, representing nearly 1 of every 6 children. Each year more than 10,000 children in the United States die from serious injury. Injury morbidity and mortality surpass all major diseases in children and young adults, making injury the most serious public health and health care problem in this population. Because failure to secure the airway, support breathing, and recognize and respond to intraabdominal and intracranial hemorrhage are known to be the leading causes of unsuccessful resuscitation in severe pediatric trauma, application of ATLS® principles to the care of injured children can have a significant impact on ultimate survival.

Types and Patterns of Injury

❓ What types of injuries do children sustain?

Motor vehicle-associated injuries are the most common cause of deaths in children of all ages, whether the child is an occupant, pedestrian, or cyclist. Deaths due to drowning, house fires, homicides, and falls follow in descending order. Child maltreatment accounts for the great majority of homicides in infants (children younger than 12 months of age), whereas firearm injuries account for the majority of homicides in children and adolescents. Falls account for the majority of all pediatric injuries, but infrequently result in death.

Blunt mechanisms of injury and children's physical characteristics result in multisystem injury being the rule rather than the exception. Table 10.1 outlines common mechanisms of injury and associated patterns of injury in pediatric patients. It should be presumed, therefore, that all organ systems may be injured until proven otherwise. **Although the condition of the majority of injured children will not deteriorate, and most injured children have no hemodynamic abnormalities, the fact remains that the condition of some children with multisystem injuries will rapidly deteriorate, and serious complications will develop. Therefore, such patients should be transferred early to a facility capable of treating children with multisystem injuries.**

The Triage Decision Scheme (see Figure 1-2) and Pediatric Trauma Score (Table 10.2) are both useful tools for the early identification of pediatric patients with multisystem injuries.

Unique Characteristics of Pediatric Patients

? *What aspects of childhood anatomy do I need to consider?*

The priorities of assessment and management of injuries in children are the same as for adults. However, the unique anatomic and physiologic characteristics of pediatric patients combine with the different mecha-

---

■ TABLE 10.1 Common Mechanisms of Injury and Associated Patterns of Injury in Pediatric Patients

MECHANISM OF INJURY	COMMON PATTERNS OF INJURY
Pedestrian struck	• Low speed: Lower extremity fractures • High speed: Multiple trauma, head and neck injuries, lower extremity fractures
Automobile occupant	• Unrestrained: Multiple trauma, head and neck injuries, scalp and facial lacerations • Restrained: Chest and abdomen injuries, lower spine fractures
Fall from a height	• Low: Upper extremity fractures • Medium: Head and neck injuries, upper and lower extremity fractures • High: Multiple trauma, head and neck injuries, upper and lower extremity fractures
Fall from a bicycle	• Without helmet: Head and neck injuries, scalp and facial lacerations, upper extremity fractures • With helmet: Upper extremity fractures • Striking handlebar: Internal abdominal injuries

---

nisms of injury to produce distinct patterns of injury. For example, most serious pediatric trauma is blunt trauma that involves the brain. As a result, apnea, hypoventilation, and hypoxia occur five times more often than hypovolemia with hypotension in seriously injured children. Therefore, treatment protocols for pediatric trauma patients emphasize aggressive management of the airway and breathing.

SIZE AND SHAPE

Because of the smaller body mass of children, the energy imparted from, for example, fenders, bumpers, and falls results in a greater force applied per unit of body area. This more intense energy is transmitted to a body that has less fat, less connective tissue, and closer proximity of multiple organs. These factors result in the high frequency of multiple injuries seen in the pediatric popula-

tion. In addition, the head is proportionately larger in young children, resulting in a higher frequency of blunt brain injuries in this age group.

SKELETON

The child's skeleton is incompletely calcified, contains multiple active growth centers, and is more pliable than an adult's. For these reasons, internal organ damage is often noted without overlying bony fracture. For example, rib fractures in children are uncommon, but pulmonary contusion is not. Other soft tissues of the thorax, heart, and mediastinum also may sustain significant damage without evidence of bony injury. The identification of skull or rib fractures in a child suggests the transfer of a massive amount of energy, and underlying organ injuries, such as traumatic brain injury and pulmonary contusion, should be suspected.

■ TABLE 10.2 Pediatric Trauma Score			
ASSESSMENT COMPONENT	SCORE		
	+2	+1	−1
Weight	>20 kg (>44 lb)	10–20 kg (22–44 lb)	<10 kg (<22 lb)
Airway	Normal	Oral or nasal airway, oxygen	Intubated, cricothyroidotomy, or tracheostomy
Systolic Blood Pressure	>90 mm Hg; good peripheral pulses and perfusion	50–90 mm Hg; carotid/femoral pulses palpable	<50 mm Hg; weak or no pulses
Level of Consciousness	Awake	Obtunded or any loss of consciousness	Coma, unresponsive
Fracture	None seen or suspected	Single, closed	Open or multiple
Cutaneous	None visible	Contusion, abrasion, laceration <7 cm not through fascia	Tissue loss, any gunshot wound or stab wound through fascia
Totals:			

Adapted with permission from Tepas JJ, Mollitt DL, Talbert JL, et al: The pediatric trauma score as a predictor of injury severity in the injured child. *Journal of Pediatric Surgery* 1987;22(1)15.

SURFACE AREA

The ratio of a child's body surface area to body volume is highest at birth and diminishes as the child matures. As a result, thermal energy loss is a significant stress factor in children. Hypothermia may develop quickly and complicate the treatment of the pediatric patient with hypotension.

PSYCHOLOGICAL STATUS

There may be significant psychological ramifications of injuries in children. In young children, emotional instability frequently leads to a regressive psychological behavior when stress, pain, and other perceived threats intervene in the child's environment. The child's ability to interact with unfamiliar individuals in strange and difficult situations is limited, making history taking and cooperative manipulation, especially if it is painful, extremely difficult. Clinicians who understand these characteristics and are willing to cajole and soothe an injured child are more likely to establish a good rapport, which facilitates a comprehensive assessment of the child's psychological and physical injuries. In addition, the presence of parents or guardians during evaluation and treatment, including resuscitation, may assist the clinician during early care of pediatric trauma patients by minimizing the injured child's natural fears and anxieties.

LONG-TERM EFFECTS

A major consideration in treating injured children is the effect that injury can have on their subsequent growth and development. Unlike adults, children must not only recover from the effects of the traumatic event, but also must continue the normal process of growth and development. The physiologic and psychological effects of injury on this process should not be underestimated, particularly in cases involving long-term function, growth deformity, or subsequent abnormal development. Children who sustain even a minor injury may have prolonged disability in cerebral function, psychological adjustment, or organ system.

Some evidence suggests that as many as 60% of children who sustain severe multisystem trauma have residual personality changes at one year after hospital discharge, and 50% show cognitive and physical handicaps. Social, affective, and learning disabilities are present in one-half of seriously injured children. In addition, childhood injuries have a significant impact on the family, with personality and emotional disturbances found in two-thirds of uninjured siblings. Frequently, a child's injuries impose a strain on the parents' marital relationship, including financial and sometimes employment hardships. Trauma may affect not only the child's survival, but also the quality of the child's life for years to come.

Bony and solid visceral injuries are cases in point: Injuries through growth centers may result in growth abnormalities of the injured bone. If the injured bone is a femur, a leg length discrepancy may result, causing a lifelong disability in running and walking. If the fracture is through the growth center of one or more thoracic vertebra, the result may be scoliosis, kyphosis, or even gibbus. In addition, massive disruption of a child's spleen may require a splenectomy. The loss of the spleen predisposes the child to a lifelong risk of overwhelming postsplenectomy sepsis and death.

Ionizing radiation, used commonly in the evaluation of injured patients, is known to increase the risk of certain malignancies and should be used only in the following circumstances:

- The information needed cannot be practically or expeditiously obtained by other means

- The information gained will change the clinical management of the patient

- The information is obtained at the lowest possible radiation "cost" to the patient

- Obtaining the information will not delay the transfer of patients who require higher levels of care

Nevertheless, the long-term quality of life for children who have sustained trauma is surprisingly robust, even though in many cases they will experience lifelong physical challenges. Most such patients report a good to excellent quality of life and find gainful employment as adults, justifying aggressive resuscitation attempts, even for pediatric patients whose initial physiologic status, e.g., Glasgow Coma Scale (GCS) score, might suggest otherwise.

EQUIPMENT

Immediately available equipment of the appropriate sizes is essential for the successful initial treatment of injured children (Table 10.3). A length-based resuscitation tape, such as the Broselow® Pediatric Emergency Tape, is an ideal adjunct for the rapid determination of weight based on length for appropriate fluid volumes, drug doses, and equipment size. By measuring the height of the child, the child's estimated weight can be determined readily. One side of the tape provides drugs and their recommended doses for the pediatric patient based on weight. The other side identifies equipment needs for

pediatric patients based on length (■ FIGURE 10-1). Clinicians should be familiar with length-based resuscitation tapes and their uses.

The American College of Surgeons Committee on Trauma, American College of Emergency Physicians, National Association of EMS Physicians, the Pediatric Equipment Guidelines Committee of the Emergency Medical Services for Children (EMSC) Partnership for Children Stakeholder Group and the American Academy of Pediatrics issued a policy statement regarding required equipment for ambulances in the July 2009 issue of *Pediatrics*.

PITFALLS

- The unique anatomic and physiologic characteristics of children occasionally lead to pitfalls in their treatment.

- The necessity of frequent reassessment must be emphasized.

Airway: Evaluation and Management

? How do I apply ATLS principles to the treatment of children?

The "A" of the ABCDEs of initial assessment is the same in children as for adults. Establishing a patent airway to provide adequate tissue oxygenation is the

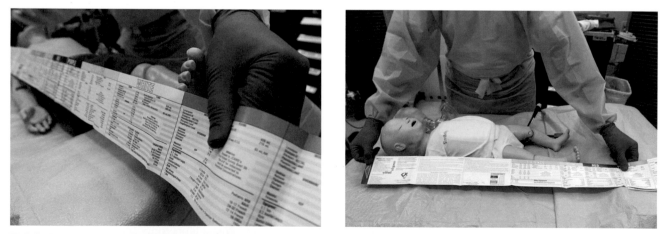

■ **FIGURE 10-1 Resuscitation Tape.** A length-based resuscitation tape, such as the Broselow® Pediatric Emergency Tape, is an ideal adjunct for the rapid determination of weight based on length for appropriate fluid volumes, drug doses, and equipment size. One side of the tape provides drugs and their recommended doses for the pediatric patient based on weight. The other side identifies equipment needs for pediatric patients based on length.

TABLE 10.3 Pediatric Equipment[1]	AIRWAY AND BREATHING							CIRCULATION			SUPPLEMENTAL EQUIPMENT		
AGE AND WEIGHT	O₂ MASK	ORAL AIRWAY	BAG-MASK	LARYNGO-SCOPE	ET TUBE	STYLET	SUCTION	BP CUFF	IV CATHETER[2]	OG/NG TUBE	CHEST TUBE	URINARY CATHETER	CERVICAL COLLAR
Premie 3 kg	Premie, newborn	Infant	Infant	0 straight	2.5–3.0	6 Fr	6–8 Fr	Premie, newborn	22–24 ga	8 Fr	10–14 Fr	5 Fr feeding	—
0–6 mos 3.5 kg	Newborn	Infant, small	Infant	1 straight	3.0–3.5	6 Fr	8 Fr	Newborn, infant	22 ga	10 Fr	12–18 Fr	6 Fr or 5–8 Fr feeding	—
6–12 mos 7 kg	Pediatric	Small	Pediatric	1 straight	3.5–4.0	6 Fr	8–10 Fr	Infant, child	22 ga	12 Fr	14–20 Fr	8 Fr	Small
1–3 yrs 10–12 kg	Pediatric	Small	Pediatric	1 straight	4.0–4.5	6 Fr	10 Fr	Child	20–22 ga	12 Fr	14–24 Fr	10 Fr	Small
4–7 yrs 16–18 kg	Pediatric	Medium	Pediatric	2 straight or curved	5.0–5.5	14 Fr	14 Fr	Child	20 ga	12 Fr	20–28 Fr	10–12 Fr	Small
8–10 yrs 24–30 kg	Adult	Medium, large	Pediatric, adult	2–3 straight or curved	5.5–6.5	14 Fr	14 Fr	Child, adult	18–20 ga	14 Fr	28–38 Fr	12 Fr	Medium

[1] Use of a length-based resuscitation tape, such as a Broselow® Pediatric Emergency Tape, is preferred.
[2] The largest IV catheter that can readily be inserted with reasonable certainty of success is preferred.

first objective. The inability to establish and/or maintain a patent airway with the associated lack of oxygenation and ventilation is the most common cause of cardiac arrest in children. Therefore, the child's airway is the first priority.

ANATOMY

The smaller the child, the greater is the disproportion between the size of the cranium and the midface. This leads to a propensity for the posterior pharynx to buckle anteriorly as a result of passive flexion of the cervical spine caused by the large occiput. Avoiding passive flexion of the cervical spine requires that the plane of the midface be maintained parallel to the spine board in a neutral position, rather than in the "sniffing position" (■ FIGURE 10-2A). Placement of a 1-inch-thick layer of padding beneath the infant's (younger than 1 year of age) or toddler's (between 1 and 3 years of age) entire torso will preserve neutral alignment of the spinal column (■ FIGURE 10-2B).

The soft tissues in an infant's oropharynx (i.e., the tongue and tonsils) are relatively large compared with the tissues in the oral cavity, which may make visualization of the larynx difficult. A child's larynx is funnel-shaped, allowing secretions to accumulate in the retropharyngeal area. The larynx and vocal cords are more cephalad and anterior in the neck. The vocal cords are frequently more difficult to visualize when the child's head is in the normal, supine, anatomical position during intubation than when it is in the neutral position required for optimal cervical spine protection. The infant's trachea is approximately 5 cm long and grows to 7 cm by about 18 months. Failure to appreciate this short length may result in intubation of the right mainstem bronchus, inadequate ventilation, accidental tube dislodgment, and/or mechanical barotrauma. Optimal endotracheal tube (ETT) depth (in cm) can be determined to be three times the appropriate tube size. For example, a 4.0 ETT would be properly positioned at 12 cm from the gums.

MANAGEMENT

In a spontaneously breathing child with a partially obstructed airway, the airway

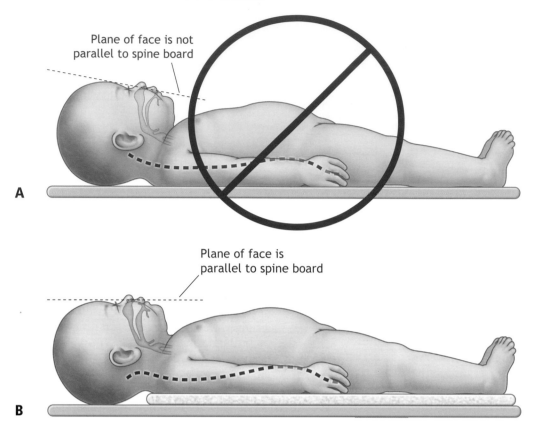

■ FIGURE 10-2 **Positioning for Airway Maintenance. (A)** Improper positioning of a child to maintain a patent airway. The disproportion between the size of the child's cranium and midface leads to a propensity for the posterior pharynx to buckle anteriorly. The large occiput causes passive flexion of the cervical spine. **(B)** Proper positioning of a child to maintain a patent airway. Avoid passive flexion of the cervical spine by keeping the plane of the midface parallel to the spine board in a neutral position, rather than in the "sniffing position." Placement of a 1-inch-thick layer of padding beneath the infant's or toddler's entire torso will preserve neutral alignment of the spinal column.

should be optimized by keeping the plane of the face parallel to the plane of the stretcher or gurney, while maintaining neutral alignment of the cervical spine. The jaw-thrust maneuver combined with bimanual in-line spinal immobilization is used to open the airway. After the mouth and oropharynx are cleared of secretions or debris, supplemental oxygen is administered. If the patient is unconscious, mechanical methods of maintaining the airway may be necessary. **Before attempts are made to mechanically establish an airway, the child should be fully preoxygenated.**

Oral Airway

An oral airway should only be inserted if a child is unconscious, since vomiting is likely if the gag reflex is intact. **The practice of inserting the airway backward and rotating it 180 degrees is not recommended for children, as trauma with resultant hemorrhage into soft tissue structures of the oropharynx may occur.** The oral airway should be gen-tly inserted directly into the oropharynx. The use of a tongue blade to depress the tongue may be helpful.

Orotracheal Intubation

Endotracheal intubation is indicated for injured children in a variety of situations, including:

- a child with severe brain injury who requires controlled ventilation
- a child in whom an airway cannot be maintained
- a child who exhibits signs of ventilatory failure
- a child who has suffered significant hypovolemia who has a depressed sensorium or requires operative intervention

Orotracheal intubation is the most reliable means of establishing an airway and administering ventilation to a child. The smallest area of the young child's

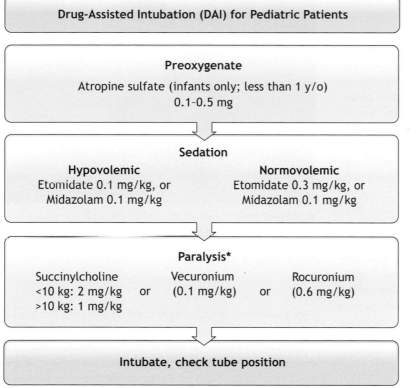

Drug-Assisted Intubation (DAI) for Pediatric Patients

Preoxygenate
Atropine sulfate (infants only; less than 1 y/o)
0.1–0.5 mg

Sedation

Hypovolemic	Normovolemic
Etomidate 0.1 mg/kg, or	Etomidate 0.3 mg/kg, or
Midazolam 0.1 mg/kg	Midazolam 0.1 mg/kg

Paralysis*

Succinylcholine		Vecuronium		Rocuronium
<10 kg: 2 mg/kg	or	(0.1 mg/kg)	or	(0.6 mg/kg)
>10 kg: 1 mg/kg				

Intubate, check tube position

* Proceed according to clinical judgment and skill/experience level.

■ **FIGURE 10-3** Algorithm for Drug-Assisted Intubation (DAI) in Pediatric Patients.

airway is at the cricoid ring, which forms a natural seal around an uncuffed endotracheal tube. Uncuffed endotracheal tubes are commonly used in infants because of the anatomic differences. However, the use of cuffed endotracheal tubes, even in toddlers and small children, provides the benefit of improving ventilation and CO_2 management, which has a positive impact on cerebral blood flow. Previous concerns about cuffed endotracheal tubes causing tracheal necrosis are no longer relevant due to improvements in the design of the cuffs. Ideally, cuff pressure should be measured as soon as is feasible, and <30 mm Hg is considered safe.

A simple technique to gauge the size of the endotracheal tube needed is to approximate the diameter of the child's external nares or the tip of the child's small finger and use a tube with a similar diameter. A length-based pediatric resuscitation tape, such as the Broselow® Pediatric Emergency Tape, also lists appropriate tube sizes of endotracheal tubes. However, be sure to have tubes readily available that are one size larger and one size smaller than the predicted size. If a stylet is used to facilitate endotracheal intubation, be sure that the tip does not extend beyond the end of the tube.

Most trauma centers use a protocol for emergency intubation, referred to as drug-assisted intubation (DAI), previously known as rapid sequence intubation (RSI). Careful attention must be paid to the child's

weight, vital signs (pulse and blood pressure), and level of consciousness to determine which branch of the Algorithm for Drug-Assisted Intubation (■ **FIGURE 10-3**) to use.

Preoxygenation should be performed in children who require an endotracheal tube for airway control. Infants have a more pronounced vagal response to endotracheal intubation than children and adults, and may experience bradycardia with direct laryngeal stimulation. Bradycardia in children (>1 year of age) is much more likely to be due to hypoxia. Atropine sulfate pretreatment should be considered for infants requiring DAI, but it is not required for children. Atropine also dries oral secretions, permitting easier visualization of landmarks for intubation. The dose of atropine is 0.01 to 0.03 mg/kg given at least 1 to 2 minutes before intubation, with a maximum single dose of 0.5 mg. Appropriate drugs for intubation sedation include etomidate (0.3 mg/kg) or midazolam (0.3 mg/kg) in infants and children with normovolemia, and etomidate (0.1 mg/kg) or midazolam (0.1 mg/kg) in children with hypovolemia. The specific antidote for midazolam is flumazenil, which should be immediately available.

This is followed by temporary chemical paralysis. Ideally, a short-acting, depolarizing, neuromuscular blocking (chemical paralytic) agent should be used, such as succinylcholine (2 mg/kg in children <10 kg;

1 mg/kg in children >10 kg). Succinylcholine has a rapid onset, a short duration of action, and may be the safest drug of choice (unless the patient has a known spinal cord injury). If a longer period of paralysis is needed—for example, in a child who needs a computed tomographic (CT) scan for further evaluation—a longer-acting, nondepolarizing, neuromuscular blocking agent, such as rocuronium (0.6 mg/kg), or vecuronium (0.1 mg/kg) may be indicated.

After the endotracheal tube is inserted, its position must be assessed clinically (see below) and, if correct, the tube carefully secured. If it is not possible to place the endotracheal tube after the child is chemically paralyzed, the child must receive ventilation with 100% oxygen administered with a self-inflating bag-mask device until a definitive airway is secured.

Orotracheal intubation under direct vision with adequate immobilization and protection of the cervical spine is the preferred method of obtaining initial airway control (■ FIGURE 10-4). Nasotracheal intubation should not be performed in children, as it requires blind passage around a relatively acute angle in the nasopharynx toward the anterosuperiorly located glottis, making intubation by this route difficult. The potential for penetrating the child's cranial vault or damaging the more prominent nasopharyngeal (adenoidal) soft tissues and causing hemorrhage also discourages the use of the nasotracheal route for airway control.

Once past the glottic opening, the endotracheal tube should be positioned 2 to 3 cm below the level of the vocal cords and carefully secured in place. A rule of thumb for the correct endotracheal tube position at the gums is 3 times the ETT size. Primary confirmation techniques, such as auscultation of both hemithoraces in the axillae, should then be performed to ensure that right mainstem bronchial intubation has not occurred and that both sides of the chest are being adequately ventilated. A secondary confirmation device, such as a real-time wave-form capnograph, a colorimetric end-tidal carbon dioxide ($ETCO_2$) detector, or an esophageal detector device (EDD), should then be used to document tracheal intubation, and a chest x-ray should be obtained to accurately identify the position of the endotracheal tube.

Because of the short length of the trachea in young children (5 cm in infants, 7 cm in toddlers), any movement of the head can result in displacement of the endotracheal tube, inadvertent extubation, right mainstem bronchial intubation, or vigorous coughing due to irritation of the carina by the tip of the endotracheal tube. These conditions may not be recognized clinically until significant deterioration has occurred. Thus, breath sounds should be evaluated periodically to ensure that the tube remains in the appropriate position and to identify the possibility of evolving ventilatory dysfunction. If there is any doubt about cor-

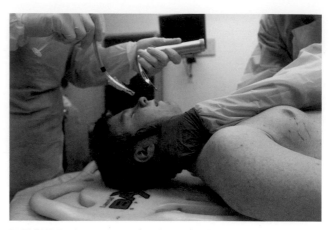

■ **FIGURE 10-4** Orotracheal intubation under direct vision with adequate immobilization and protection of the cervical spine is the preferred method of obtaining initial airway control.

rect placement of the endotracheal tube that cannot be resolved expeditiously, the tube should be removed and replaced immediately. Use of the mnemonic, "Don't be a DOPE," (D for dislodgment, O for obstruction, P for pneumothorax, E for equipment failure) may serve as a useful reminder of the common causes of deterioration in intubated patients. See Chapter 2: Airway and Ventilatory Management, and Skill Station II: Airway and Ventilatory Management, Skill II-G: Infant Endotracheal Intubation.

Cricothyroidotomy

When airway maintenance and control cannot be accomplished by bag-mask ventilation or orotracheal intubation, a rescue airway with either laryngeal mask airway (LMA), intubating LMA, or needle cricothyroidotomy is necessary. Needle-jet insufflation via the cricothyroid membrane is an appropriate, temporizing technique for oxygenation, but it does not provide adequate ventilation, and progressive hypercarbia will occur. Laryngeal mask airways are appropriate adjunct airways for infants and children, but their placement requires experience, and the airway may distend the stomach if ventilation is overly vigorous. LMA sizes range from 1 (appropriate for infants <6.5 kg), 1.5 (for 5 to 10 kg), 2 (for 10 to 20 kg), 2.5 (for 20 to 30 kg), and 3 (for between 30 and 70 kg); in patients over 70 kg, adult sizing is appropriate. See Chapter 2: Airway and Ventilatory Management, and Skill Station III: Cricothyroidotomy, Skill III-A: Needle Cricothyroidotomy.

Surgical cricothyroidotomy is rarely indicated for infants or small children. It can be performed in older children in whom the cricothyroid membrane is easily palpable (usually by the age of 12 years). See Skill Station III: Cricothyroidotomy, Skill III-B: Surgical Cricothyroidotomy.

Breathing: Evaluation and Management

BREATHING AND VENTILATION

The respiratory rate in children decreases with age. An infant breathes 30 to 40 times per minute, whereas an older child breathes 15 to 20 times per minute. Normal, spontaneous tidal volumes vary from 4 to 6 mL/kg for infants and children, although slightly larger tidal volumes of 6 to 8 mL/kg, and occasionally as high as 10 mL/kg, may be required during assisted ventilation. Although most bag-mask devices used with pediatric patients are designed to limit the pressure exerted manually on the child's airway, excessive volume or pressure during assisted ventilation substantially increases the potential for iatrogenic barotrauma because of the fragile nature of the immature tracheobronchial tree and alveoli. If an adult bag-mask device is used to ventilate a pediatric patient, the risk of barotrauma is significantly increased. Use of a pediatric bag-mask is recommended for children under 30 kg.

Hypoxia is the most common cause of cardiac arrest in the child. However, before cardiac arrest occurs, hypoventilation causes respiratory acidosis, which is the most common acid/base abnormality encountered during the resuscitation of injured children. With adequate ventilation and perfusion, a child should be able to maintain a relatively normal pH. **In the absence of adequate ventilation and perfusion, attempting to correct an acidosis with sodium bicarbonate can result in further hypercarbia and worsened acidosis.**

NEEDLE AND TUBE THORACOSTOMY

Injuries that disrupt pleural apposition—for example, hemothorax, pneumothorax, and hemopneumothorax, have similar physiologic consequences in children and adults. These injuries are managed with pleural decompression, preceded in the case of tension pneumothorax by needle decompression just over the top of the third rib in the midclavicular line. Care should be taken during this procedure when using 14- to 18-gauge over-the-needle catheters in infants and small children, since the longer needle length may cause, rather than cure, a tension pneumothorax. Chest tubes need to be proportionally smaller (see Table 10.3) and are placed into the thoracic cavity by tunneling the tube over the rib above the skin incision site, and directing it superiorly and posteriorly along the inside of the chest wall. However, the size must be large enough to drain hemothoraces. Tunneling is especially important in children because of the thinner chest wall. The site of chest tube insertion is the same in children as in adults: the fifth intercostal space, just anterior to the midaxillary line. See Chapter 4: Thoracic Trauma, and Skill Station VII: Chest Trauma Management.

Circulation and Shock: Evaluation and Management

? What physiologic differences will have an impact on my treatment of pediatric trauma patients?

Key factors in the evaluation and management of circulation in pediatric trauma patients include recognition of circulatory compromise, accurate determination of the patient's weight and circulatory volume, fluid resuscitation, blood replacement, venous access, assessments of adequacy of resuscitation such as urine output, and thermoregulation.

RECOGNITION OF CIRCULATORY COMPROMISE

Injuries in children may result in significant blood loss. A child's increased physiologic reserve allows for maintenance of systolic blood pressure in the normal range, even in the presence of shock (■ **FIGURE 10-5**).

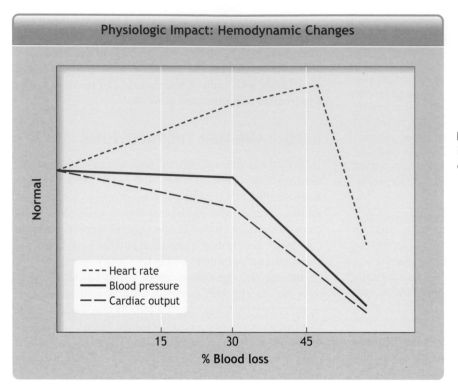

Physiologic Impact: Hemodynamic Changes

Normal

% Blood loss

----- Heart rate
—— Blood pressure
— — Cardiac output

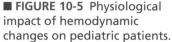

■ **FIGURE 10-5** Physiological impact of hemodynamic changes on pediatric patients.

Up to a 30% diminution in circulating blood volume may be required to manifest a decrease in the child's systolic blood pressure. This may be misleading to medical professionals who are not familiar with the subtle physiologic changes manifested by children in hypovolemic shock. Tachycardia and poor skin perfusion often are the only keys to early recognition of hypovolemia and the early initiation of appropriate fluid resuscitation. **When possible, early assessment by a surgeon is essential to the appropriate treatment of injured children.**

Although a child's primary response to hypovolemia is tachycardia, this sign also may be caused by pain, fear, and psychological stress. Other more subtle signs of blood loss in children include progressive weakening of peripheral pulses, a narrowing of pulse pressure to less than 20 mm Hg, skin mottling (which substitutes for clammy skin in infants and young children), cool extremities compared with the torso skin, and a decrease in level of consciousness with a dulled response to pain. A decrease in blood pressure and other indices of inadequate organ perfusion, such as urinary output, should be monitored closely, but generally develop later. Changes in vital organ function are outlined in Table 10.4.

The mean normal systolic blood pressure for children is 90 mm Hg plus twice the child's age in years. The lower limit of normal systolic blood pressure in children is 70 mm Hg plus twice the child's age in years.

The diastolic pressure should be about two-thirds of the systolic blood pressure. (Normal vital functions by age group are listed in Table 10.5.) Hypotension in a child represents a state of decompensated shock and indicates severe blood loss of greater than 45% of the circulating blood volume. Tachycardia changing to bradycardia often accompanies this hypotension, and this change may occur suddenly in infants. These physiologic changes must be treated by a rapid infusion of both isotonic crystalloid and blood.

DETERMINATION OF WEIGHT AND CIRCULATING BLOOD VOLUME

It is often very difficult for emergency department (ED) personnel to estimate the weight of a child, particularly if these personnel do not treat many children. The simplest and quickest method of determining a child's weight in order to accurately calculate fluid volumes and drug dosages is to ask a caregiver. If a caregiver is unavailable, a length-based resuscitation tape, such as the Broselow® Pediatric Emergency Tape, is extremely helpful. This tool rapidly provides the child's approximate weight, respiratory rate, fluid resuscitation volume, and a variety of drug dosages. A final method for estimating weight in kilograms is the formula ((2 × age) + 10).

The goal of fluid resuscitation is to rapidly replace the circulating volume. An infant's blood volume

TABLE 10.4 Systemic Responses to Blood Loss in Pediatric Patients

SYSTEM	MILD BLOOD VOLUME LOSS (<30%)	MODERATE BLOOD VOLUME LOSS (30%–45%)	SEVERE BLOOD VOLUME LOSS (>45%)
Cardiovascular	Increased heart rate; weak, thready peripheral pulses; normal systolic blood pressure (80–90 + 2 × age in years); normal pulse pressure	Markedly increased heart rate; weak, thready central pulses; absent peripheral pulses; low normal systolic blood pressure (70–80 + 2 × age in years); narrowed pulse pressure	Tachycardia followed by bradycardia; very weak or absent central pulses; absent peripheral pulses; hypotension (<70 + 2 × age in years); narrowed pulse pressure (or undetectable diastolic blood pressure)
Central Nervous System	Anxious; irritable; confused	Lethargic; dulled response to pain[1]	Comatose
Skin	Cool, mottled; prolonged capillary refill	Cyanotic; markedly prolonged capillary refill	Pale and cold
Urine Output[2]	Low to very low	Minimal	None

[1]The child's dulled response to pain with this degree of blood loss (30%–45%) may be indicated by a decreased response to IV catheter insertion.
[2]After initial decompression by urinary catheter. Low normal is 2 ml/kg/hr (infant), 1.5 ml/kg/hr (younger child), 1 ml/kg/hr (older child), and 0.5 ml/hg/hr (adolescent). IV contrast can falsely elevate urinary output.

TABLE 10.5 Vital Functions

AGE GROUP (IN MONTHS OR YEARS)	WEIGHT RANGE (IN KG)	HEART RATE (BEATS/MIN)	BLOOD PRESSURE (MM HG)	RESPIRATORY RATE (BREATHS/MIN)	URINARY OUTPUT (ML/KG/HR)
Infant 0–12 months	0–10	<160	>60	<60	2.0
Toddler 1–2 years	10–14	<150	>70	<40	1.5
Preschool 3–5 years	14–18	<140	>75	<35	1.0
School Age 6–12 years	18–36	<120	>80	<30	1.0
Adolescent ≥13 years	36–70	<100	>90	<30	0.5

can be estimated at 80 mL/kg, and a child's at 70 ml/kg. When shock is suspected, a bolus of 20 mL/kg of warmed isotonic crystalloid solution is needed. If it were to remain in the vascular space, this would represent 25% of the child's blood volume.

VENOUS ACCESS

Severe hypovolemic shock usually occurs as the result of disruption of intrathoracic or intraabdominal organs or blood vessels. Venous access is preferably established by a peripheral percutaneous route. If percutaneous access is unsuccessful after two attempts, consideration should be given to intraosseous infusion via a bone marrow needle (18 gauge in infants, 15 gauge in young children) (■ FIGURE 10-6) or insertion of a femoral venous line using the Seldinger technique

or a through-the-needle catheter of appropriate size. If these procedures fail, a doctor with skill and expertise can safely perform direct venous cutdown. However, this should be done only as a last resort, since this procedure can rarely be performed in less than 10 minutes, even in experienced hands, whereas an intraosseous needle can reliably be placed in the bone marrow cavity in less than 1 minute, even by providers with limited skill and expertise. See Skill Station IV: Shock Assessment and Management.

The preferred sites for venous access in children are:

- Percutaneous peripheral (two attempts)—Antecubital fossa(e), saphenous vein(s) at the ankle

- Intraosseous placement—(1) Anteromedial tibia, (2) distal femur

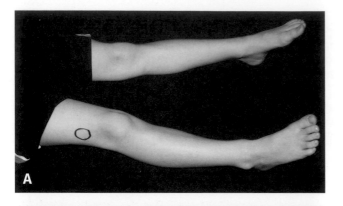

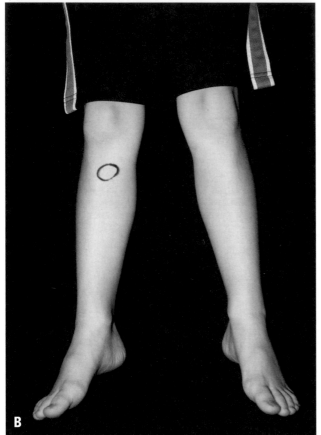

■ **FIGURE 10-6 Intraosseous Infusion, (A) Distal femur, (B) Proximal tibia.** If percutaneous access is unsuccessful after two attempts, consideration should be given to intraosseous infusion via a bone marrow needle (18 gauge in infants, 15 gauge in young children).

- Percutaneous placement—Femoral vein(s)

- Percutaneous placement—External jugular vein(s) (should be reserved for pediatric experts; do not use if there is airway compromise, or a cervical collar is applied)

- Venous cutdown—Saphenous vein(s) at the ankle

Intravenous access in young children with hypovolemia is a challenging problem, even in the most experienced hands. Intraosseous infusion, cannulating the marrow cavity of a long bone in an uninjured extremity, is an appropriate emergency access procedure. The intraosseous route is safe and efficacious, and requires far less time than venous cutdown. Intraosseous infusion should be discontinued when suitable venous access has been established.

Indications for intraosseous infusion are limited to children for whom venous access is impossible because of circulatory collapse or for whom two attempts at percutaneous peripheral venous cannulation have failed. Complications of this procedure include cellulitis, osteomyelitis, compartment syndrome, and iatrogenic fracture. The preferred site for intraosseous cannulation is the proximal tibia, below the level of the tibial tuberosity. An alternative site is the distal femur, although the contralateral proximal tibia is preferred. Intraosseous cannulation should not be performed in an extremity with a known or suspected fracture.

FLUID RESUSCITATION

Fluid resuscitation in the child is based on the child's weight, and an isotonic solution is the appropriate fluid for rapid repletion of circulating blood volume. Because the goal is to replace lost intravascular volume, it may be necessary to give three boluses of 20 mL/kg, or a total of 60 mL/kg, to achieve a replacement of the lost 25%. See Chapter 3: Shock. When considering the third 20 mL/kg bolus, the use of packed red blood cells (pRBCs) should be considered. The pRBCs are administered as a bolus of 10 mL/kg. Once blood product administration is begun, consideration should be given to the need for additional products such as plasma and platelets.

Injured children should be monitored carefully for response to fluid resuscitation and adequacy of organ perfusion. A return toward hemodynamic normality is indicated by:

- Slowing of the heart rate (<130 beats/min, with improvement of other physiologic signs; this response is age-dependent)

- Clearing of the sensorium

- Return of peripheral pulses

- Return of normal skin color

- Increased warmth of extremities

- Increased systolic blood pressure (normal is approximately 90 mm Hg plus twice the age in years)

- Increased pulse pressure (>20 mm Hg)

- Urinary output of 1 to 2 mL/kg/hour (age-dependent)

Children generally have one of three responses to fluid resuscitation. The condition of most children will be stabilized by the use of crystalloid fluid only, and blood will not be required; these children are considered "responders." Some children respond to crystalloid and blood resuscitation; these children are also considered "responders." In some children there is an initial response to crystalloid fluid and blood, but then deterioration occurs; this group is termed "transient responders." Other children do not respond at all to crystalloid fluid and blood infusion; this group is referred to as "nonresponders." The two latter groups of children (transient responders and nonresponders) are candidates for prompt infusion of additional blood products and consideration for early operation.

The resuscitation flow diagram is a useful aid in the initial treatment of injured children (■ FIGURE 10-7).

BLOOD REPLACEMENT

Failure to improve hemodynamic abnormalities following the first bolus of resuscitation fluid raises the suspicion of continuing hemorrhage, prompts the need for administra-tion of a second and perhaps a third 20 mL/kg bolus of isotonic crystalloid fluid, and requires the prompt involvement of a surgeon. When starting an additional bolus of isotonic crystalloid fluid or if at any point during the volume resuscitation the child's condition deteriorates, consideration must be given to the early use of 10 mL/kg of type-specific or O-negative warmed pRBCs.

URINE OUTPUT

Urine output varies with age. The output goal for infants up to 1 year of age is 2 mL/kg/hr, for younger children 1.5 mL/kg/hr, and for older children 1 mL/kg/hr. The lower limit of urinary output does not achieve the normal adult value of 0.5 mL/kg/hr until the adolescent has stopped growing.

Urine output combined with urine specific gravity is an excellent method of determining the adequacy of volume resuscitation. Once the circulating blood volume has been restored, the urinary output should return to normal. Insertion of a urinary catheter facilitates accurate measurement of the child's urinary output for patients receiving substantial volume resuscitation. A straight catheter, rather than one with a balloon, may be used in infants, but it is not appropriate in toddlers and children. Catheters containing temperature probes are available for children who need intensive care.

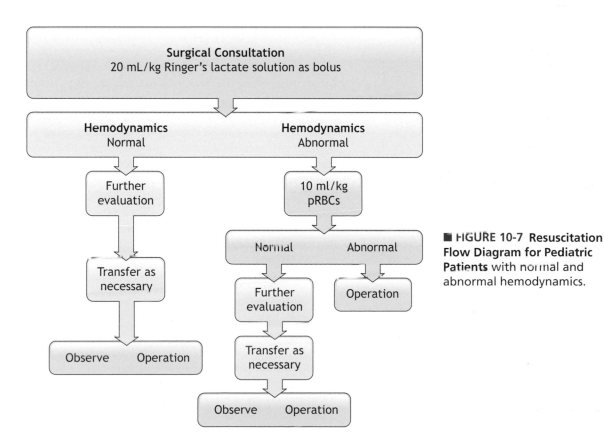

■ FIGURE 10-7 Resuscitation Flow Diagram for Pediatric Patients with normal and abnormal hemodynamics.

THERMOREGULATION

The high ratio of body surface area to body mass in children increases heat exchange with the environment and directly affects the body's ability to regulate core temperature. Increased metabolic rates, thin skin, and the lack of substantial subcutaneous tissue contribute to increased evaporative heat loss and caloric expenditure. Hypothermia may render the child's injuries refractory to treatment, prolong coagulation times, and adversely affect central nervous system (CNS) function. While the child is exposed during the initial survey and resuscitation phase, overhead heat lamps, heaters, or thermal blankets may be necessary to preserve body heat. It is advisable to warm the room as well as the intravenous fluids, blood products, and inhaled gases. Once examined during the initial resuscitation phase, it is important to cover the child's body with warm blankets to avoid unnecessary heat loss.

PITFALL

The ability of a child's body to compensate in the early phases of blood loss may create an illusion of hemodynamic normality, resulting in inadequate fluid resuscitation and rapid deterioration, which is often precipitous.

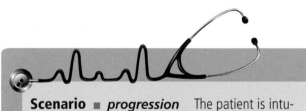

Scenario ■ *progression* The patient is intubated without difficulty and intravenous access is obtained. He is given isotonic crystalloid and O-negative blood with good response; his pulse is 100 and his blood pressure 100/60.

Cardiopulmonary Resuscitation

Children who undergo cardiopulmonary resuscitation (CPR) in the field with return of spontaneous circulation (ROSC) prior to arrival in the trauma center have roughly a 50% chance of neurologically intact survival. Children who present to an emergency department still in traumatic cardiopulmonary arrest have a uniformly dismal prognosis. Children receiving CPR for more than 15 minutes prior to arrival in an ED or with fixed pupils on arrival uniformly predict nonsurvival. In cases in which children arrive in the trauma bay with continued CPR of long duration, prolonged resuscitative efforts are typically not beneficial.

Chest Trauma

Eight percent of all injuries in children involve the chest. Chest injury also serves as a marker for other organ system injury, since more than two-thirds of children with chest injury will have multiple injuries. The mechanism of injury and the anatomy of the child's chest are directly responsible for the spectrum of injuries seen.

The vast majority of chest injuries in childhood are due to blunt mechanisms, caused principally by motor vehicles. The pliability, or compliance, of a child's chest wall allows impacting forces to be transmitted to the underlying pulmonary parenchyma, causing pulmonary contusion. Rib fractures and mediastinal injuries are not common, but, if present, they indicate a severe impacting force. The specific injuries caused by thoracic trauma in children are similar to those encountered in adults, although the frequencies of these injuries are somewhat different.

Mobility of mediastinal structures makes the child more susceptible to tension pneumothorax, the most common immediately life threatening injury in children. Pneumomediastinum is rare, and benign in the overwhelming majority of cases. Diaphragmatic rupture, aortic transection, major tracheobronchial tears, flail chest, and cardiac contusions are also seldom encountered in childhood. When identified, treatment for these injuries is the same as for adults. Significant injuries rarely occur alone and are frequently a component of major multisystem injury. Most pediatric thoracic injuries can be successfully managed using an appropriate combination of supportive care and tube thoracostomy. Thoracotomy is not generally needed in children.

The incidence of penetrating thoracic injury increases after 10 years of age. Penetrating trauma to the chest in children is managed the same way as for adults. See Chapter 4: Thoracic Trauma, and Skill Station VII: Chest Trauma Management.

Abdominal Trauma

Most pediatric abdominal injuries occur as the result of blunt trauma, primarily involving motor vehicles and falls. Serious intraabdominal injuries warrant prompt involvement by a surgeon, and hypotensive children who sustain blunt or penetrating abdominal trauma require prompt operative intervention.

ASSESSMENT

Conscious infants and young children are generally frightened by the events preceding admission to an emergency department, which may affect the abdominal examination. While talking quietly and calmly to the child, ask questions about the presence of abdominal pain and gently assess the tone of the abdominal musculature. Deep, painful palpation of the abdomen should be avoided at the onset of the examination to prevent voluntary guarding that may confuse the abdominal findings. Almost all infants and young children who are stressed and crying will swallow large amounts of air. If the upper abdomen is distended on examination, inserting a gastric tube to decompress the stomach should be a part of the resuscitation phase. Orogastric tube decompression is preferred in infants. Tenseness of the abdominal wall often decreases as gastric distention is relieved, allowing for more careful and reliable evaluation. The presence of shoulder- or lap-belt marks increases the likelihood that intraabdominal injuries are present, especially if lumbar fracture, intraperitoneal fluid, or pulse rate >120 are also detected.

Abdominal examination in unconscious patients does not vary greatly with age. Decompression of the urinary bladder facilitates abdominal evaluation. Since gastric dilation and a distended urinary bladder may both cause abdominal tenderness, abdominal tenderness must be interpreted with caution, unless these organs have been fully decompressed.

DIAGNOSTIC ADJUNCTS

Diagnostic adjuncts for assessment of abdominal trauma in children include CT, focused assessment sonography in trauma (FAST), and diagnostic peritoneal lavage.

Computed Tomography

The advent of helical CT scanning allows for extremely rapid and precise identification of injuries. CT scanning is often used to evaluate the abdomen of children who have sustained blunt trauma and have no hemodynamic abnormalities. **CT scanning should be immediately available, should be performed early, and must not delay further treatment.** The identification of intraabdominal injuries by CT scan in pediatric patients with no hemodynamic abnormalities can allow for nonoperative management by the surgeon. Early involvement of the surgeon is essential to establish a baseline that will allow the surgeon to determine whether, and when, operation is indicated. Centers that lack surgical support and where transfer of injured children is

planned are justified in foregoing the CT evaluation prior to definitive transport.

Injured children who require CT scanning as an adjunctive study often require sedation to prevent movement during the scanning process. Thus, an injured child requiring resuscitation or sedation who undergoes CT scan should be accompanied by a clinician skilled in pediatric airway management and pediatric vascular access. CT of the abdomen should routinely be performed with IV contrast agents according to local practice.

However, CT scanning is not without risk. Fatal cancers are predicted to occur in as many as 1 in 1,000 patients undergoing CT as children. Thus, the need for accurate diagnosis of internal injury must be balanced against the risk of late malignancy. Certainly every effort should be made to avoid CT scanning prior to transfer to the definitive trauma center, or to avoid repeat CT upon arrival at the trauma center, unless deemed absolutely necessary. **When CT evaluation is necessary, radiation must be kept As Low As Reasonably Achievable (ALARA). In order to achieve lowest doses possible, perform CT scans only when medically necessary, scan only when the results will change management, scan only the area of interest, and use the lowest radiation dose possible.** Criteria are now available to identify patients at low risk for head, cervical spine, and abdominal injury, who therefore do not require CT.

Focused Assessment Sonography in Trauma

Although FAST has been widely available for many years, comparatively few studies on the efficacy of ultrasound in children with abdominal injury have been reported, and it has only modest sensitivity for the detection of hemoperitoneum in young children when the most methodologically rigorous studies are analyzed. However, its use as an extension of the abdominal examination in injured children is rapidly evolving, and it offers the advantage that imaging may be repeated. FAST has been shown by some investigators to identify even small amounts of intraabdominal blood in pediatric trauma patients, a finding that is unlikely to be associated with significant injury. If large amounts of intraabdominal blood are found, significant injury is more likely to be present. However, even in these patients, operative management is indicated not by the amount of intraperitoneal blood, but by hemodynamic abnormality and its response to treatment. FAST is incapable of identifying isolated intraparenchymal injuries, which account for up to one-third of solid organ injuries in children. In summary, FAST should not be relied upon as the sole diagnostic test to rule out the presence of intraabdominal injury. If a small amount of intraabdominal fluid is found and the child is hemodynamically normal, CT should be obtained.

Diagnostic Peritoneal Lavage

Diagnostic peritoneal lavage (DPL) may be used to detect intraabdominal bleeding in children with hemodynamic abnormalities who cannot be safely transported to the CT scanner, or when CT and FAST are not readily available and the presence of blood will lead to immediate operative intervention. This is an uncommon occurrence. Most pediatric patients have self-limited intraabdominal injuries and no hemodynamic abnormalities. Therefore, blood found on a DPL would not mandate operative exploration in a child who is otherwise stable.

Warmed crystalloid solution in volumes of 10 mL/kg (up to 1000 mL) is used for DPL. Because a child's abdominal wall is relatively thin compared with that of an adult, uncontrolled penetration of the peritoneal cavity may produce iatrogenic injury to the abdominal contents, even when an open technique is used. DPL has utility in diagnosing injuries to intraabdominal viscera only; retroperitoneal organs cannot be evaluated reliably by this technique. The evaluation of the effluent from the DPL is the same in children as it is in adults.

Only the surgeon who will care for the child should perform the DPL, because DPL may interfere with subsequent abdominal examinations or imaging upon which the decision to operate may in part be based.

NONOPERATIVE MANAGEMENT

Selective, nonoperative management of solid organ injuries in children who are hemodynamically normal is performed in most trauma centers, especially those with pediatric capabilities. The presence of intraperitoneal blood on CT or FAST, the grade of injury, or the presence of a vascular blush does not necessarily mandate a laparotomy. It has been well demonstrated that bleeding from an injured spleen, liver, or kidney generally is self-limited. Therefore, a CT or FAST that is positive for blood alone does not mandate a laparotomy in a child who is hemodynamically normal or who stabilizes rapidly with fluid resuscitation. **If the child's hemodynamic condition cannot be normalized and if the diagnostic procedure performed is positive for blood, a prompt laparotomy to control hemorrhage is indicated.**

When nonoperative management is selected, children must be treated in a facility that offers pediatric intensive care capabilities and under the supervision of a qualified surgeon who specializes in the care of injured children. Intensive care must include continuous pediatric nursing staff coverage, continuous monitoring of vital signs, and immediate availability of surgical personnel and operating room resources.

Nonoperative management of confirmed solid organ injuries is a surgical decision made by surgeons, just as is the decision to operate. Therefore, the surgeon must supervise the treatment of pediatric trauma patients.

SPECIFIC VISCERAL INJURIES

A number of abdominal visceral injuries are more common in children than in adults. Injuries such as those caused by a bicycle handlebar or an elbow striking the child in the right upper quadrant or those associated with lap-belt injuries are common and result when the visceral contents are forcibly compressed between the blow on the anterior abdominal wall and the spine posteriorly. This injury also may be caused by child maltreatment.

Blunt pancreatic injuries occur from similar mechanisms, with their treatment dependent on the extent of injury. Small bowel perforations at or near the ligament of Treitz are more common in children than in adults, as are mesenteric and small bowel avulsion injuries. These particular injuries are often diagnosed late because of the vague early symptoms.

Bladder rupture is also more common in children than in adults, because of the shallow depth of the child's pelvis.

Children who are restrained by a lap belt only are at particular risk for enteric disruption, especially if they have a lap-belt mark on the abdominal wall or sustain a flexion-distraction (Chance) fracture of the lumbar spine. Any patient with this mechanism of injury and these findings should be presumed to have a high likelihood of injury to the gastrointestinal tract until proven otherwise. Penetrating injuries of the perineum, or straddle injuries, may occur with falls onto a prominent object, and may result in intraperitoneal injuries because of the proximity of the peritoneum to the perineum. Rupture of a hollow viscus requires early operative intervention.

▼ **PITFALL**

Delays in the recognition of abdominal hollow viscus injury are possible, especially when the decision is made to manage solid organ injury nonoperatively. Such an approach to the management of these injuries in children must be accompanied by an attitude of anticipation, frequent reevaluation, and preparation for immediate surgical intervention. These children should all be treated by a surgeon in a facility equipped to handle any contingencies in an expeditious manner.

Head Trauma

The information provided in Chapter 6: Head Trauma also applies to pediatric patients. This section emphasizes additional points specific to children.

Most head injuries in the pediatric population are the result of motor vehicle crashes, child maltreatment, bicycle crashes, and falls. Data from national pediatric trauma data repositories indicate that an understanding of the interaction between the CNS and extracranial injuries is imperative, because hypotension and hypoxia from associated injuries have an adverse effect on the outcome from intracranial injury. Lack of attention to the ABCDEs and associated injuries significantly increases mortality from head injury. As in adults, hypotension is infrequently caused by head injury alone, and other explanations for this finding should be investigated aggressively. In rare occasions, however, infants may lose significant amounts of blood in the subgaleal, subdural, or intraventricular spaces.

The brain of the child is anatomically different from that of the adult. It doubles in size in the first 6 months of life and achieves 80% of the adult brain size by 2 years of age. The subarachnoid space is relatively smaller, and hence offers less protection to the brain because there is less buoyancy. Thus, head momentum is more likely to impart parenchymal structural damage. Normal cerebral blood flow increases progressively to nearly twice that of adult levels by the age of 5 years, and then decreases. This accounts in part for children's severe susceptibility to cerebral hypoxia and hypercarbia.

ASSESSMENT

Children and adults may differ in their response to head trauma, which may influence the evaluation of the injured child. The principal differences include:

1. The outcome in children who suffer severe brain injury is better than that in adults. However, the outcome in children younger than 3 years of age is worse than a similar injury in an older child. Children are particularly susceptible to the effects of the secondary brain injury that may be produced by hypovolemia, with attendant reductions in cerebral perfusion, hypoxia, seizures, or hyperthermia. The effect of the combination of hypovolemia and hypoxia on the injured brain is devastating, but hypotension from hypovolemia is the worst single risk factor. **Adequate and rapid restoration of an appropriate circulating blood volume and avoidance of hypoxia are mandatory.**

2. Although an infrequent occurrence, hypotension may occur in infants as the result of blood loss into either the subgaleal, intraventricular, or epidural space. This hypovolemia, due to intracranial injury, occurs because of open cranial sutures and fontanelles in infants. Treatment is directed toward appropriate volume restoration, as is appropriate for blood loss from other body regions.

3. The infant with an open fontanelle and mobile cranial sutures has more tolerance for an expanding intracranial mass lesion or brain swelling, and signs of these conditions may be hidden until rapid decompensation occurs. **Therefore, an infant who is not in a coma but who has bulging fontanelles or suture diastases should be treated as having a more severe injury.** Early neurosurgical consultation is essential.

4. Vomiting and even amnesia are common after brain injury in children and do not necessarily imply increased intracranial pressure. However, persistent vomiting or vomiting that becomes more frequent is a concern and mandates CT of the head. Gastric decompression is essential, because of the risk of aspiration.

5. Impact seizures (seizures that occur shortly after brain injury) are more common in children and are usually self-limited. All seizure activity requires investigation by CT of the head.

6. Children tend to have fewer focal mass lesions than do adults, but elevated intracranial pressure due to brain swelling is more common. Rapid restoration of normal circulating blood volume is necessary. If hypovolemia is not corrected promptly, the outcome from head injury is made worse because of secondary brain injury. Emergency CT is vital to identify children who require emergency operation.

7. The GCS is useful when applied to the pediatric age group. However, the verbal score component must be modified for children younger than 4 years (Table 10.6).

8. Because increased intracranial pressure frequently develops in children, neurosurgical consultation to consider intracranial pressure monitoring should be obtained early in the course of resuscitation for children with:

   - A GCS score of 8 or less, or motor scores of 1 or 2

   - Multiple injuries associated with brain injury that require major volume resuscitation, immediate lifesaving thoracic or abdominal surgery, or for which stabilization and assessment is prolonged

- A CT scan of the brain that demonstrates evidence of brain hemorrhage, cerebral swelling, or transtentorial or cerebellar herniation

9. Medication dosages must be adjusted as dictated by the child's size and in consultation with a neurosurgeon. Drugs often used in children with head injuries include:

   - Phenobarbital, 10 to 20 mg/kg/dose

   - Diazepam, 0.1 to 0.2 mg/kg/dose; slow IV bolus

   - Phenytoin or fosphenytoin, 15 to 20 mg/kg, administered at 0.5 to 1.5 mL/kg/min as a loading dose, then 4 to 7 mg/kg/day for maintenance

   - Hypertonic saline 3% (Brain Trauma Foundation guidelines) 3 to 5 mL/kg

   - Mannitol, 0.5 to 1.0 g/kg (rarely required); diuresis with the use of mannitol may worsen hypovolemia and should be withheld early in the resuscitation of children with head injury unless there are incontrovertible signs of transtentorial herniation

MANAGEMENT

Management of traumatic brain injury in children involves:

1. Rapid, early assessment and management of the ABCDEs

2. Appropriate neurosurgical involvement from the beginning of treatment

3. Appropriate sequential assessment and management of the brain injury with attention directed toward the prevention of secondary brain injury—that is, hypoxia and hypoperfusion. Early endotracheal intubation with adequate oxygenation and ventilation is indicated to avoid progressive CNS damage. Attempts to orally intubate the trachea in an uncooperative child with a brain injury may be difficult and actually increase intracranial pressure. In the hands of clinicians who have considered the risks and benefits of intubating such children, pharmacologic sedation and neuromuscular blockade may be used to facilitate intubation.

   Hypertonic saline and mannitol create hyperosmolality and increased sodium levels in the brain, decreasing the brain edema and the pressure within the injured cranial vault. They have the added benefit of being rheostatic agents that improve blood flow and down-regulate the inflammatory response.

TABLE 10.6 Pediatric Verbal Score

VERBAL RESPONSE	V-SCORE
Appropriate words or social smile, fixes and follows	5
Cries, but consolable	4
Persistently irritable	3
Restless, agitated	2
None	1

4. Continuous reassessment of all parameters See Skill Station X: Head and Neck Trauma: Assessment and Management.

Spinal Cord Injury

The information provided in Chapter 7: Spine and Spinal Cord Trauma also applies to pediatric patients. This section emphasizes points specific to pediatric spinal injury.

Spinal cord injury in children is fortunately uncommon—only 5% of spinal cord injuries occur in the pediatric age group. For children younger than 10 years of age, motor vehicle crashes most commonly produce these injuries. For children aged 10 to 14 years, motor vehicles and sporting activities account for an equal number of spinal injuries.

ANATOMIC DIFFERENCES

The anatomic differences in children to be considered with regard to spinal injury include:

- Interspinous ligaments and joint capsules are more flexible.

- Vertebral bodies are wedged anteriorly and tend to slide forward with flexion.

- The facet joints are flat.

- The child has a relatively large head compared with the neck. Therefore, the angular momentum is greater, and the fulcrum exists higher in the cervical spine, which accounts for more injuries at the level of the occiput to C3.

- Growth plates are not closed, and growth centers are not completely formed.

- Forces applied to the upper neck are relatively greater than in the adult.

RADIOLOGIC CONSIDERATIONS

Pseudosubluxation frequently complicates the radiographic evaluation of a child's cervical spine. About 40% of children younger than 7 years of age show anterior displacement of C2 on C3, and 20% of children up to 16 years exhibit this phenomenon. This radiographic finding is seen less commonly at C3 on C4. Up to 3 mm of movement may be seen when these joints are studied by flexion and extension maneuvers.

When subluxation is seen on a lateral cervical spine x-ray, the clinician must ascertain whether this is a pseudosubluxation or a true cervical spine injury. Pseudosubluxation of the cervical vertebrae is made more pronounced by the flexion of the cervical spine that occurs when a child lies supine on a hard surface. To correct this radiographic anomaly, place the child's head in a neutral position by placing a 1-inch-thick layer of padding beneath the entire body from shoulders to hips, but not the head, and repeat the x-ray (see Figure 10.2). True subluxation will not disappear with this maneuver and mandates further evaluation. Cervical spine injury usually can be identified from neurologic examination findings and by detection of an area of soft tissue swelling, muscle spasm, or a step-off deformity on careful palpation of the posterior cervical spine.

An increased distance between the dens and the anterior arch of C1 occurs in approximately 20% of young children. Gaps exceeding the upper limit of normal for the adult population are seen frequently.

Skeletal growth centers can resemble fractures. Basilar odontoid synchondrosis appears as a radiolucent area at the base of the dens, especially in children younger than 5 years. Apical odontoid epiphyses appear as separations on the odontoid x-ray and are usually seen between the ages of 5 and 11 years. The growth center of the spinous process can resemble fractures of the tip of the spinous process.

Children sustain "spinal cord injury without radiographic abnormalities" (SCIWORA) more commonly than adults. A normal cervical spine series may be found in up to two-thirds of children who have suffered spinal cord injury. Thus, if spinal cord injury is suspected, based on history or the results of the neurologic examination, normal spine x-ray examination does not exclude significant spinal cord injury. **When in doubt about the integrity of the cervical spine or spinal cord, assume that an unstable injury exists, maintain immobilization of the child's head and neck, and obtain appropriate consultation.**

The indications for the use of CT scan for evaluation of the cervical spine in children are not different than in adults. CT scan may not detect the ligamentous injuries that are more common in this age group.

Spinal cord injuries in children are treated in the same way as spinal cord injuries in adults. Consultation

with a spine surgeon should be obtained early. See Chapter 7: Spine and Spinal Cord Trauma, Skill Station XI: X-Ray Identification of Spine Injuries, and Skill Station XII: Spinal Cord Injury: Assessment and Management.

Musculoskeletal Trauma

The initial priorities in the management of skeletal trauma in the child are similar to those for the adult, with additional concerns about potential injury to the growth plates. See Chapter 8: Musculoskeletal Trauma.

HISTORY

The patient's history is of vital importance. In younger children, x-ray diagnosis of fractures and dislocations is difficult because of the lack of mineralization around the epiphysis and the presence of a physis (growth plate). Information about the magnitude, mechanism, and time of the injury facilitates better correlation of the physical and x-ray findings. Radiographic evidence of fractures of differing ages should alert clinicians to possible child maltreatment, as should lower-extremity fractures in children who are too young to walk.

BLOOD LOSS

Blood loss associated with long-bone and pelvic fractures is proportionately less in children than in adults. Blood loss related to an isolated closed femur fracture that is treated appropriately is associated with an average fall in hematocrit of 4 percentage points, which is not enough to cause shock. Hemodynamic instability in the presence of an isolated femur fracture should prompt evaluation for other sources of blood loss, which usually will be found within the abdomen.

SPECIAL CONSIDERATIONS OF THE IMMATURE SKELETON

Bones lengthen as new bone is laid down by the physis near the articular surfaces. Injuries to, or adjacent to, this area before the physis has closed may potentially retard the normal growth or alter the development of the bone in an abnormal way. Crush injuries to the physis, which are often difficult to recognize radiographically, have the worst prognosis.

The immature, pliable nature of bones in children may lead to a so-called greenstick fracture. Such fractures are incomplete, with angulation maintained by cortical splinters on the concave surface. The torus, or "buckle," fracture, seen in small children, involves angulation due to cortical impaction with a radiolucent fracture line. Both types of fractures may suggest maltreatment in patients with vague, inconsistent, or conflicting histories. Supracondylar fractures at the elbow or knee have a high propensity for vascular injury as well as injury to the growth plate.

PRINCIPLES OF IMMOBILIZATION

Simple splinting of fractured extremities in children usually is sufficient until definitive orthopedic evaluation can be performed. Injured extremities with evidence of vascular compromise require emergency evaluation to prevent the adverse sequelae of ischemia. A single attempt to reduce the fracture to restore blood flow is appropriate, followed by simple splinting or traction splinting of the extremity. See Skill Station XIII: Musculoskeletal Trauma: Assessment and Management.

PITFALLS

- Many orthopedic injuries in children produce only subtle symptoms, and positive findings on physical examination are difficult to detect.

- Any evidence of unusual behavior—for example, a child who refuses to use an arm or bear weight on an extremity, must be carefully evaluated for the possibility of an occult bony or soft tissue injury.

- The caregivers are often the ones who note behavior that is out of the ordinary for the child.

- The clinician must remember the potential for child maltreatment. The history of the injury event should be viewed suspiciously when the findings do not corroborate the parent's story.

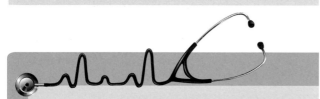

Scenario ■ continued The patient is transferred to the nearest trauma center after intubation and stabilization of his hemodynamics. Chest x-ray reveals pulmonary contusions, and a pelvic x-ray is normal.

Child Maltreatment

? How do I recognize injuries from child maltreatment?

Any child who sustains an intentional injury as the result of acts by caregivers is considered to be a battered or maltreated child. Homicide is the most common cause of injury death in the first year of life. Therefore, a history and careful evaluation of the child in whom maltreatment is suspected is critically important to prevent eventual death, especially in children who are younger than 2 years of age. Clinicians should suspect child maltreatment if:

- A discrepancy exists between the history and the degree of physical injury—for example, a young child loses consciousness or has significant injuries after falling from a bed or sofa, fractures an extremity during play with siblings or other children, or sustains a lower-extremity fracture but is too young to walk.

- A prolonged interval has passed between the time of the injury and presentation for medical care.

- The history includes repeated trauma, treated in the same or different EDs.

- The history of injury changes or is different between parents or guardians.

- There is a history of hospital or doctor "shopping."

- Parents respond inappropriately to or do not comply with medical advice—for example, leaving a child unattended in the emergency facility.

- The mechanism of injury is implausible based on the child's developmental stage (Table 10.7).

The following findings, on careful physical examination, should suggest child maltreatment and indicate more intensive investigation:

- Multicolored bruises (bruises in different stages of healing)

- Evidence of frequent previous injuries, typified by old scars or healed fractures on x-ray examination

- Perioral injuries

- Injuries to the genital or perianal area

- Fractures of long bones in children younger than 3 years of age

- Ruptured internal viscera without antecedent major blunt trauma

- Multiple subdural hematomas, especially without a fresh skull fracture

- Retinal hemorrhages

- Bizarre injuries, such as bites, cigarette burns, or rope marks

■ TABLE 10.7 Baby Milestones	
AGE	**TYPICAL SKILLS**
1 month	Lifts head when supine. Responds to sounds. Stares at faces.
2 months	Vocalizes. Follows objects across field of vision. Holds head up for short periods.
3 months	Recognizes familiar faces. Holds head steady. Visually tracks moving objects.
4 months	Smiles. Laughs. Can bear weight on legs. Vocalizes when spoken to.
5 months	Distinguishes between bold colors. Plays with hands and feet.
6 months	Turns toward sounds or voices. Imitates sounds. Rolls over in both directions.
7 months	Sits without support. Drags objects towards self.
8 months	Says "mama" or "dada" to parents. Passes objects from hand to hand.
9 months	Stands while holding on to things.
10 months	Picks things up with "pincer" grasp. Crawls well with belly off the ground.
11 months	Plays games like "patty cake" and "peek-a-boo." Stands without support for a few seconds.
12 months	Imitates the actions of others. Indicates wants with gestures.

- Sharply demarcated second- and third-degree burns
- Skull fractures or rib fractures seen in children less than 24 months of age

In many nations, clinicians are bound by law to report incidents of child maltreatment to governmental authorities, even cases in which maltreatment is only suspected. Maltreated children are at increased risk for fatal injuries, and no one is served by failing to report. The system protects clinicians from legal liability for identifying confirmed or even suspicious cases of maltreatment. Although the reporting procedures may vary, they are most commonly handled through local social service agencies or the state's health and human services department. The process of reporting child maltreatment assumes greater importance when one realizes that 50% of maltreated children who die or are dead on arrival at the hospital were victims of previous episodes of maltreatment that went unreported or were not taken seriously.

PREVENTION

The greatest pitfall related to pediatric trauma is failure to have prevented the child's injuries in the first place. Up to 80% of childhood injuries could have been prevented by the application of simple strategies in the home and the community. The ABCDEs of injury prevention have been described, and warrant special attention in a population among whom the lifetime benefits of successful injury prevention are self-evident (Box 10-1). Not only is the social and familial disruption associated with childhood injury avoided, but for every dollar invested in injury prevention, four dollars are saved in hospital care.

> ## Box 10-1 ABCDEs of Injury Prevention
>
> - **Analyze** injury data
>   —Local injury surveillance
>
> - **Build** local coalitions
>   —Hospital community partnerships
>
> - **Communicate** the problem
>   —Injuries are preventable
>
> - **Develop** prevention activities
>   —Create safer environments
>
> - **Evaluate** the interventions
>   —Ongoing injury surveillance
>
> **Source:** Pressley JC, Barlow B, Durkin M, Jacko SA, Dominguez DR, Johnson L. *J Urban Health* 2005;82:389-401.

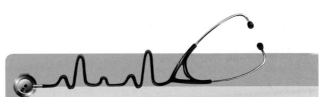

Scenario ■ conclusion   At the receiving facility, the patient undergoes CT evaluation of his head and abdomen. He has intracerebral contusions and a moderately severe splenic injury. After a prolonged intensive care unit (ICU) course, he is transferred to a rehabilitation facility. His parents receive education about bicycle helmets and are given helmets for him, his brother, and sister.

Chapter Summary

1 Unique characteristics of children include important differences in anatomy, body surface area, chest wall compliance, and skeletal maturity. Normal vital signs vary significantly with age.

2 Initial assessment and management of severely injured children is guided by the ABCDE approach. Early involvement of a general surgeon or pediatric surgeon is imperative in the management of injuries in a child. Nonoperative management of abdominal visceral injuries should be performed only by surgeons in facilities equipped to handle any contingency in an expeditious manner.

3 Child maltreatment should be suspected if suggested by suspicious findings on history or physical examination. These include discrepant history, delayed presentation, frequent prior injuries, and perineal injuries.

4 Most childhood injuries are preventable. Doctors caring for injured children have a special responsibility to promote the adoption of effective injury prevention programs and practices within their hospitals and communities.

▶ BIBLIOGRAPHY

1. American College of Surgeons Committee on Trauma, American College of Emergency Physicians, National Association of EMS Physicians, Pediatric Equipment Guidelines Committee—Emergency Medical Services for Children (EMSC) Partnership for Children Stakeholder Group and American Academy of Pediatrics Baby Center. (n.d.) Milestone chart: 1 to 6 months and Milestone chart: 7 to 12 months. http://www.babycenter.com/baby-milestones. Accessed.

2. Bratton SL, Chestnut RM, Ghajar J, et al. Guidelines for the management of severe traumatic brain injury. II. Hyperosmolar therapy. *J Neurotrauma* 2007;24 Suppl 1:S14-20. Brain Trauma Foundation; American Association of Neurological Surgeons; Congress of Neurological Surgeons; Joint Section on Neurotrauma and Critical Care, AANS/CNS, PEDIATRICS Vol. 124 No. 1 July 2009, pp. e166-e171 (doi:10.1542/peds.2009-1094).

3. Capizzani AR, Drognonowski R, Ehrlich PF. Assessment of termination of trauma resuscitation guidelines: are children small adults? *J Pediatr Surg* 2010;45:903-907.1.

4. Carney NA, Chesnut R, Kochanek PM, et al. Guidelines for the acute medical management of severe traumatic brain injury in infants, children, and adolescents. *J Trauma* 2003;54:S235-S310.

5. Chesnut RM, Marshall LF, et al. The role of secondary brain injury in determining outcome from severe head injury. *J Trauma* 1993;43:216-222.

6. Chwals WJ, Robinson AV, Sivit CJ, et al. Computed tomography before transfer to a level I pediatric trauma center risks duplication with associated radiation exposure. *J Pediatr Surg* 2008;43:2268-2272.

7. Clements RS, Steel AG, Bates AT, et al. Cuffed endotracheal tube use in paediatric prehospital intubation: challenging the doctrine? *Emerg Med J* 2007;24(1):57-58.

8. Cloutier DR, Baird TB, Gormley P, et al. Pediatric splenic injuries with a contrast blush: successful nonoperative management without angiography and embolization. *J Pediatr Surg* 2004;39(6):969-971.

9. Cook SH, Fielding JR, Phillips JD. Repeat abdominal computed tomography scans after pediatric blunt abdominal trauma: missed injuries, extra costs, and unnecessary radiation exposure. *J Pediatr Surg* 2010;45:2019-2024.

10. Cooper A, Barlow B, DiScala C, et al. Mortality and truncal injury: the pediatric perspective. *J Pediatr Surg* 1994;29:33.

11. Cooper A, Barlow B, DiScala C. Vital signs and trauma mortality: the pediatric perspective. *Pediatr Emerg Care* 2000;16:66.

12. Corbett SW, Andrews HG, Baker EM, et al. ED evaluation of the pediatric trauma patient by ultrasonography. *Am J Emerg Med* 2000;18(3):244-249.

13. Davies DA, Ein SH, Pearl R, et al. What is the significance of contrast "blush" in pediatric blunt splenic trauma? *J Pediatr Surg* 2010;45:916-920.

14. DiScala C, Sage R, Li G, et al. Child maltreatment and unintentional injuries. *Arch Pediatr Adolesc Med* 2000;154:16-22.

15. Emery KH, McAneney CM, Racadio JM, et al. Absent peritoneal fluid on screening trauma ultrasonography in children: a prospective comparison with computed tomography. *J Pediatr Surg* 2001;36(4):565-569.

16. Fastle RK, Roback MG. Pediatric rapid sequence intubation: incidence of reflex bradycardia and effects of pretreatment with atropine. *Pediatr Emerg Care* 2004;20(10):651-655.

17. Hannan E, Meaker P, Fawell L, et al. Predicting inpatient mortality for pediatric blunt trauma patients: a better alternative. *J Pediatr Surg* 2000;35:155-159.

18. Haricharan RN, Griffin RL, Barnhart DC, et al. Injury patterns among obese children involved in motor vehicle collisions. *J Pediatr Surg* 2009;44:1218-1222.

19. Harris BH, Schwaitzberg SD, Seman TM, et al. The hidden morbidity of pediatric trauma. *J Pediatr Surg* 1989;24:103-106.

20. Herzenberg JE, Hensinger RN, Dedrick DE, et al. Emergency transport and positioning of young children who have an injury of the cervical spine. *J Bone Joint Surg Am* 1989;71:15-22.

21. Holmes JF, Brant WE, Bond WF, et al. Emergency department ultrasonography in the evaluation of hypotensive and normotensive children with blunt abdominal trauma. *J Pediatr Surg* 2001;36(7):968-973.

22. Holmes JF, London KL, Brant WE, et al. Isolated intraperitoneal fluid on abdominal computed tomography in children with blunt trauma. *Acad Emerg Med* 2000;7(4):335-341.

23. Holmes JF, Gladman A, Chang CH. Performance of abdominal ultrasonography in pediatric blunt trauma patients: a meta-analysis. *J Pediatr Surg* 2007;42:1588-1594.14.

24. Holmes J, Lillis K, Monroe D, et al. Identifying children at very low risk of intra-abdominal injuries undergoing acute intervention. *Acad Emerg Med* 2011;18:S161.

25. Kuppermann N, Holmes JF, Dayan PS, et al, for the Pediatric Emergency Care Applied Research Network (PECARN): Identification of children at very low risk of clinically-important brain injuries after head trauma: a prospective cohort study. *Lancet* 2009;374:1160-1170.

26. Leonard JC, Kuppermann N, Olsen C, et al, for the Pediatric Emergency Care Applied Research Network. Factors associated with cervical spine injury in children following blunt trauma. *Ann Emerg Med* 2011;58:145-155.

27. Lutz N, Nance ML, Kallan MJ, et al. Incidence and clinical significance of abdominal wall bruising in restrained children involved in motor vehicle crashes. *J Pediatr Surg* 2004;39(6):972-975.

28. McAuliffe G, Bissonnette B, Boutin C. Should the routine use of atropine before succinylcholine in children be reconsidered? *Can J Anaesth* 1995;42(8):724-729.

29. McVay MR, Kokoska ER, Jackson RJ, et al. Throwing out the "grade" book: management of isolated spleen and liver injury based on hemodynamic status. *J Pediatr Surg* 2008;43:1072-1076.

30. Murphy JT, Jaiswal K, Sabella J, Vinson L, et al. Prehospital cardiopulmonary resuscitation in the pediatric trauma patient. *J Pediatr Surg* 2010 Jul;45(7):1413-1419.

31. Mutabagani KH, Coley BD, Zumberge N, et al. Preliminary experience with focused abdominal sonography for trauma (FAST) in children: is it useful? *J Pediatr Surg* 1999;34:48-54.

32. National Safety Council. *Injury Facts.* Itasca, IL: National Safety Council; 2007.

33. Neal MD, Sippey M, Gaines BA, et al. Presence of pneumomediastinum after blunt trauma in children: what does it really mean? *J Pediatr Surg* 2009;44:3122-1327.

34. Paddock HN, Tepas JJ, Ramenofsky ML. Management of blunt pediatric hepatic and splenic injury: similar process, different outcome. *Am Surg* 2004;70:1068-1072.

35. Paris C, Brindamour M, Ouimet A, et al. Predictive indicators for bowel injury in pediatric patients who present with a positive seat belt sign after motor vehicle collision. *J Pediatr Surg* 2010;45:921-924.

36. Patel JC, Tepas JJ. The efficacy of focused abdominal sonography for trauma (FAST) as a screening tool in the assessment of injured children. *J Pediatr Surg* 1999;34:44-47.

37. Pershad J, Gilmore B. Serial bedside emergency ultrasound in a case of pediatric blunt abdominal trauma with severe abdominal pain. *Pediatr Emerg Care* 2000;16(5):375-376.

38. Pieretti-Vanmarcke R, Vehmahos GC, Nance ML, et al. Clinical clearance of the cervical spine in blunt trauma patients younger than 3 years: a multi-center study of the American Association for the Surgery of Trauma. *J Trauma* 2009;67:543-550.

39. Pigula FA, Wald SL, Shackford SR, et al. The effect of hypotension and hypoxia on children with severe head injuries. *J Pediatr Surg* 1993;28:310-316.

40. Pressley J, Barlow B, Durkin M, et al. A national program for injury prevention in children and adolescents: the Injury Free Coalition for Kids. *J Urban Health* 2005;82:389-402.

41. Rana AR, Drogonowski R, Breckner G, et al. Traumatic cervical spine injuries: characteristics of missed injuries. *J Pediatr Surg* 2009;44:151-155.

42. Rathaus V, Zissin R, Werner M, et al. Minimal pelvic fluid in blunt abdominal trauma in children: the significance of this sonographic finding. *J Pediatr Surg* 2001;36(9):1387-1389.

43. Retzlaff T, Hirsch W, Till H, et al. Is sonography reliable for the diagnosis of pediatric blunt abdominal trauma? *J Pediatr Surg* 2010;45(5):912-915.

44. Rice HE, Frush DP, Farmer D, et al, APSA Education Committee. Review of radiation risks from computed tomography: essentials for the pediatric surgeon. *J Pediatr Surg* 2007;42:603-607.

45. Rogers CG, Knight V, MacUra KJ. High-grade renal injuries in children—is conservative management possible? *Urology* 2004;64:574-579.

46. Rothrock SG, Pagane J. Pediatric rapid sequence intubation incidence of reflex bradycardia and effects of pretreatment with atropine. *Pediatr Emerg Care* 2005;21(9):637-638.

47. Sasser SM, Hunt RC, Sullivent EE, et al. Guidelines for field triage of injured patients: recommendations of the National Expert Panel on Field Triage. *Morb Mortal Wkly Rep* 2009;58(RR-1):1-35.

48. Schwaitzberg SD, Bergman KS, Harris BW. A pediatric trauma model of continuous hemorrhage. *J Pediatr Surg* 1988;23:605-609.

49. Soudack M, Epelman M, Maor R, et al. Experience with focused abdominal sonography for trauma (FAST) in 313 pediatric patients. *J Clin Ultrasound* 2004;32(2):53-61.

50. Soundappan SV, Holland AJ, Cass DT, et al. Diagnostic accuracy of surgeon-performed focused abdominal sonography (FAST) in blunt paediatric trauma. *Injury* 2005;36(8):970-975.

51. Stylianos S. Compliance with evidence-based guidelines in children with isolated spleen or liver injury: a prospective study. *J Pediatr Surg* 2002;37:453-456.

52. Suthers SE, Albrecht R, Foley D, et al. Surgeon-directed ultrasound for trauma is a predictor of intra-abdominal injury in children. *Am Surg* 2004;70(2):164-167; discussion 167-168.

53. Tepas JJ, DiScala C, Ramenofsky ML, et al. Mortality and head injury: the pediatric perspective. *J Pediatr Surg* 1990;25:92-96.

54. Tepas JJ, Ramenofsky ML, Mollitt DL, et al. The Pediatric Trauma Score as a predictor of injury severity: an objective assessment. *J Trauma* 1988;28:425-429.

55. Tollefsen WW, Chapman J, Frakes M, et al. Endotracheal tube cuff pressures in pediatric patients intubated before aeromedical transport. *Pediatr Emerg Care* 2010 May;26(5):361-3.

56. Tourtier JP, Auroy Y, Borne M, et al. Focused assessment with sonography in trauma as a triage tool. *J Pediatr Surg* 2010;45(4):849; author reply 849.

57. van der Sluis CK, Kingma J, Eisma WH, et al. Pediatric polytrauma: short-term and long-term outcomes. *J Trauma* 1997;43(3):501-506.

58. Weiss M, Dullenkopf A, Fischer JE, et al., European Paediatric Endotracheal Intubation Study Group. Prospective randomized controlled multi-centre trial of cuffed or uncuffed endotracheal tubes in small children. *Br J Anaesth* 2009;103(6):867-873.

11 Geriatric Trauma

Special considerations in caring for elderly patients include the effects of age on physiologic functions, comorbidities, and concomitant medications. However, the priorities in evaluation and resuscitation remain the same.

Scenario A 79-year-old male is brought to the emergency department (ED) after he was found at the base of the stairs by his wife. The patient's initial vital signs are: respiratory rate 32; heart rate 64; blood pressure 110/60; Glasgow Coma Scale (GCS) score 12.

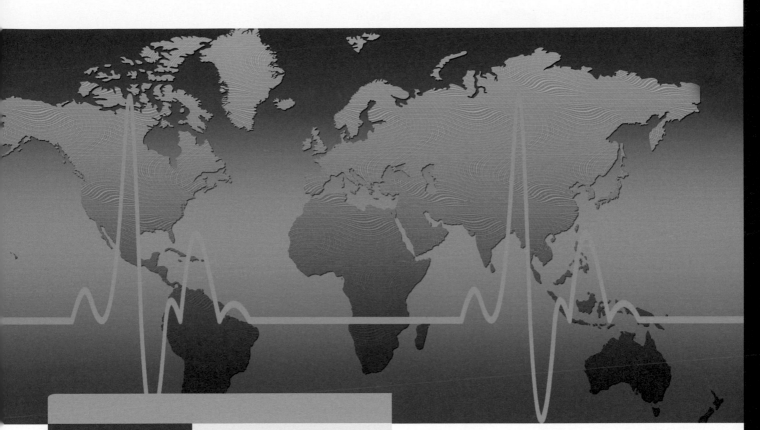

Objectives

1 Identify the unique characteristics of elderly trauma patients, including common types of injury, patterns of injury, and anatomic and physiologic differences.

2 Describe the primary management of critical injuries in geriatric patients, including the following related issues unique to geriatric patients, emphasizing the anatomic and physiologic differences from younger patients and their impact on resuscitation:

- Airway management
- Breathing and ventilation
- Shock, fluid, and electrolyte management
- Central nervous system and cervical spine injuries

3 Identify common causes and signs of elder maltreatment, and formulate a strategy for managing situations of elder maltreatment.

By 2050, it is projected that the elderly will represent 22% of the population in the United States. The rapid growth of the senior population has had a significant economic impact because of their unique medical requirements and the fact that these individuals consume more than one-third of the country's health care resources. Currently, trauma is the seventh leading cause of death in the elderly, surpassed only by heart disease, cancer, chronic obstructive pulmonary disease, stroke, diabetes, and pneumonia.

Types and Patterns of Injury

? *What are the unique characteristics of geriatric trauma?*

Although patients aged 65 and older are less likely to be injured than are younger individuals, older patients are more likely to have a fatal outcome from their injuries. This high mortality rate reflects the decreased physical reserves of the elderly due to the changes of aging, co-morbidities, and a lack of understanding of their needs by many healthcare providers. ■ FIGURE 11-1 illustrates the effects of aging on organ systems, and Box 11-1 outlines the impact of preexisting disease on trauma

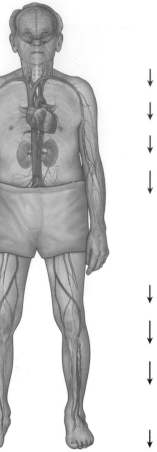

↓ Brain mass

Eye disease

↓ Depth perception

↓ Discrimination of colors

↓ Pupillary response

↓ Respiratory vital capacity

↓ Renal function

2- to 3-inch loss in height

Impaired blood flow to lower leg(s)

Degeneration of the joints

↓ Total body water

Nerve damage (peripheral neuropathy)

Stroke

Diminished hearing

↓ Sense of smell and taste

↓ Saliva production

↓ Esophageal activity

↓ Cardiac stroke volume and rate

Heart disease and high blood pressure

Kidney disease

↓ Gastric secretions

↓ Number of body cells

↓ Elasticity of skin

Thinning of epidermis

↓ 15%–30% body fat

■ **FIGURE 11-1** The effects of aging on organ systems.

Box 11-1
Relationship between Age, Preexisting Disease, and Mortality

- Mean age of patients with preexisting disease: 49.2

- Mean age of patients without preexisting disease: 30.6

- Mortality rate for older patients with preexisting disease: 9.2%

- Mortality rate for younger patients without preexisting disease: 3.2%

Source: Milzman DP, Boulanger BR, Rodriguez A, et al. Pre-existing disease in trauma patients: a predictor of fate independent of age and injury severity score. *J Trauma* 1992;31:236-244.

outcome. Milzman et al. reported that preexisting disease was more common in the older age group (mean age, 49.2) than in the younger age group (mean age, 30.0), and the mortality rate was three times greater in older patients with preexisting disease (9.2% vs 3.2%). However, more than 80% of injured older adults can return to their preexisting level of independent living after aggressive resuscitation and follow-up care.

Falls are the most common mechanism of injury encountered in older adults seen in trauma centers and are the most common cause of unintentional injury and death among the elderly. Falls account for 40% of the deaths in this age group. Both the incidence of falls and the severity of complications rise with age, and large numbers of emergency department visits and subsequent hospital admissions occur as a result of falls. Falls are most frequently caused by the accumulated effects of the aging process and environmental hazards. Changes in the central nervous and musculoskeletal systems make older people less flexible and less coordinated than younger adults. Geriatric patients are more likely to have gait disturbances.

Visual, hearing, and memory impairments place older adults at high risk for hazards that can cause falls. Falls resulting from dizziness or vertigo are extremely common.

In addition, drugs—including alcohol—cause or contribute to many falls. **Seemingly minor mechanisms of injury can produce potentially lethal injury and complications because of the effect of multiple medications, especially anticoagulants.** Warfarin (Coumadin) and clopidogrel (Plavix) are frequently prescribed to older patients. The presence of these medications with traumatic brain injury increases the likelihood of poor outcomes. Beta blockers can blunt the cardiovascular response to hypovolemia.

The effects of the aging process are a major influence on the incidence of injury and death in older adults from motor vehicle crashes. Often, the elderly have diminished visual and auditory acuity. Daylight acuity, glare resistance, and night vision decrease markedly with age. Medical conditions and their treatments may alter attention and consciousness. Because of senescent changes in the brain, judgment may be altered. **Finally, there often is decreased ability to avoid injury because of impairment from conditions such as arthritis, osteoporosis, emphysema, heart disease, and decreased muscle mass.**

Thermal injury is the third leading cause of death due to injury in the elderly, accounting for almost 2000 deaths annually in the United States. One-third of these individuals are fatally injured while under the influence of alcohol, while smoking in bed, or when exposed to heat and toxic products of combustion when trapped in a building fire. Of the remainder, the majority sustain injury because their clothing is ignited or they have prolonged contact with hot substances.

As with falls, factors associated with degenerative disease and physical impairment appear to contribute substantially to the rate of thermal injury in the elderly. Older adults who come into contact with hot surfaces or liquids or are exposed to fire often are not able to remove themselves before extensive injury occurs. Finally, preexisting cardiovascular, respiratory, and renal diseases often make it impossible for the injured person to overcome serious, but potentially survivable burns.

Airway

? How do I apply ATLS airway principles to the treatment of elderly patients?

The "A" of the ABCDE mnemonic of the primary survey is the same in the elderly as for any other injured patient. **Establishing and maintaining a patent airway to provide adequate oxygenation is the first objective.** Sup-

plemental oxygen should be administered as soon as possible, even in the presence of chronic pulmonary disease. Because of the elderly patient's limited cardiopulmonary reserve, early intubation should be considered for elderly trauma patients presenting in shock and those with chest wall injury or alteration in the level of consciousness.

Features that affect management of the airway in the elderly include dentition, nasopharyngeal fragility, macroglossia (enlargement of tongue), microstomia (small oral aperture), and cervical arthritis. Less than full dentition can interfere with achieving a proper seal on a face mask. **Consequently, whereas broken dentures should be removed, intact well-fitted dentures are often best left in place until after airway control is achieved.** Care must be taken when placing nasogastric and nasotracheal tubes because of nasopharyngeal friability, especially around the turbinates. Profuse bleeding can ensue. The oral cavity may be compromised by either macroglossia, associated with amyloidosis or acromegaly, or microstomia, such as the constricted, birdlike mouth of progressive systemic sclerosis. Arthritis can affect the temporomandibular joints and the cervical spine, making endotracheal intubation more difficult and increasing the risk of spinal cord injury with manipulation of the osteoarthritic spine. Degenerative changes and calcification in laryngeal cartilage place the elderly population at increased risk of injury from minor blows to the neck.

The principles of airway management remain the same, with endotracheal intubation as the preferred method for definitive airway control. If acute airway obstruction exists or the vocal cords cannot be visualized, surgical cricothyroidotomy should be considered as an option. See Chapter 2: Airway and Ventilatory Management, and Skill Station III: Cricothyroidotomy, Skill III-B: Surgical Cricothyroidotomy.

Breathing and Ventilation

Many of the changes that occur in the airway and lungs of elderly patients are difficult to ascribe purely to the process of aging and may be the result of chronic exposure to toxic agents such as tobacco smoke and other environmental toxins throughout life. **The loss of respiratory reserve due to the effects of aging and chronic diseases makes careful monitoring of the geriatric patient's respiratory system imperative (■ FIGURE 11-2).** Administration of supplemental oxygen is mandatory, although caution should be exercised with its use because some elderly patients rely on hypoxic drive to maintain ventilation. Oxygen administration can result in loss of this hypoxic drive, causing CO_2 retention and respiratory acidosis. In an acute trauma situation,

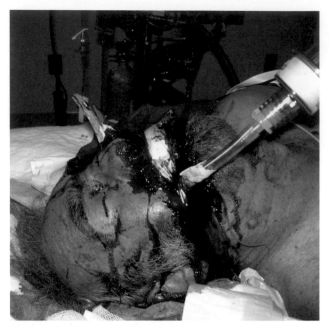

■ **FIGURE 11-2** The loss of respiratory reserve due to the effects of aging and chronic diseases makes careful monitoring of the geriatric patient's respiratory system imperative.

however, hypoxemia should be corrected by administering oxygen while accepting the risk of hypercarbia. In these situations, if respiratory failure is imminent, intubation and mechanical ventilation is necessary.

Chest injuries occur in patients of all ages with similar frequency, but the mortality rate for elderly patients is higher. Chest wall injuries with rib fractures or pulmonary contusions are common and not well tolerated. Patients older than 65 years of age with multiple rib fractures have increased rates of morbidity and mortality. Simple pneumothorax and hemothorax also are poorly tolerated, and geriatric patients with these injuries should be considered for intensive care unit (ICU) observation, as respiratory failure can be gradual or precipitous. Respiratory failure may result from the increased work of breathing combined with a decreased energy reserve. Adequate pain control and vigorous pulmonary toilet are essential for a satisfactory outcome. The balance between adequate pain control and narcotic side effects can be difficult in the elderly, and the use of epidural catheters may improve outcome in these patients. Pulmonary complications—such as atelectasis, pneumonia, and pulmonary edema—occur in the elderly with great frequency. Marginal cardiopulmonary reserve coupled with overzealous crystalloid infusion increases the potential for pulmonary edema and worsening of pulmonary contusions. Admission to the hospital usually is necessary, even with apparently minor injuries.

PITFALLS

- Failure to recognize the indications for early intubation.

- Undue manipulation of the osteoarthritic cervical spine, leading to spinal cord injury.

- Failure to recognize the serious effects of rib fractures and lung contusion, which may require mechanical ventilation.

Circulation

CHANGES WITH AGING

As the heart ages, there is progressive loss of function. By the age of 65 years, nearly 50% of the population has coronary artery stenosis. The cardiac index falls off linearly with age, and the maximal heart rate also begins to decrease after 40 years of age. The formula for maximal heart rate is 220 minus the individual's age in years. Although the resting heart rate varies little, the maximum tachycardic response decreases with age.

The cause of this diminution of function is multifaceted. With aging, total blood volume decreases and circulation time increases. There is increasing myocardial stiffness, slowed electrophysiologic conduction, and loss of myocardial cell mass. The response to endogenous catecholamine release with stress is also different, which is likely related to a reduction in responsiveness of the cellular membrane receptors. These changes predispose the aged heart to reentry dysrhythmias. Diastolic dysfunction makes the heart more dependent on atrial filling to increase cardiac output.

The kidney loses mass after the age of 50 years. This loss involves entire nephron units and is accompanied by a gradual decline in the glomerular filtration rate and renal blood flow. Levels of serum creatinine usually remain within normal limits, presumably because of a reduction in creatinine production by muscles. The aged kidney is less able to resorb sodium and excrete potassium or hydrogen ions. The maximum concentrating ability of the kidney of an individual between 80 and 90 years old is only 850 mOsm/kg, which is 70% of the ability of a 30-year-old individual's kidney. A decrease in the production of, and responsiveness of the kidney to, renin and angiotensin occurs with age. As a result, creatinine clearance in the elderly is reduced, and the aged kidney is more susceptible to injury from hypovolemia, medications, and other nephrotoxins.

EVALUATION AND MANAGEMENT

A common pitfall in the evaluation of geriatric trauma patients is the mistaken impression that "normal" blood pressure and heart rate indicate normovolemia. **Early monitoring of the cardiovascular system must be instituted.** Blood pressure generally increases with age. Thus, a systolic blood pressure of 120 mm Hg can represent hypotension in an elderly patient whose preinjury systolic blood pressure was 170 mm Hg. Early stages of shock can be masked by the absence of early tachycardia. The onset of hypotension also may be delayed. In addition, the chronic high afterload state induced by elevated peripheral vascular resistance can limit cardiac output and ultimately cerebral, renal, coronary, and peripheral perfusion.

Geriatric patients have a limited physiologic reserve and may have difficulty generating an adequate response to injury. Severely injured elderly patients with hypotension and metabolic acidosis frequently die, especially if they have sustained brain injury. Fluid requirements—once corrected for the lesser, lean body mass—are similar to those of younger patients. **Elderly patients with hypertension who are on chronic diuretic therapy may have a chronically contracted vascular volume and a serum potassium deficit; therefore careful monitoring of the administration of crystalloid solutions is important to prevent electrolyte disorders.**

Geriatric patients should be resuscitated in a manner similar to younger patients. However, they may be more sensitive to volume overload due to a higher incidence of cardiac disease. See Chapter 3: Shock.

The optimal hemoglobin level for an injured elderly patient is a point of controversy. Many authors suggest that, in people over the age of 65 years, hemoglobin concentrations of over 10 g/dL should be maintained to maximize oxygen-carrying capacity and delivery. There is little support in the literature for this position. Indiscriminate blood transfusion should be avoided because of the attendant risk of bloodborne infections, impairment of the immune host response and resulting complications, and the effect of a high hematocrit on blood viscosity, which can adversely affect myocardial function. **The indication for blood transfusion should be the same as in younger patients. Early recognition and correction of coagulation defects is crucial, including reversal of drug-induced anticoagulation.**

Because elderly patients may have significant limitation in cardiac reserve, a rapid and complete assessment for all sources of blood loss is necessary. The focused assessment sonography in trauma (FAST) examination is a rapid means of determining the presence of abnormal intraabdominal and pericardial fluid collections. Nonoperative management of blunt abdominal solid viscus injuries in elderly patients must be done by an experienced surgeon. **The risk of** nonoperative management may be greater than the risk of an early operation.

The retroperitoneum is an often-unrecognized source of blood loss. Exsanguinating retroperitoneal hemorrhage may develop in elderly patients after relatively minor pelvic or hip fractures. A patient with pelvic, hip, or lumbar vertebral fractures who demonstrates continuing blood loss without a specific source should be considered for prompt angiography and control with transcatheter embolization.

The process of aging and superimposed disease states make close monitoring mandatory, especially in cases of injury with acute intravascular volume loss and shock. The mortality rate in patients who on initial assessment appear to be uninjured or to have only minor injuries can be significant (up to 44%). Approximately 33% of elderly patients do not die from direct consequences of their injury, but from "inexplicable" sequential organ failure, which may reflect early, unsuspected states of hypoperfusion. Failure to recognize inadequate oxygen delivery creates an oxygen deficit from which the geriatric patient may not be able to recover. Because of associated coronary artery disease, hypotension and hypovolemia frequently results in impaired cardiac performance from myocardial ischemia. Thus, hypovolemic and cardiogenic shock may coexist. Early invasive monitoring with a pulmonary artery catheter may be beneficial. Hemodynamic resuscitation may require the use of inotropes after volume restoration in these patients. Prompt transfer to a trauma center may be lifesaving.

PITFALLS

- Equating normal blood pressure with normovolemia.
- Failure to recognize metabolic acidosis as a predictor of mortality.
- Failure to institute early hemodynamic monitoring.
- Failure to recognize the effects of indiscriminate blood transfusion.

Disability: Brain and Spinal Cord Injury

CHANGES WITH AGING

Brain mass decreases approximately 10% by 70 years of age. This loss is replaced by cerebrospinal fluid. Concomitantly, the dura becomes tightly adherent to the skull. Although the increased space created around the brain may serve to protect it from contusion, it also causes stretching of the parasagittal bridging veins, making them more prone to shear injury. This loss of brain volume also allows for more brain movement in response to angular acceleration and deceleration. Significant amounts of blood can collect around the brain in the subdural space of an elderly individual before overt symptoms become apparent.

Cerebral blood flow is reduced by 20% by the age of 70 years. This is further reduced if atherosclerotic disease occludes cerebral arteries. Peripheral conduction velocity slows as a result of demyelinization. Reduced acquisition or retention of information can cause clinically subtle changes in mental status. Visual and auditory acuity declines, vibratory and position sensation is impaired, and reaction time increases. In addition to complicating the evaluation process of injured elderly patients, these changes place the individual at greater risk for injury. Finally, preexisting medical conditions or their treatment may cause confusion in the elderly.

In the spine, the most dramatic changes occur in the intervertebral disks. Loss of water and protein affect the shape and compressibility of the disks. These changes shift the loads on the vertebral column to the facets, ligaments, and paraspinal muscles and contribute to degeneration of the facet joints and development of spinal stenosis. These alterations place the spine and spinal cord at increased risk for injury in geriatric patients. This risk is increased in the presence of osteoporosis, whether or not it is apparent radiographically. Finally, osteoarthritis may cause canal stenosis and segmental immobility, making cord injury more likely (■ FIGURE 11-3).

EVALUATION AND MANAGEMENT

Elderly patients with brain injury have fewer severe cerebral contusions than do younger patients. However, the elderly have a higher incidence of subdural and intraparenchymal hematomas. Subdural hematomas are nearly three times as frequent in the elderly, in part because elderly individuals are more likely to be taking anticoagulant medications for cardiac or cerebrovascular disease. **Rapid screening for anticoagulant use and subsequent correction with blood component therapy may improve outcomes.** Subdural hematoma may produce a gradual onset of neurologic decline, especially in elderly patients. Chronic subdural hematoma resulting from an earlier fall may be the cause of a subsequent fall that leads to admission to the trauma bay. A computed tomography (CT) scan of the head provides rapid, accurate, and detailed information on structural damage to the brain, skull, and supporting elements. Liberal use of this imaging technology is

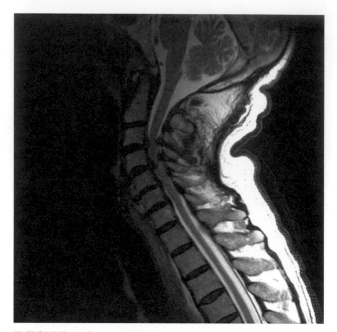

■ **FIGURE 11-3** A sagittal T$_2$-weighted image shows severe multilevel degenerative changes affecting disk spaces and posterior elements, associated with severe central canal stenosis, cord compression, and small foci of myelomalacia at the C4–C5 level.

appropriate in elderly patients with brain injury. See Chapter 6: Head Trauma.

Cervical spine injuries appear to be more common in elderly patients, although they may be occult and difficult to diagnose if osteoporosis and osteoarthritis are present. Severe osteophytic disease makes the diagnosis of cervical fracture challenging. Degeneration of intervertebral ligaments can increase the degree of subluxation that is physiologic. Preexisting spinal canal stenosis due to anterior osteophytes and posterior ligamentous hypertrophy increases the risk for central and anterior cord syndromes. These injuries often result from relatively mild extension injuries after falls or rear-end motor vehicle crashes. Magnetic resonance imaging (MRI) is particularly useful for diagnosing ligamentous injuries. See Chapter 7: Spine and Spinal Cord Trauma.

Exposure and Environment

The skin and connective tissues of elderly individuals undergo extensive changes, including a decrease in cell numbers, loss of strength, and impaired function. The epidermal keratinocytes lose a significant proportion of their proliferative ability with aging. The dermis loses as much as 20% of its thickness, undergoes a significant loss of vascularity, and has a marked decrease in the number of mast cells. **These changes result in the loss of thermal regulatory ability, decreased barrier function against bacterial invasion, and significant impairment of wound healing.**

Injured elderly patients must be protected from hypothermia. **Hypothermia not attributable to shock or exposure should alert the physician to the possibility of occult disease—in particular, sepsis, endocrine disease, or pharmacologic causes.**

The potential for invasive bacterial infection through injured skin must be recognized. Appropriate care, including assessing tetanus immunization status, to prevent infection, must be instituted early. See Tetanus Immunization (electronic version only).

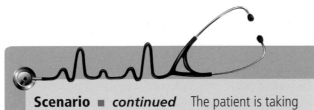

Scenario ■ *continued* The patient is taking warfarin and a beta blocker for hypertension. His chest radiograph shows multiple rib fractures, and his head CT shows a subdural hematoma with a few small intracerebral contusions.

Other Systems

Other systems that warrant special attention with regard to the treatment of elderly trauma patients include the musculoskeletal system, nutritional status, altered metabolism, and the immune system.

MUSCULOSKELETAL SYSTEM

Disorders of the musculoskeletal system are frequently the cause of presenting symptoms in the middle-aged and geriatric population. These disorders cause restrictions in daily activities and are key components in the loss of independence. Aging results in stiffening of ligaments, cartilage, intervertebral disks, and joint capsules. Deterioration of tendons, ligaments, and joint capsules leads to an increased risk of injury, spontaneous rupture, and decreased joint stability. The risk of injury increases not only for the musculoskeletal system, but also for the adjacent soft tissues.

Aging causes a decline in responsiveness to many anabolic hormones and an absolute reduction in the level of growth hormones. After the age of 25 years, muscle mass decreases by 4% every 10 years. After the age of 50 years, the rate is 10% per decade unless the levels of growth factors are low, in which case the rate of decrease approaches 35%. This is manifested by a reduction in the size and total number of muscle cells. The decrease in muscle mass is directly correlated to the decrease in strength seen with the aging process.

Osteoporosis results in a decrease of histologic normal bone with a consequent loss of strength and resistance to fractures. This disorder is endemic in the elderly population, affecting almost 50% of these individuals. The causes of osteoporosis include decrease of estrogen, loss of body mass, decreasing levels of physical activity, and inadequate intake and utilization of dietary calcium.

The consequences of these changes on the musculoskeletal system are frequently disabling and at times devastating. Injuries to ligaments and tendons affect joints and adjacent soft tissues. Osteoporosis contributes to the occurrence of spontaneous vertebral compression fractures and the high incidence of hip fractures in the elderly. The yearly incidence of these fractures approaches 1% for men and 2% for women over the age of 85 years. The ease with which fractures occur in the elderly patient magnifies the effect of force applied during injury.

Elderly individuals are particularly susceptible to fractures of the long bones, with attendant disability and associated pulmonary morbidity and mortality. Early stabilization of fractures may decrease this risk. Resuscitation should be targeted at normalizing tissue perfusion as early as possible and before fracture fixation is performed.

The most common locations of fractures in elderly patients are the ribs, proximal femur, hip, humerus, and wrist. Isolated hip fractures do not usually cause class III or IV shock. Neurovascular integrity should be assessed and compared with that of the opposite extremity.

Fractures of the humerus usually are caused by falls on an outstretched extremity. The resulting injury is a fracture of the surgical neck of the humerus. Usually, there is pain and tenderness in the shoulder or upper humerus area.

Of major importance in the evaluation of these patients is the determination of whether the fracture is impacted or nonimpacted. *Impacted fractures* demonstrate no false motion of the humerus when the shoulder is rotated gently from a flexed elbow. Patients with *nonimpacted fractures* generally experience pain on movement of the arm. These latter fractures require hospitalization for orthopedic consultation and often operation.

Colles' fracture results from a fall on the outstretched, dorsiflexed hand, causing a metaphyseal fracture of the distal radius. The classic finding of a fracture at the base of the ulnar styloid process occurs in 69% of cases. Evaluation should include careful testing of the median nerve and motor function of the finger flexors. The wrist should be examined radiographically, and all of the carpal bones should be visualized to exclude a more complex injury.

The aim of treatment for musculoskeletal injuries should be to undertake the least invasive, most definitive procedure that will permit early mobilization. Prolonged inactivity and disease often limit the ultimate functional outcome and impact survival.

NUTRITION AND METABOLISM

Caloric needs decline with age, as lean body mass and metabolic rate gradually decrease. Protein requirements actually may increase as a result of inefficient utilization. There is a widespread occurrence of chronically inadequate nutrition among the elderly, and poor nutritional status contributes to an increased complication rate. **Early and adequate nutritional support of injured elderly patients is a cornerstone of successful trauma care.**

IMMUNE SYSTEM AND INFECTIONS

Mortality from most diseases increases with age. The loss of competence of the immune system with age certainly plays a role. Thymic tissue is less than 15% of its maximum by 50 years of age. Liver and spleen size also decrease. Cell-mediated and humoral immune response to foreign antigens is decreased, whereas the response to autologous antigens is increased. It is not clear whether aging alters granulocyte function, but chronic diseases of the elderly, such as diabetes mellitus, may do so. As a consequence, elderly patients have an impaired ability to respond to bacteria and viruses, a reduced ability to respond to vaccination, and a lack of reliable response to skin antigen testing. Elderly individuals are less able to tolerate infection and more prone to multiple organ system failure. The absence of fever, leukocytosis, and other manifestations of the inflammatory response may be due to poor immune function.

PITFALLS

- Failure to recognize that minimal trauma may result in fractures and serious disability.

- Poor hemodynamic reserve combined with underestimation of blood loss from fractures may be lethal.

Scenario ■ *continued* The patient is given fresh frozen plasma to reverse the anticoagulant effects of warfarin and admitted to the intensive care unit for pulmonary care and monitoring. His pain is controlled with narcotics and, once his coagulation status is normal, an epidural catheter is placed.

Special Circumstances

? *What are the special issues to consider in treating geriatric trauma patients?*

Special circumstances that require consideration in the treatment of elderly trauma patients include medications, elder maltreatment, and end-of-life decisions.

MEDICATIONS

Concomitant disease frequently mandates the use of medications, and elderly patients are often taking several pharmacologic agents even before an injury occurs. **Drug interactions are frequently encountered, and side effects are much more common because of the narrow therapeutic range in the elderly.** Adverse reactions to some medications may even contribute to the injury-producing event. **ß-adrenergic blocking agents may limit chronotropic activity, and calcium-channel blockers may prevent peripheral vasoconstriction and contribute to hypotension.** Nonsteroidal antiinflammatory agents may contribute to blood loss because of their adverse effects on platelet function. Steroids and other drugs may further reduce the inflammatory and immune response. Long-term anticoagulant use may increase blood loss and increases the incidence of lethal brain injury. Long-term diuretic use may render elderly patients chronically hypovolemic and lead to total body deficits of potassium and sodium. Hypoglycemic agents may contribute to difficulty in control of serum glucose. **Psychotropic medications, commonly prescribed for elderly patients, may mask injuries or become problematic if discontinued abruptly.** Changes in central nervous system (CNS) function resulting from the use of these medications also may contribute to the injury. Elderly individuals frequently neglect to maintain tetanus immunization.

Pain relief in geriatric trauma patients should not be neglected after resuscitation. Narcotics are safe and effective and should be given in small, titrated intravenous doses. Antiemetic agents should be given with caution to avoid extrapyramidal effects. Potentially nephrotoxic drugs (e.g., antibiotics and radiographic dyes) must be given in doses that reflect the elderly patient's decreased renal function, contracted intravascular volume, and comorbid conditions.

PITFALLS

- Failure to take a drug history or note its impact on hemodynamics and CNS findings.
- Failure to titrate drug dosage, leading to increased incidence of side effects.

ELDER MALTREATMENT

When evaluating an injured elderly patient, consider that the injury may have been inflicted intentionally. Maltreatment of the elderly may be as common as child maltreatment. Maltreatment is defined as any willful infliction of injury, unreasonable confinement, intimidation, or cruel punishment that results in physical harm, pain, mental anguish, or other willful deprivation by a caretaker of goods or services that are necessary to avoid physical harm, mental anguish, or mental illness.

Elder maltreatment can be classified into six categories:

1. Physical maltreatment
2. Sexual maltreatment
3. Neglect
4. Psychological maltreatment
5. Financial and material exploitation
6. Violation of rights

Often, several types of maltreatment occur simultaneously. Multifaceted in cause, elder maltreatment often is not recognized and is underreported. Many cases of maltreated elderly persons involve only subtle signs (e.g., poor hygiene and dehydration) and have great potential to go undetected. Physical maltreatment occurs in up to 14% of geriatric trauma admissions, resulting in a higher mortality than in younger patients.

Physical findings suggesting elder maltreatment include:

- Contusions affecting the inner arms, inner thighs, palms, soles, scalp, ear (pinna), mastoid area, buttocks, or multiple and clustered contusions
- Abrasions to the axillary area (from restraints) or the wrist and ankles (from ligatures)
- Nasal bridge and temple injury (eyeglasses)
- Periorbital ecchymoses
- Oral injury
- Unusual alopecia pattern
- Untreated pressure ulcers or ulcers in non-lumbar/sacral areas
- Untreated fractures
- Fractures not involving the hip, humerus, or vertebra
- Injuries in various stages of evolution
- Injuries to the eyes or nose
- Contact burns and scalds
- Scalp hemorrhage or hematoma

The presence of these findings should prompt a detailed history that may be at variance with the physical findings and may uncover an intentional delay in treatment. These findings should prompt reporting to appropriate authorities and further investigation. If maltreatment is suspected or confirmed, appropriate action should be taken, including removal of the elderly patient from the abusive situation. According to the National Center on Elder Abuse, more than 1 in 10 older adults may experience some type of maltreatment, but only 1 in 5 cases or fewer are reported. This statistic holds true even though every state in United States mandates reporting of elder maltreatment. A multidisciplinary approach is required.

END-OF-LIFE DECISIONS

Many geriatric patients return to their preinjury level of function and independence after recovering from injury. Age significantly increases mortality from injury, but more aggressive care, especially early in the evaluation and resuscitation of elderly trauma patients, has been shown to improve survival. Attempts to identify which elderly trauma patients are at greatest risk for mortality have found little utility in clinical practice.

Certainly there are circumstances in which the doctor and patient, or family member(s), may choose to withdraw life-sustaining treatment and provide palliative care. This decision is particularly clear in the case of elderly patients who have sustained extensive burns or severe brain injury or when survival from the injuries sustained is unlikely. The trauma team should try to determine the patient's wishes as evidenced by a living will, advance directive, or similar document. Although no absolute guidelines can be given, the following observations may be helpful:

- The patient's right to self-determination is paramount.

- Medical intervention is appropriate only when it is in the patient's best interests.

- Medical therapy is appropriate only when its likely benefits outweigh its adverse consequences.

- The ethical issue of appropriateness of care in an environment of declining hospital resources and restrictions on finances is more challenging.

Scenario ■ conclusion   The patient recovers after a 10-day hospital stay and is discharged to a rehabilitation facility for short-term rehabilitation prior to discharge home with his family. A home safety evaluation is performed before he is discharged, focusing on fall prevention.

Chapter Summary

1 The number of elderly persons is increasing globally. Although the elderly are less likely to be injured than younger people, the mortality rate for the geriatric population is higher. Many geriatric trauma patients can be returned to their preinjury medical status and independence. Knowledge of the changes that occur with aging, an appreciation of the injury patterns seen in the elderly, and an understanding of the need for aggressive resuscitation and monitoring of injured geriatric patients are necessary for improved outcome.

2 Anatomic and physiologic changes in the elderly are associated with increased morbidity and mortality following trauma. Comorbidity increases with age. Frequent use of medications including beta blockers and anticoagulants complicate assessment and management.

3 Treatment of the geriatric trauma patient follows the same pattern as that for younger patients, but caution and a high index of suspicion for injuries specific to this age group are required for optimal treatment. Comorbidities and medications may not only cause, but also complicate injuries in the elderly. Careful volume resuscitation with close hemodynamic monitoring should guide treatment.

4 Increased awareness of elder maltreatment, including the patterns of injury, is necessary so that reporting can be improved. This should lead to earlier diagnosis and improved treatment of elderly injured patients.

BIBLIOGRAPHY

1. Alexander BH, Rivara FP, Wolf ME. The cost and frequency of hospitalization for fall-related injuries in older adults. *Am J Public Health* 1992;82:1020-1023.

2. Bergeron E, Lavoie A, Clas D, et al. Elderly trauma patients with rib fractures are at greater risk of death and pneumonia. *J Trauma* 2003;54:478-485.

3. Bouchard JA, Barei D, Cayer D, et al. Outcome of femoral shaft fractures in the elderly. *Clin Orthop* 1996;332:105-109.

4. Bulger EM, Jurkovich GJ, Farver CL, et al. Oxandrolone dose not improve outcome for chronically ventilated surgical patients. *Ann Surg* 2004;240(3):472-8.

5. Collins KM. Elder maltreatment—a review. *Arch Pathol Lab* 2006;130:1290-1296.

6. Collins KA, Bennett AT, Hanzlick R. Elder abuse and neglect. *Arch Intern Med* 2000;160:1567-1568.

7. Corwin HL, Gettinger A, Pearl RG, et al. The CRIT study: anemia and blood transfusion in the critically ill—current clinical practice in the United States. *Crit Care Med* 2004;32:39.

8. Council Report. Decisions near the end of life. *JAMA* 1992;267:2229-2233.

9. DeGoede KM, Ashton-Miller JA, Schultz AB. Fall-related upper body injuries in the older adult: a review of the biochemical issues. *J Biomech* 2003;36:1043-1053.

10. De Laet CE, Pols HA. Fractures in the elderly: epidemiology and demography. *Baillieres Best Pract Res Clin Endocrinol Metab* 2004;14:171-179.

11. Demetriades D, Sava J, Alo K, et al. Old age as a criterion for trauma team activation. *J Trauma* 2001; 51: 754-756.

12. Gillespie LD, Robertson MC, Gillespie WJ, et al. Interventions for preventing falls in older people living in the community. *Evid Based Med* 2009;14:176.

13. Gubler KD, Maier RV, Davis R, et al. Trauma recidivism in the elderly. *J Trauma* 1996;41(6):952-956.

14. Hebert PC, Wells G, Blajchman MA, et al. A multicenter, randomized, controlled clinical trial of transfusion requirements in critical care. *N Engl J Med* 1999;340:409.

15. Hebert PC, Yetisir E, Martin C, et al. Is a low transfusion threshold safe in critically ill patients with cardiovascular diseases? *Crit Care Med* 2001;29:227.

16. Horan MA, Clague JE. Injury in the aging: recovery and rehabilitation. *Br Med Bull* 1999;55:895-909.

17. Ivascu FA, Howells GA, Junn FS, Bair HA, Bendick PJ, Janczyk RJ. Predictors of mortality in trauma patients with intracranial hemorrhage on preinjury aspirin or clopidogrel. *J Trauma* 2008 Oct;65(4):785-8.

18. Karmakar MK, Ho AM-H. Acute pain management of patients with multiple fractured ribs. *J Trauma* 2003;54:615-625.

19. Koepsell TD, Wolf ME, McCloskey L, et al. Medical conditions and motor vehicle collisions in older adults. *J Am Geriatr Soc* 1994;42:695-700.

20. Lachs MS, Pillemer K. Abuse and neglect of elderly persons. *N Engl J Med* 1995;332:437-443.

21. Lotfipour S, Kaku SK, Vaca FE, et al. Factors associated with complications in older patients with isolated blunt chest trauma. *West J Emerg Med* 2009;10:79-84.

22. Mackenzie EJ, Morris JA, Edelstein SL. Effect of pre-existing disease on length of stay in trauma patients. *J Trauma* 1989;29:757-764.

23. MacKenzie EJ, Rivara FP, Jurkovich GJ, et al. A national evaluation of the effect of trauma-center care on mortality. *N Engl J Med* 2006;354(4):366-78.

24. Manton DK, Vaupel JW. Survival after the age of 80 in the United States, Sweden, France, England, and Japan. *N Engl J Med* 1995;333:1232-1235.

25. McGwin G Jr., MacLennan PA, Fife JB, et al. Preexisting conditions and mortality in older trauma patients. *J Trauma* 2004;56:1291-1296

26. McKevitt EC, Calvert E, Ng A, et al. Geriatric trauma: resource use and patient outcomes. *Can J Surg* 2003;Jun;46(3):211-215.

27. McKinley BA, Marvin RG, Cocanour CS, et al. Blunt trauma resuscitation: the old can respond. *Arch Surg* 2000;135(6):688-693, discussion 694-695.

28. McMahon DJ, Schwab CW, Kauder DR. Comorbidity and the elderly trauma patient. *World J Surg* 1996;20:1113-1119.

29. Milzman DP, Boulanger BR, Rodriguez A, et al. Pre-existing disease in trauma patients: a predictor of fate independent of age and injury severity score. *J Trauma* 1992;31:236-244.

30. Mina AA, Bair HA, Howells GA, et al. Complications of preinjury warfarin use in the trauma patient. *J Trauma* 2003;54:842-847.

31. Morris JA, Mackenzie EJ, Edelstein SL: The effect of pre-existing conditions on mortality in trauma patients. *JAMA* 1990;263:1942-1946.

32. Mosenthal AC, Livingston DH, Lavery RF, et al. The effect of age on functional outcome in mild traumatic brain injury: 6-month report of a prospective multicenter trial. *J Trauma* 2004;56:1042-1048.

33. National Center on Elder Abuse. Why Should I Care About Elder Abuse? http://www.ncea.aoa.gov/ncearoot/Main_Site/pdf/publication/NCEA_WhatIsAbuse-2010.pdf. Accessed March, 2010.

34. Osler T, Hales K, Baack B, et al. Trauma in the elderly. *Am J Surg* 1988;156:537-543.

35. Ottochian M, Salim A, DuBose J, Teixeira PG, et al. Does age matter? The relationship between age and mortality in penetrating trauma. *Injury* 2009;40:354-357.

36. Pennings JL, Bachulis BL, Simons CT, et al. Survival after severe brain injury in the aged. *Arch Surg* 1993;128:787-794.

37. Phillips S, Rond PC, Kelly SM, et al. The failure of triage criteria to identify geriatric patients with trauma: results from the Florida trauma triage study. *J Trauma* 1996;40:278-283.

38. Scalea TM, Simon HM, Duncan AO, et al. Geriatric blunt multiple trauma: improved survival with early invasive monitoring. *J Trauma* 1990;30:129-134.

39. Schwab CW, Kauder DR. Trauma in the geriatric patient. *Arch Surg* 1992;127:701-706.

40. Shabot MM, Johnson CL. Outcome from critical care in the "oldest old" trauma patients. *J Trauma* 1995;39:254-259.

41. Timberlake GA. Elder abuse. In: Kaufman HH, ed. *The Physician's Perspective on Medical Law*. Park Ridge, IL: American Association of Neurological Surgeons; 1997.

42. Utomo WK, Gabbe BJ, Simpson PM, Cameron PA. Predictors of in-hospital and 6-month functional outcomes in older patients after moderate to severe traumatic brain injury. *Injury* 2009;40:973-977.

43. van der Sluis CK, Klasen HJ, Eisma WH, et al. Major trauma in young and old: what is the difference? *J Trauma* 1996;40:78-82.

44. Wardle TD. Co-morbid factors in trauma patients. *Br Med Bull* 1999;55:744-756.

45. Zietlow SP, Capizzi PJ, Bannon MP, et al. Multisystem geriatric trauma. *J Trauma* 1994;37:985-988.

12 Trauma in Pregnancy and Intimate Partner Violence

Changes in structure and function can influence the evaluation of injured pregnant patients by altering the signs and symptoms of injury, the approach and responses to resuscitation, and the results of diagnostic tests.

Scenario A 25-year-old woman who appears to be in the third trimester of pregnancy is brought to the emergency department (ED) following a motor vehicle collision. She is unconscious and immobilized on a long spine board.

Outline

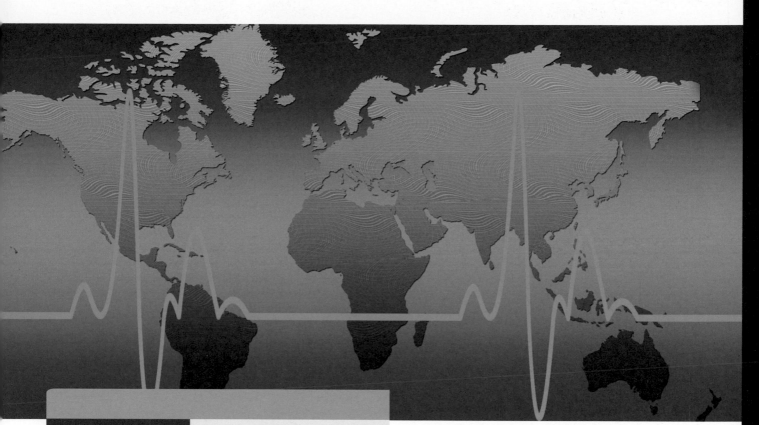

Objectives

Pregnancy causes major physiologic changes and altered anatomic relationships involving nearly every organ system of the body. These changes in structure and function can influence the evaluation of injured pregnant patients by altering the signs and symptoms of injury, the approach and responses to resuscitation, and the results of diagnostic tests. Pregnancy also can affect the patterns and severity of injury.

Clinicians who treat pregnant trauma patients must remember that there are two patients: mother and fetus. Nevertheless, initial treatment priorities for an injured pregnant patient remain the same as for the nonpregnant patient. **The best initial treatment for the fetus is the provision of optimal resuscitation of the mother.** Monitoring and evaluation techniques should allow for assessment of the mother and the fetus. If x-ray examination is indicated during critical management, it should not be withheld because of the pregnancy. **A qualified surgeon and an obstetrician should be consulted early in the evaluation of pregnant trauma patients.**

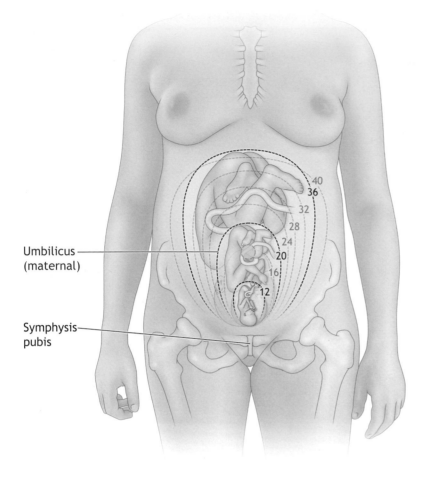

Umbilicus
(maternal)

Symphysis
pubis

■ **FIGURE 12-1 Changes in Fundal Height in Pregnancy.** As the uterus enlarges, the bowel is pushed cephalad, so that it lies mostly in the upper abdomen. As a result, the bowel is somewhat protected in blunt abdominal trauma, whereas the uterus and its contents (fetus and placenta) become more vulnerable.

Anatomic and Physiologic Alterations of Pregnancy

❓ *What changes occur with pregnancy?*

An understanding of the anatomic and physiologic alterations of pregnancy, as well as of the physiologic relationship between a pregnant patient and her fetus, is essential to serve the best interests of both patients. Such alterations include differences in anatomy, blood volume and composition, and hemodynamics, as well as changes in the respiratory, gastrointestinal, urinary, musculoskeletal, and neurologic systems.

ANATOMIC DIFFERENCES

The uterus remains an intrapelvic organ until approximately the 12th week of gestation, when it begins to rise out of the pelvis. By 20 weeks, the uterus is at the umbilicus, and at 34 to 36 weeks, it reaches the costal margin (■ **FIGURE 12-1**). During the last 2 weeks of gestation, the fundus frequently descends as the fetal head engages the pelvis. As the uterus enlarges, the bowel is pushed cephalad, so that the bowel lies mostly in the upper abdomen. As a result, the bowel is somewhat protected in blunt abdominal trauma, whereas the uterus and its contents (fetus and placenta) become more vulnerable. However, penetrating trauma to the upper abdomen during late gestation may result in complex intestinal injury because of this cephalad displacement.

During the first trimester, the uterus is a thick-walled structure of limited size, confined within the bony pelvis. During the second trimester, it enlarges beyond its protected intrapelvic location, but the small fetus remains mobile and cushioned by a generous amount of amniotic fluid. The amniotic fluid may cause amniotic fluid embolism and disseminated intravascular coagulation following trauma if the fluid gains access to the maternal intravascular space. By the third trimester, the uterus is large and thin-walled. In the vertex presentation, the fetal head is usually within the pelvis, with the remainder of the fetus exposed above the pelvic brim (■ **FIGURE 12-2**).

Pelvic fracture(s) in late gestation may result in skull fracture or serious intracranial injury to the fetus. Unlike the elastic myometrium, the placenta has little elasticity. This lack of placental elastic tissue results in vulnerability to shear forces at the uteroplacental interface, which may lead to abruptio placentae.

The placental vasculature is maximally dilated throughout gestation, yet it is exquisitely sensitive to catecholamine stimulation. **An abrupt decrease in maternal intravascular volume can result in a profound increase in uterine vascular resistance, reducing fetal oxygenation despite reasonably normal maternal vital signs.**

BLOOD VOLUME AND COMPOSITION

Plasma volume increases steadily throughout pregnancy and plateaus at 34 weeks of gestation. A smaller increase in red-blood-cell (RBC) volume occurs, resulting in a decreased hematocrit level (physiologic anemia of pregnancy). In late pregnancy, a hematocrit level of 31% to 35% is normal. Healthy pregnant patients can lose 1200 to 1500 mL of blood before exhibiting signs and symptoms of hypovolemia. However, this amount of hemorrhage may be reflected by fetal distress evidenced by an abnormal fetal heart rate.

The white-blood-cell (WBC) count increases during pregnancy. It is not unusual to see WBC counts of 12,000/mm³ during pregnancy or as high as 25,000/mm³ during labor. Levels of serum fibrinogen and other clotting factors are mildly elevated. Prothrombin and partial thromboplastin times may be shortened, but bleeding and clotting times are unchanged. Table 12.1 outlines normal laboratory values during pregnancy.

HEMODYNAMICS

Important hemodynamic factors to consider in pregnant trauma patients include cardiac output, heart rate, blood pressure, venous pressure, and electrocardiographic changes.

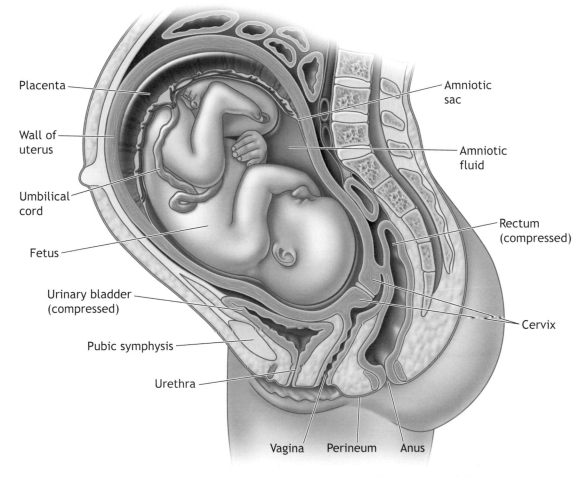

Placenta

Wall of uterus

Umbilical cord

Fetus

Urinary bladder (compressed)

Pubic symphysis

Urethra

Amniotic sac

Amniotic fluid

Rectum (compressed)

Cervix

Vagina   Perineum   Anus

■ **FIGURE 12-2 Full-Term Fetus in Vertex Presentation.** Note the displacement and compression of the abdominal viscera. Most of the viscera is displaced cephalad, which cannot be shown in this illustration.

■ TABLE 12.1 Normal Laboratory Values During Pregnancy	
Hematocrit	32%–42%
WBC count	5,000–12,000μL
Arterial pH	7.40–7.45
Bicarbonate	17–22 mEq/L
PaCO$_2$	25–30 mm Hg (3.3–4 kPa)
Fibrinogen	3.79 g/L (3rd trimester)

Cardiac Output

After the 10th week of pregnancy, cardiac output can increase by 1.0 to 1.5 L/min because of the increase in plasma volume and decrease in vascular resistance of the uterus and placenta, which receive 20% of the patient's cardiac output during the third trimester of pregnancy. This increased output may be greatly influenced by the mother's position during the second half of pregnancy. In the supine position, vena cava compression can decrease cardiac output by 30% because of decreased venous return from the lower extremities.

Heart Rate

Heart rate increases gradually by 10 to 15 beats/min during pregnancy, reaching a maximum rate by the third trimester. This change in heart rate must be considered when interpreting a tachycardic response to hypovolemia.

Blood Pressure

Pregnancy results in a 5 to 15 mm Hg fall in systolic and diastolic pressures during the second trimester. Blood pressure returns to near-normal levels at term. Some pregnant women exhibit hypotension when placed in the supine position, caused by compression of the inferior vena cava. This hypotension is corrected by relieving uterine pressure on the inferior vena cava, as described later in this chapter. Hypertension in the pregnant patient may represent preeclampsia if accompanied by proteinuria.

Venous Pressure

The resting central venous pressure (CVP) is variable with pregnancy, but the response to volume is the same as in the nonpregnant state. Venous hypertension in the lower extremities is present during the third trimester.

Electrocardiographic Changes

The axis may shift leftward by approximately 15 degrees. Flattened or inverted T waves in leads III and AVF and the precordial leads may be normal. Ectopic beats are increased during pregnancy.

RESPIRATORY SYSTEM

Minute ventilation increases primarily as a result of an increase in tidal volume. Hypocapnia (PaCO$_2$ of 30 mm Hg) is therefore common in late pregnancy. **A PaCO$_2$ of 35 to 40 mm Hg may indicate impending respiratory failure during pregnancy.** Anatomic alterations in the thoracic cavity appear to account for the decreased residual volume that is associated with diaphragmatic elevation, with increased lung markings and prominence of the pulmonary vessels seen on chest x-ray examination. Oxygen consumption is increased during pregnancy. Therefore, it is important to maintain and ensure adequate arterial oxygenation during the resuscitation of injured pregnant patients.

GASTROINTESTINAL SYSTEM

Gastric emptying is delayed during pregnancy, so early gastric tube decompression may be particularly important to avoid the aspiration of gastric contents. The intestines are relocated to the upper part of the abdomen and may be shielded by the uterus. The position of the patient's spleen and liver are essentially unchanged by pregnancy.

URINARY SYSTEM

The glomerular filtration rate and renal blood flow increase during pregnancy, whereas levels of serum creatinine and urea nitrogen fall to approximately one-half of normal prepregnancy levels. Glycosuria is common during pregnancy.

MUSCULOSKELETAL SYSTEM

The symphysis pubis widens to 4 to 8 mm, and the sacroiliac joint spaces increase by the seventh month of gestation. These factors must be considered in interpreting x-ray films of the pelvis.

The large, engorged pelvic vessels that surround the gravid uterus can contribute to massive retroperitoneal bleeding after blunt trauma with associated pelvic fractures.

NEUROLOGIC SYSTEM

Eclampsia is a complication of late pregnancy that can mimic head injury. It should be considered if seizures occur with associated hypertension, hyperreflexia, proteinuria, and peripheral edema. Expert neurologic and obstetric consultation frequently is helpful in differentiating between eclampsia and other causes of seizures.

PITFALLS

- Not understanding the anatomic and physiologic changes that occur during pregnancy
- Not recognizing that a normal $PaCO_2$ may indicate impending respiratory failure during pregnancy
- Mistaking eclampsia for head injury

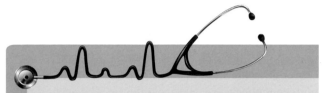

Scenario ■ *continued*   The patient is given high flow oxygen. She is unable to respond to questions, has a respiratory rate of 28, heart rate of 130, and blood pressure of 110/50. Her Glasgow Coma Scale (GCS) score is 7 (E1, V2, M4).

Mechanisms of Injury

❓ *What are the unique risks to pregnant patients?*

Most mechanisms of injury are similar to those sustained by nonpregnant patients, but certain differences must be recognized in pregnant patients who sustain blunt or penetrating injury.

BLUNT INJURY

The incidence of various types of blunt trauma in pregnancy is outlined in Table 12.2. The abdominal wall, uterine myometrium, and amniotic fluid act as buffers to direct fetal injury from blunt trauma. Nonetheless, fetal injuries may occur when the abdominal wall strikes an object, such as the dashboard or steering wheel, or when a pregnant patient is struck by a blunt instrument. Indirect injury to the fetus may occur from rapid compression, deceleration, the contrecoup effect, or a shearing force resulting in abruptio placentae.

Compared with restrained pregnant women involved in collisions, unrestrained pregnant women have a higher risk of premature delivery and fetal death. The type of restraint system affects the frequency of uterine rupture and fetal death. The use of a lap belt alone allows forward flexion and uterine compression with possible uterine rupture or abruptio placentae. A lap belt worn too high over the uterus may produce uterine rupture because of the trans-

■ TABLE 12.2 Incidence of Various Types of Blunt Trauma in Pregnancy		
TYPE OF BLUNT TRAUMA	**TOTAL NUMBER**	**PERCENTAGE**
Motor vehicle crashes/pedestrians	1098	59.6
Falls	411	22.3
Direct assaults	308	16.7
Other	24	0.1

Source: Shah AJ, Kilcline BA. Trauma in pregnancy. *Emerg Med Clin N Am* 2003;21:615-629.

mission of direct force to the uterus on impact. The use of shoulder restraints in conjunction with the lap belt reduces the likelihood of direct and indirect fetal injury, presumably because of the greater surface area over which the deceleration force is dissipated, as well as the prevention of forward flexion of the mother over the gravid uterus. Therefore, determination of the type of restraint device worn by the pregnant patient, if any, is important in the overall assessment. There does not appear to be any increase in pregnancy-specific risks from the deployment of airbags in motor vehicles.

PENETRATING INJURY

As the gravid uterus increases in size, the other viscera are relatively protected from penetrating injury, whereas the likelihood of uterine injury increases. The dense uterine musculature in early pregnancy can absorb a great amount of energy from penetrating missiles, decreasing missile velocity and lessening the likelihood of injury to other viscera. The amniotic fluid and fetus also absorb energy and contribute to slowing of the penetrating missile. The resulting low incidence of associated maternal visceral injuries accounts for the generally excellent maternal outcome in cases of penetrating wounds of the gravid uterus. However, the fetus generally fares poorly when there is a penetrating injury to the uterus.

Severity of Injury

The severity of maternal injuries determines maternal and fetal outcome. Therefore, treatment methods also depend on the severity of maternal injuries. All pregnant patients with major injuries require admission to a facility with trauma and obstetric capabilities. Even pregnant patients with minor injuries should be carefully observed, since occasionally minor injuries are associated with abruptio placentae and fetal loss.

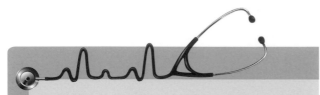

Scenario ■ continued The patient undergoes rapid sequence intubation due to her GCS score. Her heart rate is now 130, and blood pressure is 90/60. Intravenous access is obtained, and she is given 1 liter of crystalloid.

Assessment and Treatment

? How do I evaluate and treat two patients?

For optimal outcome of mother and fetus, clinicians must assess and resuscitate the mother first, and then assess the fetus before conducting a secondary survey of the mother.

PRIMARY SURVEY AND RESUSCITATION

Mother

Ensure a patent airway, adequate ventilation and oxygenation, and effective circulatory volume. If ventilatory support is required, intubation is appropriate for pregnant patients, and consideration should be given to maintaining the appropriate PCO_2 for her stage of pregnancy (e.g., approximately 30 mm Hg in late pregnancy). See Chapter 2: Airway and Ventilatory Management.

Uterine compression of the vena cava may reduce venous return to the heart, thereby decreasing cardiac output and aggravating the shock state. **The uterus should be displaced manually to the left side to relieve pressure on the inferior vena cava.** If the patient requires immobilization in a supine position, the patient or spine board can be logrolled 4 to 6 inches (or 15 degrees) to the left and supported with a bolstering device, thus maintaining spinal precautions and decompressing the vena cava (■ FIGURE 12-3).

Because of their increased intravascular volume, pregnant patients can lose a significant amount of blood before tachycardia, hypotension, and other signs of hypovolemia occur. Thus, the fetus may be in distress and the placenta deprived of vital perfusion while the mother's condition and vital signs appear stable. Crystalloid fluid resuscitation and early type-specific blood administration are indicated to support the physiologic hyper-

volemia of pregnancy. Vasopressors should be an absolute last resort in restoring maternal blood pressure, because these agents further reduce uterine blood flow, resulting in fetal hypoxia. Baseline laboratory evaluation in the trauma patient should include a fibrinogen level, as this may double in late pregnancy; a normal fibrinogen level may indicate early disseminated intravascular coagulation (DIC).

Fetus

The abdominal examination during pregnancy is critically important, as rapid identification of serious maternal injuries and fetal well-being depend on a thorough evaluation. The main cause of fetal death is maternal shock and maternal death. The second most common cause of fetal death is placental abruption. Abruptio placentae is suggested by vaginal bleeding (70% of cases), uterine tenderness, frequent uterine contractions, uterine tetany, and uterine irritability (uterus contracts when touched). In 30% of abruptions following trauma, vaginal bleeding may not occur. Uterine ultrasonography may be helpful in diagnosis, but is not definitive. Late in pregnancy, abruption may occur following relatively minor injuries.

Uterine rupture, a rare injury, is suggested by findings of abdominal tenderness, guarding, rigidity, or rebound tenderness, especially if there is profound

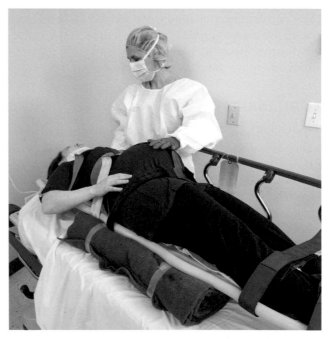

■ FIGURE 12-3 **Proper Immobilization of a Pregnant Patient.** If the patient requires immobilization in a supine position, the patient or spine board can be logrolled 4 to 6 inches (or 15 degrees) to the left and supported with a bolstering device, thus maintaining spinal precautions and decompressing the vena cava.

shock. Frequently, peritoneal signs are difficult to appreciate in advanced gestation because of expansion and attenuation of the abdominal wall musculature. Other abnormal findings suggestive of uterine rupture include abdominal fetal lie (e.g., oblique or transverse lie), easy palpation of fetal parts because of their extrauterine location, and inability to readily palpate the uterine fundus when there is fundal rupture. X-ray evidence of rupture includes extended fetal extremities, abnormal fetal position, and free intraperitoneal air. Operative exploration may be necessary to diagnose uterine rupture.

In most cases of abruptio placentae and uterine rupture, the patient reports abdominal pain or cramping. Signs of hypovolemia can accompany each of these injuries.

Initial fetal heart tones can be auscultated with Doppler ultrasound by 10 weeks of gestation. **Continuous fetal monitoring with a tocodynamometer should be performed beyond 20 to 24 weeks of gestation.** Patients with no risk factors for fetal loss should have continuous monitoring for 6 hours, whereas patients with risk factors for fetal loss or placental abruption should be monitored for 24 hours. The risk factors are maternal heart rate >110, an Injury Severity Score (ISS) >9, evidence of placental abruption, fetal heart rate >160 or <120, ejection during a motor vehicle crash, and motorcycle or pedestrian collisions.

ADJUNCTS TO PRIMARY SURVEY AND RESUSCITATION

Mother

If possible, the patient should be monitored on her left side after physical examination. Monitoring of the patient's fluid status is important in order to maintain the relative hypervolemia required in pregnancy. Monitoring should also include pulse oximetry and arterial blood gas determinations. Remember, maternal bicarbonate normally is low during pregnancy as a compensation for respiratory alkalosis.

Fetus

Obstetric consultation should be obtained, since fetal distress can occur at any time and without warning. Fetal heart rate is a sensitive indicator of both maternal blood volume status and fetal well-being. Fetal heart tones should be monitored in every injured pregnant woman. The normal range for fetal heart rate is 120 to 160 beats/min. An abnormal fetal heart rate, repetitive decelerations, absence of accelerations or beat-to-beat variability, and frequent uterine activity can be signs of impending maternal and/or fetal decompensation (e.g., hypoxia and/or acidosis) and should prompt immediate obstetric consultation.

Indicated radiographic studies should be performed, because the benefits certainly outweigh the potential risk to the fetus.

SECONDARY ASSESSMENT

The maternal secondary survey should follow the same pattern as for nonpregnant patients. See Chapter 1: Initial Assessment and Management. Indications for abdominal computed tomography, focused assessment sonography in trauma (FAST), and diagnostic peritoneal lavage (DPL) are also the same. However, if DPL is performed, the catheter should be placed above the umbilicus using the open technique. Pay careful attention to the presence of uterine contractions, which suggest early labor, or tetanic contractions, which suggest placental abruption. Evaluation of the perineum should include a formal pelvic examination, ideally performed by a clinician skilled in obstetric care. The presence of amniotic fluid in the vagina, evidenced by a pH of 7 to 7.5, suggests ruptured chorioamnionic membranes. Cervical effacement and dilation, fetal presentation, and the relationship of the fetal presenting part to the ischial spines should be noted.

Because vaginal bleeding in the third trimester may indicate disruption of the placenta and impending death of the fetus, a vaginal examination is vital. Repeated vaginal examinations should be avoided. The decision regarding an emergency cesarean section should be made with advice from an obstetrician.

Admission to the hospital is mandatory in the presence of vaginal bleeding, uterine irritability, abdominal tenderness, pain or cramping, evidence of hypovolemia, changes in or absence of fetal heart tones, or leakage of amniotic fluid. Care should be provided at a facility with appropriate fetal and maternal monitoring and treatment capabilities. **The fetus may be in jeopardy even with apparently minor maternal injury.**

DEFINITIVE CARE

Obstetric consultation should be obtained whenever specific uterine problems exist or are suspected. With extensive placental separation or amniotic fluid embolization, widespread intravascular clotting may develop, causing depletion of fibrinogen, other clotting factors, and platelets. This consumptive coagulopathy can emerge rapidly. In the presence of life-threatening amniotic fluid embolism and/or disseminated intravascular coagulation, uterine evacuation should be accomplished on an urgent basis, along with replacement of platelets, fibrinogen, and other clotting factors, if necessary.

Consequences of fetomaternal hemorrhage include not only fetal anemia and death, but also isoimmunization if the mother is Rh-negative. Because as little as 0.01 mL of Rh-positive blood will sensitize 70% of Rh-negative patients, the presence of fetomaternal hemorrhage in an Rh-negative mother should warrant Rh immunoglobulin therapy. Although a positive Kleihauer-Betke test (a maternal blood smear allowing detection of fetal RBCs in the maternal circulation) indicates fetomaternal hemorrhage, a negative test does not exclude minor degrees of fetomaternal hemorrhage that are capable of sensitizing the Rh-negative mother. **All pregnant Rh-negative trauma patients should receive Rh immunoglobulin therapy unless the injury is remote from the uterus (e.g., isolated distal extremity injury).** Immunoglobulin therapy should be instituted within 72 hours of injury.

PITFALLS

- Failure to recognize the need to displace the uterus to the left side in a hypotensive pregnant patient.

- Failure to recognize need for Rh immunoglobulin therapy in an Rh-negative mother.

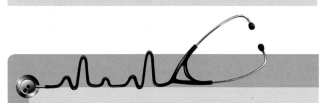

Scenario ■ continued The uterus is displaced to the left; the patient does not respond to crystalloid resuscitation, and her heart rate increases to 140. A FAST exam is done, which shows intraabdominal fluid. She is given Rh immunoglobulin therapy and antibiotics, and is taken emergently to the operating room.

Perimortem Cesarean Section

There are few data to support perimortem cesarean section in pregnant trauma patients who experience hypovolemic cardiac arrest. Remember, fetal distress can be present when the mother has no hemodynamic abnormalities, and progressive maternal instability compromises fetal survival. At the time of maternal hypovolemic cardiac arrest, the fetus already has suffered prolonged hypoxia. For other causes of maternal cardiac arrest, perimortem cesarean section occasionally may be successful if performed within 4 to 5 minutes of the arrest.

Intimate Partner Violence

? How do I recognize intimate partner violence?

Intimate partner violence is a major cause of injury to women during cohabitation, marriage, and pregnancy regardless of ethnic background, cultural influences, or socioeconomic status. Seventeen percent of injured pregnant patients experience trauma inflicted by another person, and 60% of these patients experience repeated episodes of intimate partner violence. According to estimates from the U.S. Department of Justice, 2 million to 4 million incidents of intimate partner violence occur per year, and almost one-half of all women over their lifetimes are physically and/or psychologically abused in some manner. Worldwide, between 10%–69% of women report having been assaulted by an intimate partner.

Suspicion of intimate partner violence should be documented, and reported. These attacks can result in death and disability. They also represent an increasing number of ED visits. Although the majority of victims are women, men make up approximately 40% of all reported cases of intimate partner violence in the United States.

Indicators that suggest the presence of intimate partner violence include:

- Injuries inconsistent with the stated history

- Diminished self-image, depression, or suicide attempts

- Self-abuse

- Frequent ED or doctor's office visits

- Symptoms suggestive of substance abuse

- Self-blame for injuries

- Partner insists on being present for interview and examination and monopolizes discussion

These indicators raise the suspicion of the potential for intimate partner violence and should serve to initiate further investigation. The three questions in Box 12-1, when asked in a nonjudgmental manner and without the patient's partner being present, can identify 65% to 70% of victims of intimate partner violence. Suspected cases of intimate partner violence should be handled through local social service agencies or the state health and human services department.

Box 12-1 Intimate Partner Violence Screen

1 Have you been kicked, hit, punched, or otherwise hurt by someone within the past year? If so, by whom?

2 Do you feel safe in your current relationship?

3 Is there a partner from a previous relationship who is making you feel unsafe now?

Reprinted with permission from Feldhaus KM, Koziol-McLain J, Amsbury HL, et al. Accuracy of 3 brief screening questions for detecting partner violence in the emergency department. *JAMA* 1997;277:1357-1361.

Scenario ■ conclusion The patient undergoes emergent splenectomy, and an intraoperative cesarean section is performed. She undergoes a head computed tomography (CT) postoperatively, which identifies small intraparenchymal contusions with a moderate amount of subarachnoid blood. She recovers after a prolonged intensive care unit (ICU) course and is able to go home to a healthy baby boy.

Chapter Summary

1 Important and predictable anatomic and physiologic changes occur during pregnancy that can influence the assessment and treatment of injured pregnant patients. Attention also must be directed toward the fetus, the second patient of this unique duo, after its environment is stabilized. A qualified surgeon and an obstetrician should be consulted early in the evaluation of pregnant trauma patients.

2 The abdominal wall, uterine myometrium, and amniotic fluid act as buffers to direct fetal injury from blunt trauma. As the gravid uterus increases in size, the remainder of the abdominal viscera are relatively protected from penetrating injury, whereas the likelihood of uterine injury increases.

3 Appropriate volume resuscitation should be given to correct and prevent maternal and fetal hypovolemic shock. Assess and resuscitate the mother first, and then assess the fetus before conducting a secondary survey of the mother.

4 A search should be made for conditions unique to the injured pregnant patient, such as blunt or penetrating uterine trauma, abruptio placentae, amniotic fluid embolism, isoimmunization, and premature rupture of membranes.

5 Minor degrees of fetomaternal hemorrhage are capable of sensitizing the Rh-negative mother. All pregnant Rh-negative trauma patients should receive Rh immunoglobulin therapy unless the injury is remote from the uterus.

6 Presence of indicators that suggest intimate partner violence should serve to initiate further investigation and protection of the victim.

BIBLIOGRAPHY

1. ACEP Clinical Policies Committee and Clinical Policies Subcommittee on Early Pregnancy. American College of Emergency Physicians. Clinical policy: critical issues in the initial evaluation and management of patients presenting to the emergency department in early pregnancy. *Ann Emerg Med* 2003;41:122-133.

2. Adler G, Duchinski T, Jasinska A, et al. Fibrinogen fractions in the third trimester of pregnancy and in puerperium. *Thromb Res* 2000;97:405–410.

3. Berry MJ, McMurray RG, Katz VL. Pulmonary and ventilatory responses to pregnancy, immersion, and exercise. *J Appl Physiol* 1989;66(2):857-862.

4. Buchsbaum HG, Staples PP Jr. Self-inflicted gunshot wound to the pregnant uterus: report of two cases. *Obstet Gynecol* 1985;65(3):32S-35S.

5. Connolly AM, Katz VL, Bash KL, et al. Trauma and pregnancy. *Am J Perinatol* 1997;14:331-336.

6. Curet MJ, Schermer CR, Demarest GB, et al. Predictors of outcome in trauma during pregnancy: identification of patients who can be monitored for less than 6 h. *J Trauma* 2000;49:18-25.

7. Dahmus M, Sibai B. Blunt abdominal trauma: are there any predictive factors for abruption placentae or maternal-fetal distress? *Am J Obstet Gynecol* 1993;169:1054-1059.

8. Eisenstat SA, Sancroft L. Domestic violence. *N Engl J Med* 1999;341:886-892.

9. Esposito TJ. Trauma during pregnancy. *Emerg Med Clin North Am* 1994;12:167-199.

10. Esposito T, Gens D, Smith L, et al. Trauma during pregnancy. *Arch Surg* 1991;126:1073-1078.

11. Feldhaus KM, Koziol-McLain J, Amsbury HL, et al. Accuracy of 3 brief screening questions for detecting partner violence in the emergency department. *JAMA* 1997;277:1357-1361.

12. George E, Vanderkwaak T, Scholten D. Factors influencing pregnancy outcome after trauma. *Am Surg* 1992;58:594-598.

13. Goodwin T, Breen M. Pregnancy outcome and fetomaternal hemorrhage after noncatastrophic trauma. *Am J Obstet Gynecol* 1990;162:665-671.

14. Grisso JA, Schwarz DF, Hirschinger N, et al. Violent injuries among women in an urban area. *N Engl J Med* 1999;341:1899-1905.

15. Hamburger KL, Saunders DG, Hovey M. Prevalence of domestic violence in community practice and rate of physician inquiry. *Fam Med* 1992;24:283-287.

16. Hellgren M. Hemostasis during normal pregnancy and puerperium. *Semin Thromb Hemost* 2003;29(2):125-130.

17. Higgins SD, Garite TJ. Late abruptio placenta in trauma patients: implications for monitoring. *Obstet Gynecol* 1984;63:10S-12S.

18. Hoff W, D'Amelio L, Tinkoff G, et al. Maternal predictors of fetal demise in trauma during pregnancy. *Surg Gynecol Obstet* 1991;172:175-180.

19. Hyde LK, Cook LJ, Olson LM, et al. Effect of motor vehicle crashes on adverse fetal outcomes. *Obstet Gynecol* 2003;102:279-286.

20. Ikossi DG, Lazar AA, Morabito D, et al. Profile of mothers at risk: an analysis of injury and pregnancy loss in 1,195 trauma patients. *J Am Coll Surg* 2005;200:49-56.

21. Kissinger DP, Rozycki GS, Morris JA, et al. Trauma in pregnancy—predicting pregnancy outcome. *Arch Surg* 1991;125:1079-1086.

22. Klinich KD, Schneider LW, Moore JL et al. Investigations of crashes involving pregnant occupants. *Annu Proc Assoc Adv Automot Med* 2000;44:37-55.

23. Kyriacou DN, Anglin D, Taliaferro E, et al. Risk factors for injury to women from domestic violence. *N Engl J Med* 1999;341:1892-1898.

24. Lee D, Contreras M, Robson SC, et al. Recommendations for the use of anti-D immunoglobulin for Rh prophylaxis. British Blood Transfusion Society and Royal College of Obstetricians and Gynaecologists. *Transfus Med* 1999;9:93-97.

25. Mattox KL, Goetzl L. Trauma in pregnancy. *Crit Care Med* 2005;33:S385-S389.

26. Metz TD, Abbott JT. Uterine trauma in pregnancy after motor vehicle crashes with airbag deployment: a 30-case series. *J Trauma* 2006;61:658-661.

27. Minow M. Violence against women—a challenge to the Supreme Court. *N Engl J Med* 1999;341:1927-1929.

28. Mollison PL. Clinical aspects of Rh immunization. *Am J Clin Pathol* 1973;60:287.

29. Nicholson BE, ed. Family violence. *J South Carolina Med Assoc* 1995;91:409-446.

30. Pearlman MD, Tintinalli JE, Lorenz RP. Blunt trauma during pregnancy. *N Engl J Med* 1991;323:1606-1613.

31. Pearlman M, Tintinalli J, Lorenz R. A prospective controlled study of outcome after trauma during pregnancy. *Am J Obstet Gynecol* 1990;162:1502-1510.

32. Rose PG, Strohm PL, Zuspan FP. Fetomaternal hemorrhage following trauma. *Am J Obstet Gynecol* 1985;153:844-847.

33. Rothenberger D, Quattlebaum F, Perry J, et al. Blunt maternal trauma: a review of 103 cases. *J Trauma* 1978;18:173-179.

34. Schoenfeld A, Ziv E, Stein L, et al. Seat belts in pregnancy and the obstetrician. *Obstet Gynecol Surv* 1987;42:275-282.

35. Scorpio R, Esposito T, Smith G, et al. Blunt trauma during pregnancy: factors affecting fetal outcome. *J Trauma* 1992;32:213-216.

36. Sela HY, Weiniger, CF, Hersch, et al. The pregnant motor vehicle accident casualty. Adherence to basic workup and admission guidelines. *Ann Surg* 2011;254(2).

37. Shah AJ, Kilcline BA. Trauma in pregnancy. *Emerg Med Clin North Am* 2003;21:615-629.

38. Sims CJ, Boardman CH, Fuller SJ. Airbag deployment following a motor vehicle accident in pregnancy. *Obstet Gynecol* 1996;88:726.

39. Sisley A, Jacobs LM, Poole G, et al. Violence in America: a public health crisis—domestic violence. *J Trauma* 1999;46:1105-1113.

40. Statement on Domestic Violence. *Bull Am Coll Surg* 2000;85:26.

41. Timberlake GA, McSwain NE. Trauma in pregnancy, a ten-year perspective. *Am Surg* 1989;55:151-153.

42. Towery RA, English TP, Wisner DW. Evaluation of pregnant women after blunt injury. *J Trauma* 1992;35:731-736.

43. Tsuei BJ. Assessment of the pregnant trauma patient. *Injury* 2006;37:367-373.

44. Weinberg L, Steele RG, Pugh R, et al. The pregnant trauma patient. *Anaesth Int Care* 2005;33:167-180.

45. Wolf ME, Alexander BH, Rivara FP, et al. A retrospective cohort study of seatbelt use and pregnancy outcome after a motor vehicle crash. *J Trauma* 1993;34:116-119.

46. www.who.int/violence_injury_prevention/violence/world_report/factsheets/en/ipvfacts.pdf. Accessed 5/14/12.

RESOURCE

National Coalition Against Domestic Violence, PO Box 18749, Denver, CO 80218-0749; 303-839-1852; 303-831-9251 (fax).

13 Transfer to Definitive Care

If definitive care cannot be provided at a local hospital, the patient requires transfer to a hospital that has the resources and capabilities to care for him or her.

Scenario A 27-year-old male is brought to an 80-bed rural hospital following a motor vehicle collision. Although the hospital has a computed tomography (CT) scanner and ultrasound capability, it does not have neurosurgical capabilities. The patient's vital signs are: systolic blood pressure 90 mm Hg; heart rate 120; shallow breathing; and Glasgow Coma Scale (GCS) score 6.

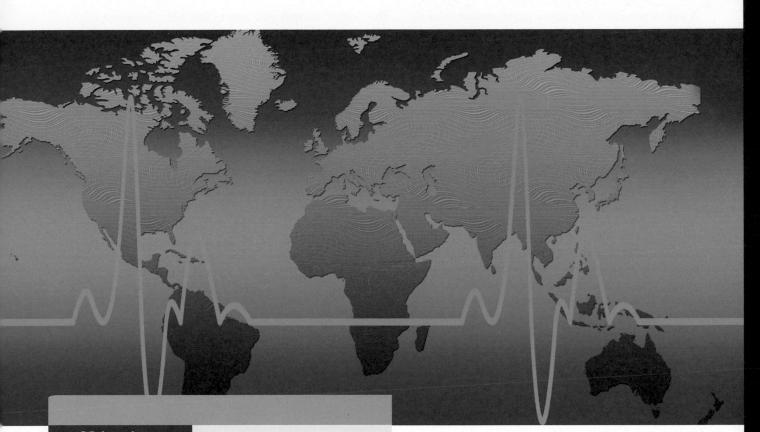

Objectives

1. Identify injured patients who require transfer from a primary care institution to a facility capable of providing the necessary level of trauma care.

2. Initiate procedures to optimally prepare trauma patients for safe transfer to a higher-level trauma care facility via the appropriate mode of transportation.

The Advanced Trauma Life Support® course is designed to train clinicians to be proficient in assessing, stabilizing, and preparing trauma patients for definitive care. Definitive care, whether support and monitoring in an intensive care unit (ICU) or operative intervention, requires the presence and active involvement of a surgeon and trauma team. If definitive care cannot be provided at a local hospital, the patient requires transfer to a hospital that has the resources and capabilities to care for him or her. Ideally, this facility should be a verified trauma center, the level of which depends on the patient's needs.

The decision to transfer a patient to another facility depends on the patient's injuries and the local resources. Decisions as to which patients should be transferred and when transfer should occur are based on medical judgment. Evidence supports the view that trauma outcome is enhanced if critically injured patients are treated in trauma centers. **Therefore, trauma patients should be transferred to the closest appropriate hospital, preferably a verified trauma center.** See American College of Surgeons (ACS) Committee on Trauma, Resources for Optimal Care of the Injured Patient; Guidelines for Trauma System Development and Trauma Center Verification Processes and Standards.

A major principle of trauma management is to do no further harm. Indeed, the level of care of trauma patients should consistently improve with each step, from the scene of the incident to the facility that can provide the patient with the necessary, proper treatment. All providers who care for trauma patients must ensure that the level of care never declines from one step to the next.

Determining the Need for Patient Transfer

The vast majority of patients receive their total care in a local hospital, and movement beyond that point is not necessary. **It is essential that clinicians assess their own capabilities and limitations, as well as those of their institution, to allow for early differentiation between patients who may be safely cared for in the local hospital and those who require transfer for definitive care.** Once the need for transfer is recognized, arrangements should be expedited and not delayed for diagnostic procedures (e.g., diagnostic peritoneal lavage [DPL] or CT scan) that do not change the immediate plan of care.

TIMELINESS OF TRANSFER

? *When should I transport the patient?*

Patient outcome is directly related to the time elapsed between injury and properly delivered definitive care. In institutions in which there is no full-time, in-house emergency department (ED) coverage, the timeliness of transfer is partly dependent on the how quickly

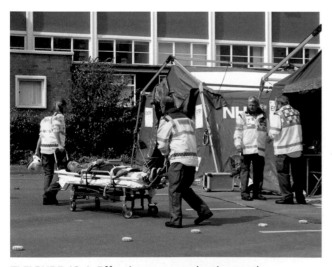

■ **FIGURE 13-1** Effective communication and coordination with the prehospital system should be developed and fine-tuned with regular exercises.

the doctor on call can reach the ED. Consequently, effective communication with the prehospital system should be developed to identify patients who require the presence of a doctor in the ED at the time of arrival (■ FIGURE 13-1). In addition, the attending doctor must be committed to respond to the ED prior to the arrival of critically injured patients. Identification of patients who require prompt attention can be based on physiologic measurements, specific identifiable injuries, and mechanism of injury.

The timing of interhospital transfer varies based on the distance of transfer, the available skill levels for transfer, circumstances of the local institution, and intervention that is necessary before the patient can be transferred safely. If the resources are available and the necessary procedures can be performed expeditiously, life-threatening injuries should be treated before patient transport. This treatment may require operative intervention to ensure that the patient is in the best possible condition for transfer. **Intervention prior to transfer is a surgical decision.**

PITFALL

Delaying transfer for diagnostic tests that will not change the need for transfer and only delay definitive care.

TRANSFER FACTORS

? *Whom do I transport?*

To assist clinicians in determining which patients may require care at a higher-level facility, the ACS Committee on Trauma recommends using certain physiologic indices, injury mechanisms and patterns, and historical information. These factors also help clinicians decide which stable patients might benefit from transfer. Criteria for interhospital transfer when a patient's needs exceed available resources are outlined in Table 13.1. It is important to note that these criteria are flexible and must take into account local circumstances.

Certain clinical measurements of physiologic status are useful in determining the need for transfer to an institution that provides a higher level of care. Patients who exhibit evidence of shock, significant physiologic deterioration, or progressive deterioration in neurologic status require the highest level of care and will likely benefit from timely transfer (■ FIGURE 13-2).

Stable patients with blunt abdominal trauma and documented liver or spleen injuries may be candidates for nonoperative management. Implicit in such prac-

■ TABLE 13.1 Interhospital Transfer Criteria	
CLINICAL CIRCUMSTANCES THAT WARRANT INTERHOSPITAL TRANSPORT WHEN THE PATIENT'S NEEDS EXCEED AVAILABLE RESOURCES:	
Category	**Specific Injuries and Other Factors**

Central Nervous System	• Head injury
	  –Penetrating injury or depressed skull fracture
	  –Open injury with or without cerebrospinal fluid (CSF) leak
	  –GCS score <15 or neurologically abnormal
	  –Lateralizing signs
	• Spinal cord injury or major vertebral injury

Chest	• Widened mediastinum or signs suggesting great vessel injury • Major chest wall injury or pulmonary contusion • Cardiac injury • Patients who may require prolonged ventilation
Pelvis/Abdomen	• Unstable pelvic-ring disruption • Pelvic-ring disruption with shock and evidence of continuing hemorrhage • Open pelvic injury • Solid organ injury
Extremities	• Severe open fractures • Traumatic amputation with potential for replantation • Complex articular fractures • Major crush injury • Ischemia
Multisystem Injuries	• Head injury with face, chest, abdominal, or pelvic injury • Injury to more than two body regions • Major burns or burns with associated injuries • Multiple, proximal long-bone fractures
Comorbid Factors	• Age >55 years • Children < 5 years of age • Cardiac or respiratory disease • Insulin-dependent diabetes • Morbid obesity • Pregnancy • Immunosuppression
Secondary Deterioration (Late Sequelae)	• Mechanical ventilation required • Sepsis • Single or multiple organ system failure (deterioration in central nervous, cardiac, pulmonary, hepatic, renal, or coagulation systems) • Major tissue necrosis

Adapted with permission, ACS Committee on Trauma. *Resources for Optimal Care of the Injured Patient.* Chicago, IL: ACS; 2006.

tice is the immediate availability of an operating room and a qualified surgical team. A general or trauma surgeon should supervise nonoperative management, regardless of the patient's age. Such patients should not be treated expectantly at facilities that are not prepared for urgent operative intervention; they should be transferred to a trauma center.

Patients with specific injuries, combinations of injuries (particularly those involving the brain), or historical findings that indicate high-energy-transfer injury may be at risk for death and are candidates for early transfer to a trauma center. High-risk criteria suggesting the necessity for early transfer are also outlined in Table 13.1.

Treatment of combative and uncooperative patients with an altered level of consciousness is difficult and fraught with hazards. These patients are often immobilized in the supine position with wrist/leg restraints. If sedation is required, the patient should be intubated. Therefore, before administering any sedation, the treating doctor must:

1. Ensure that the patient's ABCDEs are appropriately managed.

2. Relieve the patient's pain if possible (e.g., splint fractures and administer small doses of narcotics intravenously).

3. Attempt to calm and reassure the patient.

Remember, benzodiazepines, fentanyl (Sublimaze), propofol (Diprivan), and ketamine (Ketaset) are all hazardous in patients with hypovolemia, patients who

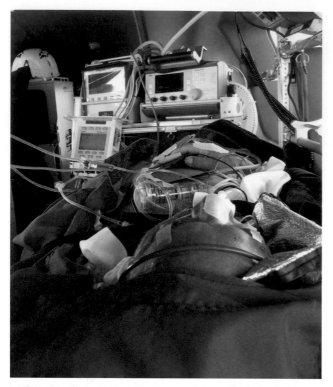

■ **FIGURE 13-2** Patients who exhibit evidence of shock, significant physiologic deterioration, or progressive deterioration in neurologic status require the highest level of care and will likely benefit from timely transfer.

are intoxicated, and patients with head injuries. **Pain management, sedation, and intubation should be accomplished by the individual most skilled in these procedures.** See Chapter 2: Airway and Ventilatory Management.

Abuse of alcohol and/or other drugs is common to all forms of trauma and is particularly important to identify, because these substances can alter pain perception and mask significant physical findings. Alterations in the patient's responsiveness can be related to alcohol and/or drugs, but the absence of cerebral injury should never be assumed in the presence of alcohol or drugs. If the examining doctor is unsure, transfer to a higher-level facility may be appropriate.

Death of another individual involved in the incident suggests the possibility of severe, occult injury in survivors. **In these cases, a thorough and careful evaluation of the patient, even in the absence of obvious signs of severe injury, is mandatory.**

PITFALL

Inadequate preparation for transport, increasing the likelihood that deterioration of the patient will occur during transfer.

Transfer Responsibilities

Specific transfer responsibilities are held by both the referring doctor and the receiving doctor.

REFERRING DOCTOR

? Where should I send the patient?

The referring doctor is responsible for initiating transfer of the patient to the receiving institution and selecting the appropriate mode of transportation and level of care required for optimal treatment of the patient en route. The referring doctor should consult with the receiving doctor and should be thoroughly familiar with the transporting agencies, their capabilities, and the arrangements for patient treatment during transport.

Stabilizing the patient's condition before transfer to another facility is the responsibility of the referring doctor, within the capabilities of his or her institution. Initiation of the transfer process should begin while resuscitative efforts are in progress.

Transfer agreements must be established to provide for the consistent and efficient movement of patients between institutions. These agreements allow for feedback to the referring hospital and enhance the efficiency and quality of the patient's treatment during transfer (■ FIGURE 13-3).

PITFALL

Inadequate or inappropriate communication between referring and accepting care providers resulting in loss of information critical to the patient's care.

RECEIVING DOCTOR

The receiving doctor must be consulted with regard to the transfer of a trauma patient. He or she must ensure that the proposed receiving institution is qualified, able, and willing to accept the patient, and is in agreement with the intent to transfer. The receiving doctor should assist the referring doctor in making arrangements for the appropriate mode and level of care during transport. If the proposed receiving doctor and facility are unable to accept the patient, they should assist in finding an alternative placement for the patient.

The quality of care rendered en route is of vital importance to the patient's outcome. Only by direct communication between the referring and receiving doctors can the details of patient transfer be clearly

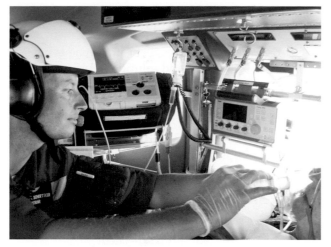

■ **FIGURE 13-3 Transfer Agreements.** Establishment of transfer agreements provide for the consistent and efficient movement of patients between institutions, and enhance the efficiency and quality of the patient's treatment during transfer.

delineated. If adequately trained emergency medical personnel are not available, a nurse or doctor should accompany the patient. All monitoring and management rendered en route should be documented.

Scenario ■ *continued* The patient is intubated, intravenous access is established, and resuscitation with crystalloid is begun. A chest x-ray confirms good position of the endotracheal tube, the patient's heart rate and blood pressure improve, and a pelvic x-ray does not demonstrate any fracture. A right thigh deformity is noted on secondary survey. A call is made to the nearest Level 1 trauma center.

Modes of Transportation

? *How should I transport the patient?*

Do no further harm is the most important principle when choosing the mode of patient transportation. Ground, water, and air transportation can be safe and effective in fulfilling this principle, and no one form is intrinsically superior to the others. Local factors such as availability, geography, cost, and weather are the main determining factors as to which to use in a given circumstance.

The interhospital transfer of a critically injured patient is potentially hazardous unless the patient's condition is optimally stabilized before transport, transfer personnel are properly trained, and provision has been made for managing unexpected crises during transport (■ **FIGURE 13-4**). To ensure safe transfers, trauma surgeons must be involved in training, continuing education, and quality improvement programs designed for transfer personnel and procedures. Surgeons also should be actively involved in the development and maintenance of systems of trauma care.

PITFALL

Failure to anticipate deterioration in the patient's neurologic condition or hemodynamic status during transport.

Transfer Protocols

Where protocols for patient transfer do not exist, the following guidelines are suggested:

INFORMATION FROM REFERRING DOCTOR

The doctor who has determined that patient transfer is necessary should speak directly to the surgeon accepting the patient at the receiving hospital. The following information must be provided:

- Patient identification
- Brief history of the incident, including pertinent prehospital data
- Initial findings in the ED
- Patient's response to the therapy administered

INFORMATION TO TRANSFERRING PERSONNEL

Information regarding the patient's condition and needs during transfer should be communicated to the transporting personnel. This information includes, but is not limited to:

- Airway maintenance
- Fluid volume replacement
- Special procedures that may be necessary
- Revised Trauma Score, resuscitation procedures, and any changes that may occur en route

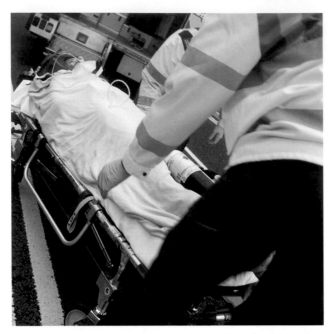

■ **FIGURE 13-4** The interhospital transfer of a critically injured patient is potentially hazardous unless the patient's condition is optimally stabilized before transport, transfer personnel are properly trained, and provision has been made for managing unexpected crises during transport.

DOCUMENTATION

A written record of the problem, treatment given, and patient status at the time of transfer, as well as certain physical items, must accompany the patient (■ **FIGURE 13-5**). A facsimile transmission may be used to avoid delay in transfer.

TREATMENT PRIOR TO TRANSFER

Patients should be resuscitated and attempts made to stabilize their conditions as completely as possible based on the following suggested outline:

1. Airway
   a. Insert an airway or endotracheal tube, if needed.
   b. Provide suction.
   c. Insert a gastric tube to reduce the risk of aspiration.

2. Breathing
   a. Determine rate and administer supplementary oxygen.
   b. Provide mechanical ventilation when needed.
   c. Insert a chest tube if needed.

3. Circulation
   a. Control external bleeding.
   b. Establish two large-caliber intravenous lines and begin crystalloid solution infusion.
   c. Restore blood volume losses with crystalloid fluids or blood and continue replacement during transfer.
   d. Insert an indwelling catheter to monitor urinary output.
   e. Monitor the patient's cardiac rhythm and rate.

4. Central nervous system
   a. Assist respiration in unconscious patients.
   b. Administer mannitol, if needed.
   c. Immobilize any head, neck, thoracic, and lumbar spine injuries.

5. Diagnostic studies (When indicated; obtaining these studies should not delay transfer.)
   a. Obtain x-rays of chest, pelvis, and extremities.
   b. Sophisticated diagnostic studies, such as CT and aortography, are usually not indicated.
   c. Order hemoglobin or hematocrit, type and crossmatch, and arterial blood gas determinations for all patients; also order pregnancy tests for females of childbearing age.
   d. Determine cardiac rhythm and hemoglobin saturation (electrocardiograph [ECG] and pulse oximetry).

6. Wounds (Performing these procedures should not delay transfer.)
   a. Clean and dress wounds after controlling external hemorrhage.
   b. Administer tetanus prophylaxis.
   c. Administer antibiotics, when indicated.

7. Fractures
   a. Apply appropriate splinting and traction.

The flurry of activity surrounding the initial evaluation, resuscitation, and preparations for transfer of trauma patients often takes precedence over other logistic details. This may result in the failure to include certain items in the information that is sent with the patient, such as x-ray films, laboratory reports, or narrative descriptions of the evaluation process and treatment rendered at the local hospital. A checklist is helpful in this regard to make sure that all important components of care have been addressed (see Figure 13-5). Checklists can be printed or stamped on an x-ray jacket or the patient's medical record to remind the referring doctor to include all pertinent information.

TRANSFER FORM

County General Hospital

Patient Information

Name _____   Next of kin _____

Address _____   Address _____

City _____ State _____ Zip _____   City _____ State _____ Zip _____

Age _____ Sex _____ Weight _____   Phone # _____ / _____ – _____

Phone # _____ / _____ – _____   Relationship to patient _____

Date and Time

Date _____ / _____ / _____

Time of injury _____ AM/PM

Time admitted to ED _____ AM/PM

Time admitted to OR _____ AM/PM

Time transferred _____ AM/PM

AMPLE History

_____

_____

_____

_____

_____

Condition on Admission

HR _____ Rhythm _____

BP _____ / _____ RR _____ Temp _____

Probable diagnoses _____

_____

_____

_____

_____

Management During Transport

_____

Information in transfer materials

_____ MIST _____ AMPLE

Checklist

Airway: ___ Endotracheal tube ___ C-spine protection

Breathing: ___ Oxygen ___ SAO_2 ___ $EtCO_2$ ___ Chest tubes

Diagnostic: ___ X-Rays (chest, pelvis)   ___ Laboratory

Equipment: ___ ECG ___ BP ___ SAO_2 ___ IV ___ T°
        ___ Indwelling catheter ___ Splints ___ Gastric tube

Circulation: ___ Volume ___ Blood
        ___ Drugs

Family notification: ___

Referral Information:

Doctor _____

Hospital _____

Phone # _____ / _____ – _____

Receiving Information:

Doctor _____

Hospital _____

Phone # _____ / _____ – _____

■ **FIGURE 13-5 Sample Transfer Form.** This form includes all of the information that should be sent with the patient to the receiving doctor and facility.

TREATMENT DURING TRANSPORT

The appropriate personnel should transfer the patient, based on the patient's condition and potential problems. Treatment during transport typically includes:

- Monitoring vital signs and pulse oximetry
- Continued support of cardiorespiratory system
- Continued blood-volume replacement
- Use of appropriate medications as ordered by a doctor or as allowed by written protocol
- Maintenance of communication with a doctor or institution during transfer
- Maintenance of accurate records during transfer

While preparing for transport and while it is underway, remember that, if air transport is used, changes in altitude lead to changes in air pressure, which may result in increases in the size of pneumothoraces and gastric distention. Hence, placement of a chest tube or gastric tube should be carefully considered. Similar cautions pertain to any air-filled device. For example, during prolonged flights, it may be necessary to decrease the pressure in air splints or endotracheal tube balloons.

PITFALL

Endotracheal tubes may become dislodged or malpositioned during transport. The necessary equipment for reintubation must accompany the patient, and the transfer personnel must be capable of performing the procedure.

Transfer Data

The information accompanying the patient should include both demographic and historical information pertinent to the patient's injury. Uniform transmission of information is enhanced by the use of an established transfer form, such as the example shown in Figure 13-5. In addition to the information already outlined, space should be provided for recording data in an organized, sequential fashion—vital signs, central nervous system (CNS) function, and urinary output—during the initial resuscitation and transport period. See Sample Trauma Flow Sheet.

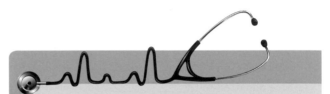

Scenario ■ *continued* The patient is reevaluated on arrival at the Level 1 trauma center; his airway is secured, and he has bilateral breath sounds. His heart rate is 110 and blood pressure 100/60; his GCS is 3T. A CT scan shows a subdural hematoma and a moderate splenic injury. Plain radiographs confirm a right femur fracture.

Chapter Summary

1 Patients whose injuries exceed an institution's capabilities for definitive care should be identified early during assessment and resuscitation. Individual capabilities of the treating doctor, institutional capabilities, and indications for transfer should be known. Transfer agreements and protocols should be in place to support definitive care.

2 Optimal preparation for transfer includes attention to ATLS® principles and clear documentation. The referring doctor and receiving doctor should communicate directly. Transfer personnel should be adequately skilled to administer the required patient care en route.

BIBLIOGRAPHY

1. American College of Surgeons Committee on Trauma. *Resources for Optimal Care of the Injured Patient.* Chicago, IL: ACS; 2006.

2. Bledsoe BE, Wesley AK, Eckstein M, et al. Helicopter scene transport of trauma patients with nonlife-threatening injuries: a meta-analysis. *J Trauma* 2006;60:1257-1266.

3. Champion HR, Sacco WJ, Copes WS, et al. A revision of the trauma score. *J Trauma* 1989;29:623-629.

4. Mullins PJ, Veum-Stone J, Helfand M, et al. Outcome of hospitalized injured patients after institution of a trauma system in an urban area. *JAMA* 1994;271:1919-1924.

5. Scarpio RJ, Wesson DE. Splenic trauma. In: Eichelberger MR, ed. Pediatric Trauma: Prevention, Acute Care, Rehabilitation. St. Louis, MO: Mosby Yearbook; 1993:456-463.

6. Schoettker P, D'Amours S, Nocera N, et al. Reduction of time to definitive care in trauma patients: effectiveness of a new checklist system. *Injury* 2003;34:187-190.

7. Sharar SR, Luna GK, Rice CL, et al. Air transport following surgical stabilization: an extension of regionalized trauma care. *J Trauma* 1988;28:794-798.

Appendices

Ocular Trauma *(Optional Lecture)*

Objectives

1. Obtain patient and event histories.

2. Perform a systematic examination of the orbit and its contents.

3. Identify eyelid injuries that can be treated by the primary care doctor and those that must be referred to an ophthalmologist for treatment.

4. Explain how to examine the eye for a foreign body and how to remove superficial foreign bodies to prevent further injury.

5. Identify corneal abrasion and describe its proper management.

6. Identify hyphema and describe its initial management and the necessity for referral to an ophthalmologist.

7. Identify eye injuries that require referral to an ophthalmologist.

8. Identify ruptured-globe injury and describe its initial management prior to referral to an ophthalmologist.

9. Evaluate and treat eye injuries that result from chemicals.

10. Evaluate a patient with an orbital fracture and describe its initial management and the necessity for referral.

11. Identify retrobulbar hematoma and explain the necessity for immediate referral.

Introduction

The initial assessment of a patient with an ocular injury requires a systematic approach. The physical examination should proceed in an organized, step-by-step manner. It does not require extensive, complicated instrumentation in the multiple-trauma setting. Rather, simple therapeutic measures often can save the patient's vision and prevent serious sequelae before an ophthalmologist is available. This appendix provides pertinent information regarding the early identification and treatment of ocular injuries that will enhance the clinicians' basic knowledge and may save their patients' vision.

Assessment

Key factors in the assessment of patients with ocular trauma include patient history, history of the injury incident, initial symptoms, and results of physical examination.

Patient History

Obtain a history of any preexisting ocular disease. Key questions include:

1. Does the patient wear corrective lenses?

2. Is there a history of glaucoma or previous eye surgery?

3. What medications does the patient use (e.g., pilocarpine)?

History of Injury Incident

Obtain a detailed description of the circumstances surrounding the injury. This information often raises the index of suspicion for certain potential injuries and their sequelae, such as the higher risk of infection from certain foreign bodies (e.g., wood vs. metallic). Key questions include:

1. Was there blunt trauma?

2. Was there penetrating injury? (In motor vehicular crashes there is potential for glass and metallic foreign bodies.)

3. Was there a missile injury?

4. Was there a possible thermal, chemical, or flash burn?

Initial Symptoms

Key questions regarding the patient's initial symptoms include:

1. What were the initial symptoms?

2. Did the patient report pain or photophobia?

3. Was there an immediate decrease in vision that has remained stable, or is it progressive?

Physical Examination

The physical examination must be systematic so that function and anatomic structures are evaluated. As with injuries to other organ systems, the pathology also may evolve with time, and the patient must be reevaluated periodically. A directed approach to the ocular examination, beginning with the most external structures in an "outside-to-inside" manner, ensures that injuries are not missed.

Visual Acuity   Visual acuity is evaluated first by any means possible and recorded (e.g., patient counting fingers at 3 feet [0.9 m]).

Eyelid   The most external structures to be examined are the eyelids. The eyelids should be assessed for: (1) edema; (2) ecchymosis; (3) evidence of burns or chemical injury; (4) laceration(s)—medial, lateral, lid margin, canaliculi; (5) ptosis; (6) foreign bodies that contact the globe; and (7) avulsion of the canthal tendon.

Orbital Rim   Gently palpate the orbital rim for any step-off deformity or crepitus. Subcutaneous emphysema can result from a fracture of the medial orbit into the ethmoids or a fracture of the orbital floor into the maxillary antrum.

Globe   The eyelids should be retracted to examine the globe without applying pressure to the globe. Specially designed retractors are available for this purpose. Cotton-tipped applicators can also be used; they should be placed gently against the superior and inferior orbital rims, enabling the eyelids to be rolled open. Then assess the globe anteriorly for any displacement from a retrobulbar hematoma and for any posterior or inferior displacement due to an orbit fracture. Also assess the globes for normal ocular movement, diplopia, and evidence of entrapment.

Pupil   Assess the pupils for roundness, regular shape, equality, and reaction to light stimulus. It is important to test for an afferent pupil defect. Optic nerve trauma usually results in the failure of both pupils to constrict when light is directed at the affected eye.

Cornea   Assess the cornea for opacity, ulceration, and foreign bodies. Fluorescein and a blue light can facilitate this assessment.

Conjunctiva   Assess the conjunctivae for chemosis, subconjunctival emphysema (indicating probable fracture of the orbit into the ethmoid or maxillary sinus), subconjunctival hemorrhage, and foreign bodies.

Anterior Chamber   Examine the anterior chamber for hyphema (blood in the anterior chamber). The depth of the anterior chamber can be assessed by shining a light into the eye from the lateral aspect of the eye. If the light does not illuminate the entire surface of the iris, a shallow anterior chamber should be suspected. This condition can result from an anterior penetrating wound. A deep anterior chamber can result from a posterior penetrating wound of the globe.

Iris   The iris should be reactive and regular in shape. Assess the iris for iridodialysis (a tear of the iris) and iridodonesis (a floppy or tremulous iris).

Lens   The lens should be transparent. Assess the lens for possible anterior displacement into the anterior chamber, partial dislocation with displacement into the posterior chamber, and dislocation into the vitreous.

Vitreous   The vitreous should be transparent, allowing for easy visualization of the fundus. Visualization may be difficult if vitreous hemorrhage has occurred. In this situation, a black rather than red reflex is seen on ophthalmoscopy. Vitreous bleeding usually indicates a significant underlying ocular injury. The vitreous also should be assessed for an intraocular foreign body.

Retina   The retina is examined for hemorrhage, possible tears, and detachment. A detached retina is opalescent, and the blood columns are darker.

Specific Injuries

Common traumatic ocular injuries include eyelid injury, corneal injury, anterior chamber injury, injury to the iris, injury to the lens, vitreous injuries, injury to the retina, globe injury, chemical injury, fractures, retrobulbar hematoma, and fat emboli.

Eyelid Injury

Eyelid injuries often result in marked ecchymosis, making examination of injuries to the globe and lid difficult. However, a more serious injury to the underlying structures must be excluded. Look beneath the lid as well to exclude damage to the globe. Lid retractors or cotton-tipped applicators can be used if necessary to forcibly open the eye to inspect the globe. Ptosis may result from edema, damage to the levator palpebrae, or oculomotor nerve injury.

Lacerations of the upper and lower lids that are horizontal, superficial, and do not involve the levator in the upper lid may be closed by the examining clinician using interrupted 6-0 skin sutures. The clinician also should examine the eye beneath the lid to rule out damage to the globe.

Lid injuries that require treatment by an ophthalmologist include:

- Wounds involving the medial canthus that may have damaged the medial canaliculus

- Injuries to the lacrimal sac and nasal lacrimal duct, which can lead to obstruction if not properly repaired

- Deep horizontal lacerations of the upper lid that may involve the levator and result in ptosis if not repaired correctly

- Lacerations of the lid margin that are difficult to close and can lead to notching, entropion, or ectropion

These wounds may be covered with a saline dressing pending emergency ophthalmologic consultation.

Foreign bodies of the lid result in profuse tearing, pain, and a foreign-body sensation that increases with lid movement. The conjunctiva should be inspected, and the upper and lower lids should be everted to examine the inner surface. Topical anesthetic drops may be used, but only for initial examination and removal of the foreign body.

Penetrating foreign bodies should not be disturbed and are removed only in the operating room by an ophthalmologist or appropriate specialist. If the patient requires transport to another facility for treatment of this injury or others, consult an ophthalmologist regarding management of the eye during transport.

Corneal Injury

Corneal abrasions result in pain, foreign-body sensation, photophobia, decreased visual acuity, and chemosis. The injured epithelium stains with fluorescein.

Corneal foreign bodies sometimes can be removed with irrigation. However, if the foreign body is embedded, the patient should be referred to an ophthalmologist. Corneal abrasions are treated with antibiotic drops or ointment to prevent ulcers. Clinical studies have demonstrated no advantage to patching in terms of patient comfort or time required for the abrasion to heal. The patient should be instructed to instill the drops or ointment and should be followed up within 24 to 48 hours.

Anterior Chamber Injury

Hyphema is blood in the anterior chamber, which may be difficult to see if there is only a small amount. In extreme cases, the entire anterior chamber is filled. The hyphema can often be seen with a penlight. Hyphema usually indicates severe intraocular trauma.

Glaucoma develops in 7% of patients with hyphema. Corneal staining also may occur. Remember, hyphema can be the result of serious underlying ocular injury. Even in the case of a small bleed, spontaneous rebleeding often occurs within the first 5 days, which may lead to total hyphema. Therefore, the patient must be referred to an ophthalmologist. The affected eye will be patched, and the patient usually is hospitalized, and reevaluated frequently. Pain after hyphema usually indicates rebleeding and/or acute glaucoma.

Injury to the Iris

Contusion injuries of the iris can cause traumatic mydriasis or miosis. There may be disruption of the iris from the ciliary body, causing an irregular pupil and hyphema.

Injury to the Lens

Contusion of the lens can lead to later opacification or cataract formation. Blunt trauma can cause a break of the zonular fibers that encircle the lens and anchor it to the ciliary body. This results in subluxation of the lens, possibly into the anterior chamber, causing shallowing of the chamber. In cases of posterior subluxation, the anterior chamber deepens. Patients with these injuries should be referred to an ophthalmologist.

Vitreous Injury

Blunt trauma may also lead to vitreous hemorrhage. This usually is secondary to retinal vessel damage and bleeding into the vitreous, resulting in sudden, profound loss of vision. Funduscopic examination may be impossible, and the red reflex, seen with an ophthalmoscope light, is lost. A patient with this injury should be placed on bed rest with the eye shielded and referred to an ophthalmologist.

Injury to the Retina

Blunt trauma also can cause retinal hemorrhage. The patient may or may not have decreased visual acuity, depending on involvement of the macula. Superficial retinal hemorrhages appear cherry red in color, whereas deeper lesions appear gray.

Retinal edema and detachment can occur with head trauma. In such cases, a white, cloudy discoloration is observed. Retinal detachments appear "curtain-like." If the macula is involved, visual acuity is affected. An acute retinal tear usually occurs in conjunction with blunt trauma to an eye with preexisting vitreoretinal pathology. Retinal detachment most often occurs as a late sequela of blunt trauma, with the patient describing light flashes and a curtain-like defect in peripheral vision.

A rupture of the choroid initially appears as a beige area at the posterior pole. Later it becomes a yellow-white scar. If it transects the macula, vision is seriously and permanently impaired.

Globe Injury

A patient with a ruptured globe has marked visual impairment. The eye is soft because of decreased intraocular pressure, and the anterior chamber may be flattened or shallow. If the rupture is anterior, ocular contents may be seen extruding from the eye.

The goal of initial management of the ruptured globe is to protect the eye from any additional damage. As soon as a ruptured globe is suspected, the eye should not be manipulated any further. A sterile dressing and eye shield should be applied carefully to prevent any pressure to the eye that may cause further extrusion of the ocular contents. The patient should be instructed not to squeeze the injured eye shut. If not contraindicated by other injuries, the patient may be sedated while awaiting transport or treatment. Do not remove foreign objects, tissue, or clots before placing the dressing. Do not use topical analgesics—only oral or parenteral, if not contraindicated by any other injuries.

An *intraocular foreign body* should be suspected if the patient reports sudden, sharp pain with a decrease in visual acuity, particularly if the eye might have been struck by a small fragment of metal, glass, or wood. Inspect the surface of the globe carefully for any small lacerations and possible sites of entry. These may be difficult to find. In the anterior chamber, tiny foreign bodies may be hidden by blood or in the crypt of the iris. A tiny iris perforation may be impossible to see directly, but with a pen light the red reflex may be detected through the defect (if the lens and vitreous are not opaque).

Chemical Injury

Chemical injuries require immediate intervention in order to preserve sight. Acid precipitates proteins in the tissue and sets up somewhat of a natural barrier against extensive tissue penetration. However, alkali combines with lipids in the cell membrane, leading to disruption of the cell membranes, rapid penetration of the caustic agent, and extensive tissue destruction. Chemical injury to the cornea causes disruption of stromal mucopolysaccharides, leading to opacification.

The treatment for chemical injuries to the eyes involves copious and continuous irrigation. Attempts should not be made to neutralize the agent. Intravenous solutions (e.g., crystalloid solution) and tubing can be used to improvise continuous irrigation. Blepharospasm is extensive, and the lids must be manually opened during irrigation. Analgesics and sedation should be used, if not contraindicated by coexisting injuries. Thermal injuries usually occur to the lids only and rarely involve the cornea. However, burns of the globe occasionally occur. A sterile dressing should be applied and the patient referred to an ophthalmologist. Exposure of the cornea must be prevented or it may perforate, and the eye may be lost.

Fractures

Blunt trauma to the orbit may cause rapid compression of the tissues and increased pressure within the orbit. One of the weakest points is the orbital floor, which may fracture, allowing orbital contents to herniate into the antrum—leading to the use of the term "blowout."

Clinically, the patient presents with pain, swelling, and ecchymosis of the lids and periorbital tissues. There may be subconjunctival hemorrhage. Facial asymmetry and possible enophthalmos can be evident or masked by surrounding edema. Limitation of ocular motion and diplopia secondary to edema or entrapment of the orbital contents may be noted. Palpation of the rims may reveal a fracture step-off deformity.

Subcutaneous and/or subconjunctival emphysema may occur when the fracture is into the ethmoid or maxillary sinuses. Hypesthesia of the cheek occurs secondary to injury of the infraorbital nerve. Examine the orbital floor and look for soft-tissue density in the maxillary sinus or an air fluid level (blood). Computed tomographic scans are almost essential for adequate evaluation.

Treatment of fractures may be delayed up to 2 weeks. Watchful waiting may help to avoid unnecessary surgery by allowing the edema to decrease. Indications for orbital blowout repair include persistent diplopia in a functional field of gaze, enophthalmos greater than 2 mm, and fracture involving more than 50% of the orbital floor.

Retrobulbar Hematoma

A retrobulbar hematoma requires immediate treatment by an ophthalmologist. The resulting increased pressure within the orbit compromises the blood supply to the retina and optic nerve, resulting in blindness if not treated. If possible, the head should be elevated, with no direct pressure placed on the eye.

Summary

Thorough, systematic evaluation of the injured eye results in few significant injuries being missed. Once injuries have been identified, treat the eye injury using simple, systematic measures; prevent further damage; and help preserve sight until the patient is in an ophthalmologist's care.

Bibliography

1. Arbour JD, Brunette I, Boisjoly HM, et al. Should we patch corneal erosions? *Arch Ophthalmol* 1997;115:313-317.

2. Campanile TM, St Clair DA, Benaim M. The evaluation of eye patching in the treatment of traumatic corneal epithelial defects. *J Emerg Med* 1997;15:769-774.

3. Flynn CA, D'Amico F, Smith G. Should we patch corneal abrasions? A meta-analysis. *J Fam Pract* 1998;47:264-270.

4. Hart A, White S, Conboy P, et al. The management of corneal abrasions in accident and emergency. *Injury* 1997;28:527-529.

5. Patterson J, Fetzer D, Krall J, et al. Eye patch treatment for the pain of corneal abrasion. *South Med J* 1996;89:227-229.

6. Poon A, McCluskey PJ, Hill DA. Eye injuries in patients with major trauma. *J Trauma* 1999;46:494-499.

7. Sastry SM, Paul BK, Bain L, Champion HR: Ocular trauma among major trauma victims in a regional trauma center. *J Trauma* 1993;34:223-226.

8. Tasman WS. Posterior vitreous detachment and peripheral retinal breaks. *Trans Am Acad Ophthalmol Otolaryngol* 1968;72:217.

Hypothermia and Heat Injuries

Objectives

1 Identify the problems encountered with injuries due to exposure.

2 Describe the differences between accidental hypothermia and therapeutic hypothermia.

3 Explain the danger of hypothermia in the injured patient.

4 Define the two levels of heat injury: heat exhaustion and heat stroke.

Introduction

Patients may be exposed to the environment and sustain additional injuries or complications due to this exposure, without sustaining burns or frostbite. The environmental exposure may be the only injury, but the exposure can complicate traumatic injuries. This appendix describes the two extremes of environmental exposure and the potential resulting injuries.

Cold Injury: Systemic Hypothermia

Hypothermia is defined as a core body temperature below 35°C (95°F). In the absence of concomitant traumatic injury, hypothermia may be classified as *mild* (35°C to 32°C, or 95°F to 89.6°F), *moderate* (32°C to 30°C, or 89.6°F to 86°F), or s*evere* (below 30°C, or 86°F). This drop in core temperature can be rapid, as in immersion in near-freezing water, or slow, as in exposure to more temperate environments.

Older adults are particularly susceptible to hypothermia because of their impaired ability to increase heat production and decrease heat loss by vasoconstriction. Children also are more susceptible because of their relative increased body-surface area (BSA) and limited energy sources.

The risk of hypothermia is of special concern in trauma patients, as they are exposed for examinations, given room temperature fluid boluses, and may be given medication that affects their ability to maintain core body temperature (e.g., paralytics).

Hypothermia is common in the severely injured, but further loss of core temperature can be limited with the administration of only warmed intravenous fluids and blood, judicious exposure of the patient, and maintenance of a warm environment. Because determination of the core temperature, preferably esophageal, is essential for the diagnosis of systemic hypothermia, special thermometers capable of registering low temperatures are required in those suspected of hypothermia.

Signs

In addition to a decrease in core temperature, a depressed level of consciousness is the most common feature of hypothermia. Patients with hypothermia are cold to the touch and can appear gray and cyanotic. Vital signs, including heart rate, respiratory rate,

317

and blood pressure, are all variable, and the absence of respiratory or cardiac activity is not uncommon in patients who eventually recover. **Because of severe depression of the respiratory rate and heart rate, signs of respiratory and cardiac activity are easily missed unless careful assessment is conducted.**

Management

Immediate attention is devoted to the ABCDEs, including the initiation of cardiopulmonary resuscitation (CPR) and establishment of intravenous access if the patient is in cardiopulmonary arrest. Care must be taken to identify the presence of an organized cardiac rhythm; if one exists, sufficient circulation in patients with markedly reduced metabolism is likely present, and vigorous chest compressions can convert this rhythm to fibrillation. In the absence of an organized rhythm, CPR should be instituted and continued until the patient is rewarmed or there are other indications to discontinue CPR. However, the exact role of CPR as an adjunct to rewarming remains controversial.

Prevent heat loss by removing the patient from the cold environment and replacing wet, cold clothing with warm blankets. Administer oxygen via a bag-reservoir device. The patient should be treated in a critical care setting whenever possible, and cardiac monitoring is required. A careful search for associated disorders (e.g., diabetes, sepsis, and drug or alcohol ingestion) or occult injuries should be conducted, and the disorders should be treated promptly. Blood should be drawn for complete blood count (CBC), electrolytes, blood glucose, alcohol, toxins, creatinine, amylase, and blood cultures. Abnormalities should be treated accordingly; for example, hypoglycemia requires intravenous glucose administration.

Determination of death can be very difficult in patients with hypothermia. Patients who appear to have suffered a cardiac arrest or death as a result of hypothermia should not be pronounced dead until full efforts have been made to rewarm them. **Remember the axiom: "You are not dead until you are warm and dead."** An exception to this rule is a patient with hypothermia who has sustained an anoxic event while still normothermic and who has no pulse or respiration, or one who has a serum potassium level greater than 10 mmol/L.

The appropriate rewarming technique depends on the patient's temperature and his or her response to simpler measures, as well as the presence or absence of concomitant injuries. For example, treat mild and moderate exposure hypothermia with passive external rewarming in a warm room using warm blankets, ambient overhead heaters, warmed forced-air blankets, and warmed intravenous fluids. Severe hypothermia may require active core rewarming methods, starting with bladder irrigation with a three-way foley, adding warmed humidification to ventilation, and proceeding to invasive surgical rewarming techniques such as peritoneal lavage, thoracic/pleural lavage, arteriovenous rewarming, and cardiopulmonary bypass, all of which are best accomplished in a critical care setting. Cardiopulmonary bypass is the most effective method of rewarming patients with severe hypothermia.

Physiologic Effects of Hypothermia

Cardiac output falls in proportion to the degree of hypothermia, and cardiac irritability begins at approximately 33°C (91.4°F). Ventricular fibrillation becomes increasingly common as the temperature falls below 28°C (82.4°F), and at temperatures below 25°C (77°F) asystole can occur. Cardiac drugs and defibrillation are not usually effective in the presence of acidosis, hypoxia, and hypothermia. In general, these treatment methods should be postponed until the patient is warmed to at least 28°C (82.4°F). Given the high potential for cardiac irritablity, it is inadvisable to insert a subclavian or internal jugular line in hypothermic patients due to the risk of triggering an uncontrollable cardiac arrythmia. Bretylium tosylate is the only dysrhythmia agent known to be effective; however, it is no longer manufactured. Lidocaine is ineffective in patients with hypothermia who have ventricular fibrillation. Dopamine is the single inotropic agent that has some degree of action in patients with hypothermia. Administer 100% oxygen while the patient is being rewarmed. Arterial blood gases are probably best interpreted "uncorrected," that is, the blood warmed to 37°C (98.6°F), with the values used as guides to administering sodium bicarbonate and adjusting ventilation parameters during rewarming and resuscitation. Attempts to actively rewarm the patient should not delay transfer to a critical care setting.

Heat Injuries

Heat exhaustion (HE) and heat stroke (HS), the most serious forms of heat injury, are common and preventable conditions. Excessive core temperature initiates a cascade of inflammatory pathologic events that leads to mild heat exhaustion and, if untreated, eventually to multi-organ failure and death. The severity of HS correlates with the duration of hyperthermia. Rapid reduction of body temperature is associated with improved survival. Other causes of hyperthermia need to be ruled out, especially in patients on psychotropic drugs or with a history of recent exposure to anesthetics.

Types of Heat Injuries

Heat exhaustion is a common disorder caused by excessive loss of body water, electrolyte depletion, or both.

It represents an ill-defined spectrum of symptoms, including headache, nausea, vomiting, light-headedness, malaise, and myalgia. It is distinguished from HS by having mental function that is essentially intact and a core temperature usually less than 39°C (102.2°F).

Heat stroke (HS) is a life-threatening disease, generally defined as hyperthermia ≥ 40°C (104°F) with associated dehydration, hot flushed dry skin, and central nervous system dysfunction, resulting in delirium, convulsions, and coma. HS is associated with a systemic inflammatory response, which may lead to multiple organ dysfunction and disseminated intravascular coagulation (DIC).

There are two forms of HS. Classic, or non-exertional HS, frequently occurs during environmental heat waves and primarily affects elderly and/or ill patients. Exertional HS usually occurs in healthy, young, and physically active people who are engaged in strenuous exercise in hot and humid environments. HS occurs when the core body temperature rises and the thermoregulatory system fails to respond adequately. Children left in poorly ventilated automobiles parked in the sun can also develop HS.

The mortality of HS varies and ranges from 33% to as high as 80% in patients with classic HS. Those individuals who do survive may sustain permanent neurological damage. Patients with HS present with tachycardia and tachypnea. They may be hypotensive or normotensive with wide pulse pressure. Core body temperature is ≥ 40°C (104°F). Skin is usually warm and dry or clammy and diaphoretic. Liver and muscle enzymes level will be elevated in virtually all cases.

Pathophysiology

The human body is able to maintain a core body temperature at about 37°C (98.6°F), despite being exposed to a wide range of environmental conditions, through multiple physiological responses that serve to balance heat production and dissipation. Heat is both generated by metabolic processes and gained from the environment.

The first response to an elevated core temperature is peripheral vasodilation, increasing loss through radiation. However, if the ambient air temperature is greater than that of body temperature, hyperthermia will be exacerbated. To dissipate heat when the ambient temperature exceeds 37°C (98.6°F), sweating is required. Ambient temperature and relative humidity can affect the efficiency of heat dissipation. The average person can produce 1.5 L of sweat per hour, increasing to 2.5 L in well-trained athletes. Cutaneous vasodilatation may increase peripheral blood flow from 5% to up to 20% of total cardiac output.

The efferent information sent to the temperature-sensitive neurons in the pre-optic anterior hypothalamus results in a thermoregulatory response. This response includes not only autonomic changes, such as an increase in skin blood flow and sweating, but also behavioral changes, such as removing clothing or moving to a cooler area. Proper thermoregulation depends on adequate hydration. The normal cardiovascular adaptation to severe heat stress is an increase in cardiac output up to 20 L/min. This response can be impaired by salt and water depletion, cardiovascular disease, or medication that interferes with cardiac function, resulting in increased susceptibility to HS. When the normal physiological response fails to dissipate heat, the core body temperature increases steadily until it reaches 41 to 42°C (105.8°F to 107.6°F), or critical maximum temperature.

At the cellular level, exposure to excessive heat can lead to denaturation of proteins, phospholipids, and lipoprotein, and liquefaction of membrane lipids. This results in cardiovascular collapse, multi-organ failure, and ultimately death. A coordinated inflammatory reaction to heat stress involves endothelial cells, leukocytes, and epithelial cells in an attempt to protect against tissue injury and promote healing. A variety of cytokines are produced in response to endogenous or environmental heat. Cytokines mediate fever and leukocytosis, and increase synthesis of acute phase proteins. Endothelial cell injury and diffuse microvascular thrombosis are prominent features of HS, leading to DIC. Fibrinolysis is also highly activated. Normalization of the core body temperature inhibits fibrinolysis, but not the activation of coagulation. This pattern resembles that seen in sepsis.

HS and its progression to multi-organ dysfunction are due to a complex interplay among the acute physiological alterations associated with hyperthermia (e.g., circulatory failure, hypoxia, and increased metabolic demand), the direct cytotoxicity of heat, and the inflammatory and coagulation responses of the host.

Management

Special attention to airway protection, adequate ventilation, and fluid resuscitation are essential to treating heat injuries, as pulmonary aspiration and hypoxia are important causes of death. Initially, 100% oxygen should be administered; after cooling, further oxygen delivery should be guided by arterial blood gas results.

Patients with an altered level of consciousness, significant hypercapnia, or persistent hypoxia should be intubated and mechanically ventilated. Arterial blood gas, electrolytes, creatinine, and blood urea nitrogen levels should be obtained as early as possible. Renal failure and rhabdomyolysis are frequently seen in HS patients. A chest x-ray should be performed. Hypoglycemia, hyperkalemia, and acidosis should be treated by standard methods. Hypokalemia may become apparent and necessitate potassium replacement, particularly as acidemia is corrected. Seizures may be treated with benzodiazepines.

Prompt correction of hyperthermia by immediate cooling and support of organ-system function are the two main therapeutic objectives in patients with HS.

Cooling measures are started as soon as practical and continue en route. Water spray and airflow over the patient is ideal in the prehospital setting, with application of ice packs to areas of high blood flow (groin, neck, axilla) as an alternative. Rapid reduction of body temperature is associated with improved survival. Although there is general agreement on the need for rapid and effective cooling of hyperthermic patients with HS, there is controversy over the best method of achieving it. The cooling method based on conduction, namely immersion in iced water started within minutes of the onset of exertional HS, is fast, safe and effective in young, healthy and well-trained military personnel or athletes.

In mass casualty events with classic HS, the body-cooling unit (BCU) can achieve excellent cooling rates with improved survival. The BCU involves spraying patients with water at 15°C (59°F), and circulating warm air that reaches the skin at 30 to 35°C (86°F to 95°F). This technique is well tolerated and allows for optimal monitoring and resuscitation of unconscious and hemodynamically unstable patients. Non-invasive and well-tolerated cooling modalities, such as ice packs, wet gauze sheets, and fan alone or in combination, could represent reasonable alternatives, since they are easily applied and readily accessible. Survival and outcomes in HS are directly related to the time required to initiate therapy and cool patients to ≤ 39°C (102.2°F).

Summary

The injuries due to heat and cold exposure are not only burns or frostbite, but can result in systemic alterations in temperature regulation and homeostasis. It is important to understand the etiology and treatment of exposure injuries.

Bibliography

Cold Injuries

1. Castellani JW, Young AJ, Ducharme MB, et al. American College of Sports Medicine position stand: prevention of cold injuries during exercise. [Review]. *Med Sci Sports Exer* 2006;38(11):2012-2029.

2. Hildebrand F, Giannoudis PV, van Griensven M, et al. Pathophysiologic changes and effects of hypothermia on outcome in elective surgery and trauma patients. *Am J Surg* 2004;187(3):363-371.

3. Konstantinidis A, Inaba K, Dubose J, et al. The impact of nontherapeutic hypothermia on outcomes after severe traumatic brain injury. *J Trauma* 2011;71(6):1627-1631.

4. Larach MG. Accidental hypothermia. *Lancet* 1995; 345(8948):493-498.

5. Mallett ML. Accidental hypothermia. *QJM* 2002;95(12): 775-785.

Heat Injuries

1. Glazer JL. Management of heatstroke and heat exhaustion. *Am Fam Physician* 2005;71(11):2133-2140.

2. Yeo TP. Heat stroke: a comprehensive review. *AACN Clin Issues* 2004;15(2):280-293.

Austere and Armed Conflict Environments *(Optional Lecture)*

Introduction

Disasters occur globally from natural, technological, and human conflict causes. No community is immune: Even the most sophisticated hospitals can become austere facilities after a disaster, with limited resources available to provide care to overwhelming casualties. The disaster scene can be dangerous, with risks that include structural collapse, exposed utilities, and flooding. Effective disaster management is not business as usual; it requires a different mindset that recognizes the need for casualty population management and explicit healthcare worker safety. "Adapt and overcome" is the model slogan for readiness.

ATLS had its origins in a Nebraska field following a plane crash in which the injured received inadequate care in an austere environment. Although commonly seen through the lens of plentiful resources, ATLS provides a framework for mass casualty care in austere and conflict-ridden environments with limited resources. Further depth can be found in the ACS Disaster Management and Emergency Preparedness (DMEP) course.

Mass Casualty Care

A mass casualty event exists when casualties exceed the resources to provide complete individual care, typically in a situation of incomplete information and uncertainty regarding event evolution. In disaster, the care paradigm shifts from the greatest good for the individual to the greatest good for the greatest number of casualties. This is different from everyday trauma care, in which all resources are mobilized for the good of an individual injured patient. In the context of disaster, decisions made for one casualty can have an effect on decisions for other casualties, because of resource limitations and the situation.

Casualty disposition in the aftermath of disaster relates to the intersection of casualty, resource, and situation considerations. *Casualty* characteristics include immediately life-threatening injuries, simplicity of interventions to manage threats to life, injury severity, and survivability. Inability to survive is both absolute (e.g., 100% third-degree body surface area burns) and relative (e.g., extensive injuries consume resources for one casualty that could be used to save more than one casualty).

Resource considerations include what is available (e.g., space, staff, supplies, systems) for care and evacuation (transportation, roads), as well as the timeline for resupply and casualty evacuation.

The *situation* involves event progression, secondary events (i.e., additional events in sequence with the inciting event, to include secondary bombs, structural collapse after an explosion, and flooding after levees break), and environmental conditions (i.e., time of day, weather, and geography).

Tools for Effective Mass Casualty Care

Incident command and triage are essential tools for effective mass casualty care. *Incident command* is a system management tool that transforms existing organizations across planning, operations, logistics, and finance/administration functions for integrated and coordinated response. There is an incident commander who has responsibility for the overall response to ensure the safety of responders, save lives, stabilize the incident, and preserve property and the environment. Casualty clinical care falls under the Operations element of incident command. Casualties in a disaster require more basic than specialty care; thus, healt care specialty skills are not needed initially, yet these health professionals remain important in more dedifferentiated (i.e., general) roles in disaster response. Specialty physicians, for example, may be part of the workforce pool for logistics and casualty transport.

Triage is a system decision tool used to sort casualties for treatment priority, given casualty needs, resources, and the situation. The triage goal is to do "the best for most," rather than "everything for everyone." Effective triage is an iterative process done across all settings of casualty care. At each setting, an experienced acute care professional should serve as the triage officer. Triage is not a one-time decision; it is a dynamic sequence of decisions. Casualties, resources, and situations change, leading to refined triage decisions.

The triage decision at the scene first defines who is living and moves these casualties to safety away from the scene to a casualty collection point. The next triage decision determines who is critically injured, i.e., who has immediately life-threatening injuries. A scene triage system that uses motor response to command as a quick "sift" is helpful in finding these critically injured. Those casualties who can walk to another collection point or who can wave an arm or a leg in response to command most likely do not have life-threatening injuries. Those who do not move are critically injured or dead. Among the critically injured, some may survive and some may not survive. Triage decisions differentiate casualties to a greater degree as casualties move away from the scene to other settings and healt care facilities.

The five triage categories are:

1. Immediate (RED): immediately life-threatening injuries
2. Delayed (YELLOW): injuries requiring treatment within 6 hours
3. Minimal (GREEN): walking wounded and psychiatric
4. Expectant (BLUE): injuries greater than life or resources
5. Dead (GREY)

Each casualty category should have a defined area for collection and management. Immediate casualties should gain entrance to the emergency room.

The ATLS primary survey provides the framework for initial casualty assessment and intervention. Simple clinical assessments and interventions are paramount in austere and war-related environments. Creative solutions involve improvisation of materials to address life-threatening physiology. An initial airway intervention might stop at side-positioning and an oral airway in an unconscious patient, when endotracheal tubes and the resources to manage the casualty post-intubation are not available. Surgical airway might be considered, using tubes that are readily available, such as a hollow pen casing. Cervical spine immobilization can be performed with rolled blankets or casualty shoes. The best oxygenation might be room air, i.e., 21%. Absent stethoscopes and blood pressure cuffs, assessment for tension pneumothorax might be performed with ear to chest and a pulse check (carotid 60 torr; femoral 70 torr; radial 80 torr). Needle decompression requires longer needles in muscular or obese individuals. Field chest tubes can be managed with a "Heimlich value," constructed as the cut finger of a rubber glove over a tube.

Circulation is addressed first and foremost by stopping the bleeding. Tourniquets, fashioned from belts, clothing, or cables, can manage bleeding from mangled and amputated extremities well and free the hands of responders to manage additional casualties. Vascular access and volume are secondary considerations to rapid cessation of bleeding. In conscious casualties, oral fluids might be appropriate for hypovolemic management. Scalp lacerations can be managed with rapid whip stitch. Long-bone extremity fractures can be reduced and splinted with improvised materials from the scene to reduce hemorrhage, and pelvis fractures can be reduced with a sheet.

Casualty care is phased in over time as resources become available and casualties move to settings with greater resources. As opposed to trauma patient care, which moves quickly from primary survey and resuscitation to secondary survey and definitive care, casualty care defers secondary survey and definitive care in favor of identifying and managing as many casualties as possible with life-threatening injuries. Put another way, secondary survey and definitive care are discontinuous from the primary survey and resuscitation. Beyond the focused assessment sonography in trauma (FAST) exam, there is little role for radiological imaging and laboratory studies in the first phases of mass casualty response.

Damage control surgery is an extension of the phased approach to care and has been used extensively in civilian and war settings. The application of damage control principles to include the use of temporary shunts to restore blood flow across major vascular injuries is used to limit operative times in patients whose physiology precludes definitive repair. In comparison to the intact, resource-rich environment, severely injured trauma patients treated in austere environments may have damage control principles applied, not because of physiology, but because of resource considerations. For example, a patient with bowel injury who would have an anastamosis in an intact setting, might have the enterotomies controlled temporarily with a stapler or suture and the abdomen left open due to multiple other casualties waiting for an operating room.

Tactical Combat Casualty Care

Tactical combat casualty care (TCCC) applies ATLS principles in an actively hostile combat environment. Care begins at the point of injury with casualty self-care. When under fire, the priorities are return of fire and casualty safety. Few medical interventions can be applied when under fire. Stopping the bleeding is one of these interventions, with direct pressure, hemostatic gauze, and tourniquets providing effective temporizing hemostasis. Exsanguination is the most common cause of preventable death in combat, and ATLS principles are applied in this context as CAB interventions (circulation, airway, breathing). Note that assessment moves quickly through ABC to get to C interventions, with reevaluation of A and B in a safer environment amenable to such assessment.

War Wounds

War injuries result from high velocity guns and high energy explosives. High velocity gunshot wounds result from the linear and cavitating (radial) energy of the round, and cause tissue devitalization and destruction beyond the path of the round. High energy explosions, from military ordnance and improvised explosive devices (IEDs), cause mult-dimensional blast injuries across four mechanisms: primary blast from the supersonic pressure wave; secondary blast from fragments; tertiary blast from blunt or penetrating impact in the environment; and quaternary blast as burns or crush. Head, body, and eye armor offer significant protection, yet leave the extremities, face, and neck exposed. A prominent injury pattern includes multiple traumatic amputations and traumatic brain injury. As the energy from explosive devices increases in response to body armor, the devastation to tissues increases dramatically.

Wound management includes hemorrhage control and debridement of devitalized tissue. Energy tracks along tissue planes and strips soft tissue from bone. There may be skip areas of viable tissue with more proximal devitalized tissue. Tissue is assessed for color, consistency, contractility, and circulation (bleeding). Tissue that does not bleed with cutting and is dark, mushy, and non-contractile is no-viable and should be widely debrided. All combat wounds are dirty and should be left open; a negative-pressure device is a useful adjunct for wound coverage. Effective debridement is a process that involves serial wound assessment for injury progression and further excision of devitalized tissue. Wounds may heal ultimately by secondary intention or with delayed closure once all aspects of infection are ruled out.

Challenges in Austere and Armed Conflict Environments

Communication remains a dominant challenge in disaster response across all environments. Normal communication systems are often down, and multiple agencies and organizations, each with their own procedures and taxonomies, are brought together under stress with limited inter-operability. Application of incident command improves communication. Duplicate and rehearsed communication plans should be routinely practiced for disaster preparation.

Normal *transportation* options are limited, and any vehicle can be used to move casualties, including buses, cars, and boats.

Safety and security are challenged due to environmental and conflict conditions. These should be emphasized, planned, and practiced in drills.

Austere conditions and environments can lead to disordered body temperature regulation and *heat injury,* eincluding heat cramps, exhaustion, and stroke. Prevention of heat casualties includes acclimation for 3-5 days, alternating work and rest cycles, and emphasis on regular fluid and electrolyte replacement. Early recognition of heat casualty symptoms may prevent progression.

Psychosocial issues dominate in long-term recovery from disasters and can be more pressing in austere and war-torn environments. Resiliency can be enabled prior to disaster with healthy behaviors and organizational practice. Healthcare personnel are at risk for psychosocial stress disorders from a disaster; such stress can be attenuated through awareness and debriefings.

Summary

The principles of ATLS provide a framework by which to evaluate and treat life-threatening injuries in victims of traumatic injury. The ability to apply these principles in environments in which the traditional level of care is disrupted, or in which resources are limited or overwhelmed, requires the ability to apply a common sense adaptation of the principles taught in this course. Optimal outcomes in these settings requires that healt care professionals give forethought to the ways in which their skill sets should be employed and to anticipate the challenges associated with such settings.

Disaster Management and Emergency Preparedness
(Optional Lecture)

Objectives

1 Define the terms multiple casualty incident (MCI) and mass casualty event (MCE).

2 Explain the differences between MCIs and MCEs.

3 Describe the "all hazards" approach to disaster management and emergency. preparedness, including its application to acute injury care.

4 Identify the four phases of disaster management and describe the key elements of each phase with respect to acute injury care.

5 Describe the incident command system that has been adopted in your specific practice area.

Introduction

Disasters may be defined, from a medical perspective, as incidents or events in which the needs of patients overextend or overwhelm the resources needed to care for them. Although disasters usually strike without warning, **emergency preparedness**—the readiness for and anticipation of the contingencies that follow in the aftermath of disasters—enhances the ability of the health care system to respond to the challenges imposed. Such preparedness is the institutional and personal responsibility of every health care facility and professional. Adherence to the highest standards of quality medical practice that are consistent with the available medical resources serves as the best guideline for developing disaster plans. Commonly, the ability to respond to disaster situations is compromised by the excessive demands placed on resources, capabilities, and organizational structures.

Multiple casualty incidents (MCIs), or disasters in which patient care resources are overextended but are not overwhelmed, can stress local resources such that triage focuses on identifying the patients with the most life-threatening injuries.

Mass casualty events (MCEs) are events in which patient care resources are overwhelmed and cannot be immediately supplemented. Triage by necessity focuses on identifying those patients with the greatest probability of survival.

Note that MCIs and MCEs are both called MCIs by many experts. The ATLS course distinguishes between the terms because their different circumstances mandate alternative strategies for triage and treatment, The balance to be determined is between what is needed versus what is available in terms of human and material resource. **Any given hospital must determine its own thresholds, recognizing that the hospital disaster plan must address both MCIs and MCEs.**

Like most disciplines, disaster management and emergency preparedness experts have developed a nomenclature unique to their field. Box D-1 is a glossary of all key terms in this appendix.

Box D-1 Key Disaster Management and Emergency Preparedness Terminology

Acute Care The early care of victims of disasters that is provided in the field and in the hospital (i.e., emergency department, operating room, intensive care unit, acute care unit inpatient units) prior to recovery and rehabilitation.

Acute Care Specialists Physicians who provide acute care to victims of disasters, including, but not limited to, emergency medicine physicians, trauma surgeons, critical care medicine physicians, anesthesiologists, and hospitalists—both adult and pediatric.

Area of Operations ("Warm Zone") The geographic subdivision established around a disaster site into which only qualified personnel—for example, hazardous material (HAZMAT) technicians and emergency medical services (EMS) providers—are permitted.

Casualty Collection Point (CCP) A sector within the external perimeter of an area of operations ("warm zone") where casualties who exit the Search and Rescue (SAR) area ("hot zone") via a decontamination corridor are gathered prior to transport off site.

Chemical, Biological, Radiological, Nuclear, and Explosive (CBRNE), including incendiary, agents Human-made hazardous materials (HAZMATs) that may be the cause of human-made disasters, whether unintentional or intentional.

Decontamination Corridor A fixed or deployable facility where hazardous materials (HAZMATs) are removed from a patient, and through which the patient must pass before transport, either out of a Search and Rescue (SAR) area ("hot zone"), or into a hospital.

Disaster A natural or human-made incident or event, whether internal (originating inside the hospital) or external (originating outside the hospital) in which the needs of patients overextend or overwhelm the resources needed to care for them.

Emergency Medical Services (EMS) Emergency medical responders (EMRs), including emergency medical technicians (EMTs) and paramedics, who provide prehospital care under medical direction as part of an organized response to medical emergencies.

Emergency Operations Center (EOC) The headquarters of Unified Incident Command (UIC) for a region or system, established in a safe location outside the area of operations ("warm zone"), usually at a fixed site, and staffed by emergency managers.

Emergency Preparedness The readiness for and anticipation of the contingencies that can follow in the aftermath of natural or human-made disasters. Preparedness is the institutional and personal responsibility of every health care facility and professional.

Emergo Train System (ETS) An organizational structure used chiefly in Europe and Australasia to help coordinate an in-field or in-hospital disaster response. (Note: Nations and hospitals typically adopt their own versions of this system.)

External Perimeter The outer boundary of an Area of Operations ("warm zone") that is established around a disaster site to separate geographic subdivisions that are safe for the general public ("cold zones") from those that are safe only for qualified personnel.

Hazardous Materials (HAZMATs) Chemical, biological, radiological, nuclear, and explosive (CBRNE), including incendiary, agents that pose potential risks to human life, health, welfare, and safety.

Hospital Incident Command System (HICS) An organizational structure used chiefly in the Americas to help coordinate an in-hospital disaster response. (Note: Nations and hospitals typically adopt their own versions of this system.)

Hazard Vulnerability Analysis (HVA)   An analysis of the probability and severity of the risks of various hazardous materials (HAZMATs), industrial mishaps, natural disasters, and weather systems that pose potential risks to community health and safety.

Incident Command or Incident Commander (IC)   The final authority and overall coordinator or supervisor for the management of any disaster response.

Incident Command Post (ICP)   The headquarters for Incident Command (IC), established in a safe location within the area of operations ("warm zone"), but at a safe distance from the Search and Rescue (SAR) area ("hot zone"), for any disaster.

Incident Command System (ICS)   An organizational structure that provides overall direction for the management of the disaster response.

Internal Perimeter   The outer boundary of a Search and Rescue (SAR) area ("hot zone") that isolates this area from the surrounding Area of Operations ("warm zone").

Mass Casualty Event (MCE)   A disaster in which patient care resources are overwhelmed and cannot immediately be supplemented.

Mitigation   Activities that health care facilities and professionals undertake in an attempt to lessen the severity and impact of a potential disaster.

Medical Response Team   A team of 1 to 4 health care professionals, led by an acute care specialist, that provides emergency medical care to an individual patient.

Minimum Acceptable Care   The lowest appropriate level of medical and surgical treatment required to sustain life and limb until additional assets can be mobilized.

Multiple Casualty Incident (MCI)   A disaster in which patient care resources are overextended but not overwhelmed

Personal Protective Equipment (PPE)   Special clothing worn by disaster response personnel to avoid self-contamination by hazardous materials (HAZMATs).

Preparation   Activities that health care facilities and providers undertake to build capacity and identify resources that may be used if a disaster occurs.

Recovery   Activities that are designed to assist health care facilities and professionals resume normal operations after a disaster situation is resolved.

Response   Activities that health care facilities and professionals undertake in evaluating and treating victims of an actual disaster.

Search and Rescue (SAR) Area ("Hot Zone")   A sector within the internal perimeter of an area of operations for a disaster in which humans are directly affected by the hazard.

Surge Capability   The extra assets that can actually be deployed—for example, beds that can actually be staffed and ventilators and monitors that can actually be used—in a disaster.

Unified Incident Command (UIC)   The locus of incident command for an entire region or system, where incident commanders from all involved public safety and public health disciplines meet to direct the overall strategy of the incident response to mass casualty events (MCEs).

Weapons of Mass Destruction (WMDs)   Hazardous materials (HAZMATs) used, or intended to be used, for the explicit purpose of harming or destroying human life.

The Need

Disaster management and emergency preparedness constitute key knowledge areas that prepare ATLS providers to apply ATLS principles during natural and human-made disasters. Successful application of these principles during the chaos that typically comes in the aftermath of such catastrophes requires both familiarity with the disaster response and knowledge of the medical conditions likely to be encountered. Terror events constitute a minority of all disasters, but nearly all terror events cause physical injury, three-fourths of which are due to blast trauma and most of the rest to gunshot wounds. As such, the understanding and application of ATLS principles are essential in the evaluation and treatment of all disaster victims.

The Approach

Disasters are unpredictable because of their nature, location, and timing. An "all hazards" approach is used in contemporary disaster management. This approach is based on a single, common, initial emergency response protocol that is flexible and has branch points that lead to specific actions depending on the type of disaster encountered. **The fundamental principle of disaster management is to do the greatest good for the greatest number.**

Phases of Disaster Management

The public health approach to disaster and mass casualty management consists of four distinct phases:

1. Preparation
2. Mitigation
3. Response
4. Recovery

In most nations, local and regional disaster response plans are developed in accordance with national response plans. Emergency medicine, trauma care, public health, and disaster medicine experts must be involved in all four phases of management with respect to the medical components of the operational plan.

Preparation

Preparation involves the activities a hospital undertakes to identify risks, build capacity, and identify resources that may be used if a disaster occurs. These activities include a risk assessment of the area, the development of a simple, yet flexible, disaster plan that is regularly reviewed and revised as necessary, and provision of training that is necessary to allow these plans to be implemented when indicated.

Simple Disaster Plans   A basic and readily understood approach to MCIs and MCEs is the key to effective disaster and emergency management. Plans that are too complex or cumbersome to remember or implement are destined to fail. All plans must include training in disaster management and emergency preparedness appropriate to the educational preparation of the individuals being trained and to the specific function they will be asked to perform.

Community Planning   Disaster planning, whether at the local, regional, or national level, involves a wide range of individuals and resources. All plans:

- Should involve **acute care specialists** (e.g., emergency medicine physicians, trauma surgeons, critical care medicine physicians, anesthesiologists, and hospitalists, both adult and pediatric) and local hospitals, as well as officials of the local police, fire, **emergency medical services (EMS),** homeland security, emergency management, public health, and governmental agencies charged with **hazardous material (HAZMAT)** management and disaster preparation.

- Should be frequently tested and reevaluated.

- Must provide for a means of communication considering all contingencies, such as loss of telephone land lines and cellular circuits.

- Must provide for storage of equipment, supplies, and any special resources that may be necessary based on local **hazard vulnerability analysis (HVA)**.

- Must provide for all levels of assistance—from first aid through definitive care to rehabilitation.

- Must prepare for the transportation of casualties to other facilities by prior agreement should the local facility become saturated or unusable.

- Must consider the urgent needs of patients already hospitalized for conditions unrelated to the disaster.

Hospital Planning   Although a regional approach to planning is ideal for the management of mass casualties, circumstances may require each hospital to function with little or no outside support. Earthquakes, floods, riots, or nuclear contamination may require the individual hospital to operate in isolation. The crisis may be instantaneous or it may develop slowly. Situations may exist that disrupt the infrastructure of society and prevent access to the medical facility. For this reason, it is vital that each hospital develop a disaster plan that accurately reflects its HVA. Once a state of disaster has been declared, the hospital disaster plan should be put into effect. Specific procedures should be automatic and include:

- Establishment of an **incident command post (ICP)**.

- Notification of on-duty and off-duty personnel.

- Preparation of decontamination, triage, and treatment areas.

- Classification of in-hospital patients to determine whether additional resources can be acquired to care for them or whether they must be discharged or transferred.

- Checking of supplies (e.g., blood, fluids, medication) and other materials (e.g., food, water, power, communications) essential to sustain hospital operations.

- Activation of decontamination facilities and staff and application of decontamination procedures, if necessary.

- Institution of security precautions, including hospital lockdown if necessary, to avoid potential contamination and subsequent hospital closure.

- Establishment of a public information center and provision of regular briefings to inform family, friends, the media, and the government.

Departmental Planning Effective disaster planning builds on existing strengths to address identified weaknesses. Since patient care can best be delivered to individual patients by providers working in small teams, every hospital department with responsibility for the care of injured patients must identify its **medical response teams** in advance. These teams must be provided with specific instructions as to where to go and what to do in the event of an internal or external disaster. Such instructions should not be overly complex. They should also be readily accessible in the event of a disaster—for example, printed on the back of hospital identification cards or posted on wall charts. They should also be very specific in terms of the job action to be performed: Job action sheets predicated on the incident command system (ICS) are an effective model to employ.

Personal Planning Family disaster planning constitutes a vital part of pre-event hospital disaster preparation for both the hospital and its employees. Most health care providers have family responsibilities, and will be at best uncomfortable, and at worst unable, to meet their employment responsibilities in the event of a disaster if the health and safety of their families is uncertain. Hos-

pitals can assist health care providers in meeting their responsibilities to the hospital and to their families in a number of ways, and it is obviously to the advantage of both for hospitals to ensure that employees' family needs are met. Among these needs are assistance in identifying alternative resources for the care of dependent children and adults and ensuring that all employees develop family disaster plans, since all hospital-specific response plans depend on mobilization of additional staff, whose first duty in any disaster will be to ensure their own and their families' health and safety.

Hospital Disaster Training All health care providers must be trained in the principles of disaster management and emergency preparedness. Training in disaster management includes both operational and medical components. The ATLS provider should be well versed in the fundamental elements of the local, regional, and national disaster plans, and understand the role of medical care in the overall management plan. It is essential to realize that, although the purpose of all disaster management is to ensure the safety and security of the maximum number of human lives, the medical component is but one element of the operational plan at both the hospital and the community levels.

Beyond this basic understanding, it is also vital that the ATLS provider have a working understanding of the application of ATLS principles in disaster situations. It is important to recognize that the approach to the patient injured in a disaster is no different from the approach to the patient injured in the course of everyday activities: Airway, Breathing, Circulation, Disability, and Exposure. Rather, it is the application of this basic approach that may be altered, which is best summarized by the phrase, "Care ordinary, circumstances extraordinary." For example, the fact that the ATLS provider may need to care for multiple victims more or less simultaneously, and may not have sufficient equipment or assistance to carry out all needed tasks in a timely manner, requires that routine standards of care may need to be altered such that disaster medicine must focus on the minimum acceptable standard of care required for salvage of life and limb, not the highest possible standard of care normally offered to severely injured patients.

It is vital that the ATLS provider obtain sufficient basic education to initiate the medical care of multiple victims not only of natural disasters, but of situations involving HAZMAT. These include **weapons of mass destruction (WMDs), chemical, biological, radiological, nuclear, and explosive (CBRNE)** agents, and incendiary agents. Training in austere environment operations, such as when resources are constrained, is essential. Although brief outlines of such treatment are provided in this appendix, additional training in disaster medical care is currently beyond the scope of the ATLS provider course, but can be obtained through participation in the appropriate national disaster management courses, including the ACS COT Disaster Management and Emergency Preparedness (DMEP) course. http://www.facs.org/trauma/disaster/index.html

Mitigation

Mitigation involves the activities a hospital undertakes in attempting to lessen the severity and impact of a potential disaster. These include adoption of an incident command system for managing internal (originating inside the hospital) and external (originating outside the hospital) disasters, and the exercises and drills necessary to successfully implement, test, and refine the hospital disaster plan. *There is no substitute for adequate training and drilling.*

Incident Command System

An **incident command system (ICS)** is vital to operational success during disasters and must be known to all personnel within every health care facility and agency. The ICS establishes clear lines of responsibility, authority, reporting, and communication for all personnel, thereby maximizing collaboration and minimizing conflicts during the disaster response.

The effective ICS includes both vertical and horizontal reporting relationships, to ensure that urgent decisions can be made without the need for prior confirmation by incident commanders, which consumes valuable time. In MCEs that affect an entire region or system, the effective ICS must be fully integrated with the **unified incident command (UIC)** serving the entire region or system, which is comprised of all involved public health and safety agencies, key officials from which should be co-located in the region's or system's **Emergency Operations Center (EOC)**.

A hierarchical approach to incident command, such as the **Hospital Incident Command System (HICS),** developed under the auspices of the California EMS Authority, (http://www.emsa.ca.gov/hics/hics.asp), is favored in the Americas. A more collaborative and medically centered approach to incident command, such as the **Emergo Train System (ETS),** promulgated by the Linköping University Trauma Center in Sweden (http://www.emergotrain.com), is favored in Europe and Australasia. Most nations adopt one of the two approaches for **incident command (IC)** in developing their response plans, adapting them to fit local needs and resources. The models used by these two systems are shown in Table D.1.

Regardless of the ICS system used, IC is responsible for all aspects of the disaster response under its jurisdiction. As soon as possible after a disaster is declared by IC, an **incident command post (ICP),** previously known as the incident command center, must be established, with reliable communication links to all functional units—operational/logistic and medical. The ICP must be established in a secure location, distant from, but with ready access to, the site of primary patient care activity, whether field or hospital. In the field, it should be located within the **area of operations ("warm zone")** bounded by an **external perimeter**, and must be sited uphill, upwind, and upstream of the **search and rescue (SAR)** area **("hot zone")** bounded by an **internal perimeter**, from which **decontamination corridors** lead to **casualty collection points (CCPs).** In the hospital, it should be located at a safe distance from decontamination areas, patient care areas, family support areas, and potential hazards, such as contaminated ventilation and drainage, but close enough to patient care and family support areas so that messages can be transmitted in person if electronic communications fail.

Frequent Disaster Drills

As in trauma resuscitation, medical management of mass casualties can be provided to individual patients only by individual providers, working in small medical response teams, led by a senior acute care specialist. It is crucial to an effective disaster medical response that such teams have been drilled, not simply trained, in disaster medical care, under circumstances that are as realistic as possible. Disaster drills should always emphasize the disasters expected on the basis of the hospital's HVA. The purpose of disaster drills and exercises is not only to train emergency medical responders to provide care to disaster victims, but also to identify gaps in the hospital disaster plan so they can be closed prior to the occurrence of an actual internal or external disaster. In addition, they should involve scenarios that emphasize

■ TABLE D.1 Commonly Used Models for Incident Command Systems[a]	
HICS FUNCTIONAL JOB ACTIONS[b]	**ETS FUNCTIONAL JOB ACTIONS[c]**
Incident command (hospital)	Field
• Command staff	• Ambulance incident command
• Public information	• Medical incident command
• Liaison	
• Safety	**Hospital**
• Medical/technical	• Logistics command
• Finance and administration	• Medical command
• Logistics	
• Operations	
• Planning and intelligence	

[a]Regardless of the system being used, like structures are used in-field and in-hospital.
[b]http://www.emsa.ca.gov/hics/hics.asp
[c]http://www.emergotrain.com

the needs of special populations, such as burn patients, pediatric patients, geriatric patients, and disabled patients, which may require the mobilization and deployment of population-specific resources. The types of disaster drills and exercises hospitals should hold are described in Box D-2. It is wise to proceed from simple drills to complex exercises as staff members gain familiarity with the ICS and experience with the problems likely to arise during a disaster.

Response

Response involves activities a hospital undertakes in treating victims of an actual disaster. These include activation of the hospital disaster plan, including the ICS, and management of the disaster as it unfolds, implementing schemes for patient decontamination, triage, surge capacity and **surge capability.** Given the increased level of activity in disaster events, traffic control is needed to ensure an uninterrupted forward flow of communications, patients, supplies, and personnel. The medical disaster response must also address the needs of special populations, including children, elders, the disabled, and the dispossessed.

Prehospital Care   The prehospital (EMS) response to disasters typically occurs in four stages:

1. Chaos phase, typically lasting 15 to 20 minutes
2. Organizational phase, usually lasting 1 to 2 hours
3. Site-clearing and evacuation stage of variable length, depending on disaster type, complexity of SAR efforts, and number of evacuees
4. Gradual recovery

All SAR efforts at the scene should be the responsibility of HAZMAT technicians specifically trained for this purpose, and must proceed as rapidly and safely as possible. The potential for a "second hit" designed to injure first responding personnel, including volunteers, must be considered. Since the first respon-sibility of field providers is to protect themselves, first-response personnel, including EMS professionals, should not enter the disaster scene until it has been declared safe and secure by the appropriate authorities. Appropriate **personal protective equipment (PPE)** is mandatory for all health care personnel in direct contact with patients.

In-Hospital Care   Once the hospital disaster plan is activated, the first priority of IC is to ensure sufficient resources to mount an effective disaster response. This includes mobilization and deployment of adequate staff, facilities, and equipment to meet anticipated needs. Early discharge of eligible patients from hospital inpatient and fast track units; cancellation of elective operations and outpatient clinics; accurate determination of each unit's surge capability, not merely its capacity; and identification and mobilization of alternative care sites are all important functions. Pre-printed job action sheets should be made available to staff for each functional job description within the ICS, to serve as a tangible reminder of the tasks each staff member is expected to undertake.

Patient Decontamination   Hospital disaster care begins with decontamination, the principles and methods for which are shown in Box D-3. Ninety percent of hazardous materials to which disaster victims may have been exposed can be eliminated simply by removal of outer garments contaminated with hazardous materials. However, it may not be possible for HAZMAT teams or first responders to perform decontamination under all circumstances. Moreover, many patients are likely to transport themselves to the closest hospital, and will arrive at the emergency department before being decontaminated, demanding urgent care.

For this reason, hospitals must rapidly and conscientiously determine the likelihood of contamination and proceed accordingly. Although the safest course might be to consider all disaster patients contaminated

Box D-2 Types of Disaster Drills and Exercises

- **Disaster Drill** Supervised activity with a limited focus to test a procedure that is a limited component of a facility's overall disaster plan.

- **Tabletop Exercise** Written and verbal scenarios that evaluate the effectiveness of a facility's overall disaster plan and coordination.

- **Functional Exercise** Simulation of a disaster in the most realistic manner possible without moving real people or real equipment to a real site.

- **Field Exercise** Culmination of previous drills and exercises that tests the mobilization of as many of the response components as possible in real time, using real people and real equipment.

Box D-3 Principles and Methods of Decontamination

Gross (Primary) Decontamination

■ Performed in the field or outside the hospital after removal of clothing

■ Patient is hosed with a fine mist spray under moderate pressure

■ Washes away most remaining contaminants

Technical (Secondary) Decontamination

Self-decontamination with soap and water under a warm shower bath

OR

Assisted Decontamination with Soap and Water via a Warm Sponge Bath

■ Eradicates almost all residual contaminants, suffices for radioactive agents

■ Additional cleansing with dilute chlorine bleach may be recommended if susceptible biologic agents or chemical agents are suspected

Remember, "Dilution is the solution to pollution."

---

until public safety officials determine otherwise, this approach slows patient throughput and can result in further deterioration of high-risk patients. Another approach is to segregate patients who transport themselves to the hospital in a holding area outside the hospital until HAZMAT teams determine the nature of the event, recognizing that such patients are far less likely to deteriorate than patients transported by ambulance. Either way, hospitals must plan for decontamination of potentially contaminated patients before they can enter the emergency department. Failure to do so can result in contamination and subsequent quarantine of the entire facility. Involvement of hospital security, and local police, may be necessary if lockdown is required to prevent presumptively contaminated patients from entering the emergency department or hospital before they can be effectively decontaminated.

Disaster Triage Scheme A method for rapid identification of victims requiring priority treatment is essential. The goal of treatment in MCIs is to treat the sickest patients first, whereas the goal in MCEs is to save the greatest number of lives. As such, triage schemes in MCEs should adopt an approach that separates patients with minor injuries from those with more serious injuries, before proceeding with evaluation and sustentative treatment of patients with major injuries. Patients who may not survive receive comfort care only after other patients have been treated.

Overtriage and undertriage can substantially affect the medical disaster response. Overtriage slows system throughput, and undertriage delays medically necessary care. Both increase the fatality rate among patients who may potentially survive. Therefore, triage should be performed by an experienced clinician with specific knowledge of the conditions affecting

most patients. In addition, all injured patients should be continually reevaluated and reassessed.

Effective Surge Capability The initial disaster response is invariably a local response, as regional or national assets cannot typically be mobilized for 72 hours. Thus, local, regional, and national disaster plans must presume that hospitals will be able to deploy sufficient staff, equipment, and resources to care for an increase, or "surge," in patient volume that is approximately 20 percent higher than its baseline, an estimate that reflects recent worldwide experience with limited MCEs.

The term *surge capacity* is more often used in disaster plans than *surge capability*, but the ATLS course uses the latter term, as it is more inclusive than the former term. This is because surge capacity too often is used to refer only to the number of additional beds or assets (e.g., ventilators and monitors) that might be pressed into service on the occasion of an MCE. By contrast, surge capability refers to the number of additional beds that can actually be staffed or ventilators and monitors that can actually be operated. In large urban areas, many staff may work multiple jobs, and may unknowingly be part of more than one hospital's disaster plan. In addition, most hospital staff are working parents, who must consider the needs of their families and relatives, in addition to those of their workplaces.

Alternative Care Standards In MCEs, it can be expected that during the first 24 to 72 hours of the disaster there will be insufficient local assets to provide a level of care comparable to that routinely provided in local hospital emergency departments or intensive care units. If scarce resources, particularly intensive resources, are devoted to the first several critically ill or injured patients who require them, it will be difficult, if not impossible, to later redirect them to others in greater need.

To maximize these resources, hospital disaster plans must strive to provide the largest possible number of patients with the **minimum acceptable care,** defined as the lowest appropriate level of medical and surgical treatment required to sustain life and limb until additional assets can be mobilized. Since each disaster response presents health care providers with a different mix of patient needs and available resources, no single description of a minimum acceptable standard of care is applicable to every facility or every disaster circumstance. The selection of patients to receive scarce or intensive resources will present the trauma specialist with an ethical dilemma and potentially a later legal problem. General criteria should be developed before the disaster event, based on demographic and geographic circumstances as well as the community HVA. It is wise to develop such criteria in collaboration with the hospital's legal counsel, bioethics committee, and pastoral care department to ensure consistency with the community standard of legal, ethical, and moral values. They should then be included as part of the facility's disaster plan.

Traffic Control System   Controlling the flow of information (communications), equipment (supplies), patients (transport), and personnel (providers, relatives, the public, and the press) is of paramount importance in a medical disaster response. These are the issues most often cited in after-action reports as causes of disaster mismanagement. The unidirectional flow of patients from the emergency department to inpatient units must be ensured, since emergency department beds will be made available for later-arriving patients as they are emptied.

Redundant communications systems, reliable supply chains, and redoubtable security measures are also vital components of an effective disaster medical and operational response. These assets must be tested on a regular basis through drills and exercises that realistically reflect the disaster scenarios that are most likely to be encountered by a particular facility, whatever its location.

Special Needs Populations   Special needs populations include children, especially those who are technology-dependent; elders, especially those who are bedridden, including the nursing home population; the disabled, both physically and emotionally, for whom assistance will be illness- or injury-specific; and the dispossessed, including the poor and the homeless, who will be difficult to reach by traditional means for purposes of disaster education and treatment. Specific response plans are needed to ensure that their special needs are met.

Pathophysiology and Patterns of Injury   As with all trauma, disasters result in recognizable patterns of injury that are based on the properties of the particular wounding agent and the unique pathophysiology that results from each such agent. Although detailed descriptions of the pathophysiology and patterns of injury encountered in the acute disaster response are beyond the scope of this appendix, 100% of all natural disasters and 98% of all terror events worldwide involve physical trauma. Thus, the principles of ATLS are ideally suited to the early care of patients with blunt and penetrating injuries observed in disasters. Certain additional factors must also be considered in the early and later care of seriously injured disaster patients, including the possibility that chemical, radiologic, and biologic injuries may coexist with blast injuries. Members of the medical team should be familiar with the basics of decontamination and initial treatment of all patients injured by WMDs, not only those injured by bomb blasts and gunshot wounds. WMDs may be the sole agent used, or may be added as adulterants to explosive devices to construct a "dirty bomb." If present, WMDs can complicate the care of individuals who have suffered blast trauma, although their effectiveness in such scenarios may be limited by the effects of the blast. Descriptions of WMD agents and care of WMD injuries other than contagious illnesses are summarized in Boxes D-4 through D-10. **Remember, the emergency care of these patients becomes even more complex in the face of MCEs, with their associated needs for disaster triage, additional staff, and adequate supplies.** The treatment of contagious illnesses, which typically present with fever and rash or influenza-like symptoms days after exposure, is microbe-dependent.

Recovery

Recovery involves activities designed to help facilities resume operations after an emergency. The local public health system plays a major role in this phase of disaster management, although health professionals will provide routine health care to the affected community consistent with available resources, in terms of operable facilities, usable equipment, and credentialed personnel. **Acute care** physicians who provide care for neglected injuries and chronic illnesses may find both the medical and organizational skills required for the early care of the trauma patient useful in the days after the response phase subsides. The principles of ATLS—that is, treatment of the greatest threat to life first, without waiting for a definitive diagnosis, and causing the patient no harm, are no less useful in the austere environments that may follow natural or human-made disasters.

Box D-4 Special Considerations in the Care of Blast Injury

Early Care

Airway

■ Lateral recovery position (field care of facial trauma without cervical spine injury)

■ Modified HAINES (**H**igh **A**rm **IN** **E**ndangered **S**pine— lateral recovery position + head on outstretched arm) position (field care of facial trauma with cervical spine injury)

Breathing

■ Supplemental oxygen (blast lung)

■ Needle decompression (tension pneumothorax)

Circulation

■ Tourniquets (field care of bleeding from traumatic amputations)

■ HemCon (chitosan), QuikClot (zeolite) (field care of bleeding from soft tissues)

■ Hypotensive resuscitation (field care of patients in shock)

■ Damage control laparotomy/thoracotomy

■ Completion amputations for unsalvageable mangled extremities

■ Liberal use of fasciotomies and escharotomies (to avoid compartment syndromes)

■ Active and passive rewarming (to avoid hypothermic coagulopathies)

■ Preferential use of fresh whole blood, if available (for treatment of coagulopathies)

■ Administration of recombinant factor VIIa (rVIIa) (for treatment of coagulopathies)

■ Judicious crystalloid fluid resuscitation (for combined blast lung and blast burn)

Later Care

■ Compartment syndrome despite fasciotomy (especially during aeromedical transport)

■ Early recognition and repair of vascular injury (intimal tears caused by shock wave)

■ Wound management (reopening, irrigation, debridement, reclosure of dirty wounds)

■ Tertiary survey (should be performed by different team of examiners)

■ Documentation (essential for providers in subsequent echelons of care)

■ Feedback (all providers must learn of outcome for care to improve)

Box D-5 Chemical Agents Commonly Associated with Human-Made Disasters

Nerve (Cholinergic) Agents

■ Tabun (GA)

■ Sarin (GB)

■ Soman (GD)

■ VX (an oily, brown liquid; all other nerve agents are gases)

Blood (Asphyxiant and Hemolytic) Agents

■ Hydrogen cyanide (AC)

■ Cyanogen chloride (CK)

■ Arsine (SA)

Choking (Pulmonary) Agents

■ Chlorine (CL)

■ Phosgene (CG)

■ Diphosgene (DP)

■ Ammonia

Blister (Vesicant) Agents

■ Mustards (HD, HN, HT)

■ Lewisite (L)

■ Phosgene oxime (CX)

Incapacitating (Psychogenic) Agents

■ Agent 15

■ BZ

Box D-6 Special Considerations in the Care of Chemical Injuries

Nerve (Cholinergic) Agents (GA, GB, GD, VX)

■ Pathophysiology: form complexes with AChE→↑ ACh; victim drowns in secretions

■ Sx: cholinergic crisis (both muscarinic and nicotinic effects; see Box D.7)

■ Rx: atropine (dries secretions); pralidoxime* [2-PAM] (inactivates complexes)

■ *Note: A benzodiazepine should also be given if seizure activity is evident.*

Blood (Asphyxiant and Hemolytic) Agents (AC, CK and SA)

■ Pathophysiology:
  —AC, CK: CN- replaces O_2 in Cya_3
  —SA: acute hemolysis ± renal failure

■ Sx: telltale odor in association with cardinal signs
  —AC, CK: almonds, in association with LOC
  —SA: garlic, in association with hematuria, jaundice

■ Rx:
  —AC, CK: OHCbl (→CNCbl) [or $NaNO_2$ (Hb→MetHb)] + $Na_2S_2O_3$
  —SA: supportive

■ *Note: OHCbl has largely replaced $NaNO_2$ in treatment of AC, CK exposure.*

Choking (Pulmonary) Agents

■ Pathophysiology: chemical pneumonia, severe tracheobronchitis and alveolitis†

■ Sx: telltale odor in association with shortness of breath
  —CL: bleach
  —CG, DP: green corn, mown hay
  —NH_3: ammonia

■ Rx: supportive

■ *Note: Dry oxygen in CL exposure may lessen HCl damage to tracheobronchial tree.*

Blister (Vesicant) Agents

■ Pathophysiology: severe/painful/blistering cutaneous/pulmonary/mucous burns

■ Sx: telltale odor in association with epithelial damage
  —HD, HN, HT: garlic, mustard, onions
  —L: geraniums
  —CX: pepper

■ Rx: aggressive decontamination, wound care

■ *Note: Administer British anti-Lewisite (BAL) in L exposure.*

Incapacitating (Psychogenic) Agents (Agent 15, BZ)

■ Pathophysiology: agent specific

■ Sx: bizarre behavior

■ Rx: await recovery

*GD-AChE complexes age rapidly; pralidoxime must be given as soon as possible
†Phosgene is fatal if pulmonary edema develops in 2–4 hr

Pitfalls

The four common pitfalls in the disaster medical response are always the same—communications, supplies, security, and volunteers—leading many disaster experts to ask why humans seem incapable of learning from the mistakes made in past disaster events. Although the exact dates, times, and places of future disasters are unknown, the lessons learned from previous disasters are invaluable in teaching us how to better prepare for them.

It can be expected that land and mobile telecommunications systems will be overwhelmed. Communications systems must be fully interoperable and overly redundant, both in terms of duplicate equipment and disparate modes. Capability for both vertical and horizontal communications must be ensured. Supplies needed for disasters must be sequestered and stored in high, dry, safe, and secure areas. Security must be ensured for providers, patients, supplies, and systems needed for disaster care, such as communications and transport. Volunteers, well meaning as they may be, must be properly trained and credentialed to participate in a disaster response, and must participate only as part of a properly planned and organized disaster response, since they otherwise place both themselves, and the intended recipients of their aid, in danger.

Box D-7 Classic Toxidromes Associated with Cholingeric Crisis due to Nerve Agents

SLUDGEM*	DUMBELS*	MTW(t)HF†
Salivation	**D**iarrhea, **D**yspnea, **D**iaphoresis	**M**ydriasis
Lacrimation	**U**rination	**T**achycardia
Urination	**M**iosis	**W**eakness
Defecation	**B**radycardia, **B**ronchorrhea, **B**ronchospasm	(t)**H**ypertension
Gastrointestinal	**E**mesis	**F**asciculations
Emesis	**L**acrimation	
Miosis	**S**alivation, **S**ecretions, **S**weating	

*Muscarinic effects (treated with atropine)
†Nicotinic effects

Box D-8 Radioactive Agents Commonly Associated with Human-Made Disasters

Ionizing Radiation

- Particles:
  - Alpha (a) [He^{++} nucleus]
  - Beta (b) [energized e$^-$]
- Rays:
  - x [high energy photon waves]
  - Gamma (g) [high energy photon waves]

Likely Agents

- "Dirty bomb":
  - Low level radioactive waste (^{137}Cs, ^{192}Ir) of medical or industrial origin
- Nuclear accident:
  - Pressure water reactor: ^{133}Xe, ^{135}Xe, ^{88}Kr (based on Three Mile Island experience)
  - Graphite reactor: ^{133}I, ^{131}I, ^{132}Te, ^{137}Cs, ^{90}Sr (based on Chernobyl experience)
  - Note: Pressure water reactors are most common; graphite reactors are now obsolete.

Radiation Dosimetry

- For b, x, and g emitters, 1 R (Roentgen) = 1 rad (radiation absorbed dose) [or 0.01 Gy]
- For a or n emitters, 1 rad x Q* = # rem† (Roentgen equivalent man) [or 0.01 Sv]
- Note: In most circumstances, 1 R = 1 rad [OR 0.01 Gy] = 1 rem [OR 0.01 Sv].
- Note: "Rad" and "rem" are preferred in the Americas, "Gy" and "Sv" elsewhere.

*Q = quality factor (b, x, g emitters: 1; inhaled/ingested a emitters: 20; n emitters: 3-20)
† It is this unit that denotes extent of biological damage (background dose = 360 mSv/yr)

Box D-9 Special Considerations in the Care of Radiation and Nuclear Injuries

Ionizing Radiation

- Pathophysiology:

  – Strips electrons from atomic nuclei, damaging cellular DNA; rapidly dividing tissues (gastrointestinal, hematopoietic, epidermal) are most susceptible to ionizing radiation

  – *Note: Radioactive atoms emit particles (or rays) during decay; risk of exposure depends upon energy of emissions ("dirty bomb": low; nuclear accident: high).*

- Sx:

  – Specific to dose and type, distance to source, density of shielding; asymptomatic <50 rad (0.5 Sv), ß burns >100 rad (1 Sv), acute radiation syndrome >200 rad (2 Sv)

  – *Note: The more rapid the symptom onset, the higher the dose; patients who develop gastrointestinal symptoms within 4 hours of exposure rarely survive.*

- Rx:

  – α and β: external [± internal] decon + supportive care; χ and γ : supportive care (treat external contamination as dirt; no risk to provider from patient χ or γ exposure)

  – *Note: Do NOT delay resuscitation for decontamination, as risk to provider is nil; perform operations by day 3 to avoid wound complications 2° RES‡ failure.*

‡ RES = reticuloendothelial system

Box D-10 Classic Toxidromes Associated with Acute Radiation Syndrome

Stage I: (Chiefly Gastrointestinal)

- Onset: minutes to hours*; duration: 48–72 hr
- Presentation: nausea, vomiting; also diarrhea, cramps

Stage II (Chiefly Hematopoietic†)

- Onset: hours to days; duration: 1½–2 wk
- Presentation: asymptomatic → bone marrow suppression

Stage III (Multisystem Involvement)

- Onset: 3–5 weeks; duration: variable
- Presentation‡: CNS/CVS (>15 Sv); CRS/GIT (>5 Sv); RES (>1 Sv)

Stage IV (Gradual Recovery)

- Onset: weeks; duration: weeks to months
- Presentation: leading cause of death before recovery is sepsis

*Acute radiation syndrome is fatal if gastrointestinal symptoms develop within 2–4 hours

† Hematopoietic (RES) derangements interfere with healing, may last weeks to months

‡ CNS = central nervous system, CVS = cardiovascular system, CRS = cardiorespiratory system, GIT = gastrointestinal tract

Summary

The medical disaster response occurs within the context of the public health disaster response—preparation, mitigation, response, and recovery. Preparation requires both the conviction that a disaster will occur, and the commitment to be ready when it happens, and must ensure both that a simple plan is developed and that all are educated in its implementation. Mitigation is the key to the success of the disaster response, since it provides the framework within which medical care must be rendered—for example, incident command systems and effective disaster drills and exercises. Response is the essence of disaster management. It comprises both prehospital and in-patient care, and must embrace the minimal acceptable standard of care needed to provide the greatest good for the greatest number. It requires a sound understanding of pathophysiology and patterns of injury for care to be delivered expeditiously and deterioration anticipated and avoided. Recovery is mainly the province of public health personnel, but it depends on support from acute care physicians for treatment of untreated injuries and chronic illnesses that may develop or become exacerbated in the aftermath of the acute response. The psychosocial issues that will arise must be recognized and dealt with to ensure adequate recovery of the individuals and community involved in the incident.

Bibliography

1. American Academy of Pediatrics (Foltin GL, Schonfeld DJ, Shannon MW, eds.). *Pediatric Terrorism and Disaster Preparedness: A Resource for Pediatricians.* AHRQ Publication No. 06-0056-EF. Rockville, MD: Agency for Healthcare Research and Quality; 2006. http://www.ahrq.org/research/pedprep/resource.htm. Accessed February 26, 2008.

2. auf der Heide E. *Disaster Response: Principles of Preparation and Coordination.* Chicago, IL: CV Mosby; 1989.

3. Committee on Trauma, American College of Surgeons. *Disaster Management and Emergency Preparedness Course.* Chicago: American College of Surgeons, 2009.

4. DiPalma RG, Burris DG, Champion HR, Hodgson MJ. Blast injuries. *N Engl J Med* 2005;352:1335-1342.

5. Frykberg ER, Tepas JJ. Terrorist bombings: lessons learned from Belfast to Beirut. *Ann Surg* 1988;208:569-576.

6. Gutierrez de Ceballos JP, Turegano-Fuentes F, Perez-Diaz D, Sanz-Sanchez M, Martin-Llorente C, Guerrero-Sanz JE. Casualties treated at the closest hospital in the Madrid, March 11, terrorist bombings. *Crit Care Med* 2005;33(1 Suppl);S107-S112.

7. Gutierrez de Ceballos JP, Turegano-Fuentes F, Perez-Diaz D, Sanz-Sanchez M, Martin-Llorente C, Guerrero-Sanz JE. 11 March 2004: the terrorist bomb explosions in Madrid, Spain-an analysis of the logistics, injuries sustained and clinical management of casualties treated at the closest hospital. *Crit Care* 2005;9:104-111.

8. Hirshberg A, Scott BG, Granchi T, Wall MJ, Mattox KL, Stein M. How does casualty load affect trauma care in urban bombing incidents? A quantitative analysis. *J Trauma* 2005;58(4):686-693; discussion 694-695.

9. Holden PJ. The London attacks—a chronicle: Improvising in an emergency. *N Engl J Med* 2005;353(6):541-543.

10. Jacobs LM, Burns KJ, Gross RI. Terrorism: a public health threat with a trauma system response. *J Trauma* 2003;55(6):1014-1021.

11. Kales SN, Christiani DC. Acute chemical emergencies. *N Engl J Med* 2004;350(8):800-808.

12. Klein JS, Weigelt JA. Disaster management: lessons learned. *Surg Clin North Am* 1991;71:257-266.

13. Mettler FA, Voelz GL. Major radiation exposure—what to expect and how to respond. *N Engl J Med* 2002;346(20):1554-1561.

14. Multiple authors. Perspective: The London attacks-a chronicle. *N Engl J Med* 2005;353:541-550.

15. Musolino SV, Harper FT. Emergency response guidance for the first 48 hours after the outdoor detonation of an explosive radiological dispersal device. *Health Phys* 2006;90(4):377-385.

16. National Disaster Life Support Executive Committee, National Disaster Life Support Foundation and American Medical Association. *Advanced, Basic, Core, and Decontamination Life Support Provider Manuals.* Chicago, IL: American Medical Association, 2012.

17. Pediatric Task Force, Centers for Bioterrorism Preparedness Planning, New York City Department of Health and Mental Hygiene (Arquilla B, Foltin G, Uraneck K, eds.). *Children in Disasters: Hospital Guidelines for Pediatric Preparedness.* 3rd ed. New York: New York City Department of Health and Mental Hygiene, 2008. http://www.nyc.gov/html/doh/downloads/pdf/bhpp/hepp-peds-childrenindisasters-010709.pdf. Accessed May 1, 2012.

18. Roccaforte JD, Cushman JG. Disaster preparation and management for the intensive care unit. *Curr Opin Crit Care* 2002;8(6):607-615.

19. Sever MS, Vanholder R, Lameire N. Management of crush-related injuries after disasters. *N Engl J Med* 2006;354(10):1052-1063.

Triage Scenarios

Introduction

This is a self-assessment exercise, to be completed *before* you arrive for the course. Please read through the introductory information on the following pages before reading the individual scenarios and answering the related questions. This skill station is conducted in a group discussion format during the course, in which your participation is expected. Upon completion of this session, your instructor will review the answers.

The goal of this station is to apply trauma triage principles in multiple patient scenarios.

Definition of Triage

Triage is the process of prioritizing patient treatment during mass-casualty events.

Principles of Triage

Do the Most Good for the Most Patients Using Available Resources

This is the central guiding principle that underlies all other triage principles, rules, and strategies. Multiple-casualty events, by definition, do not exceed the resources available. Mass-casualty events, however, do exceed available medical resources and require triage; the care provider, site, system, and/or facility is unable to manage the number of casualties using standard methods. Standard of care interventions, evacuations, and procedures cannot be completed (for each injury) for every patient within the usual time frame. The principles of triage are applied when the number of casualties exceeds the medical capabilities that are immediately available to provide usual and customary care.

Make a Decision

Time is of the essence during triage. The most difficult aspect of this process is making medical decisions without complete data. The triage decision maker (or triage officer) must be able to rapidly assess the scene and the numbers of casualties, focus on individual patients for short periods, and make immediate triage determinations for each patient. Triage decisions are typically made by deciding which patients' injuries constitute the greatest immediate threat to life. As such, the airway, breathing, circulation, and disability priorities of ATLS are the same priorities used to make triage decisions. That is, in general, airway problems are more rapidly lethal than breathing problems, which are more rapidly lethal than circulation problems, which are more rapidly lethal than neurologic injuries. All available information, including vital signs, when available, should be used to make each triage decision.

Triage Occurs at Multiple Levels

Triage is not a one-time, one-place event or decision. Triage first occurs at the scene or site of the event as decisions are made regarding which patients to treat first and the sequence in which patients will be evacuated. Next, triage typically occurs just outside the hospital to determine where patients will be transported within the facility (emergency department, operating room, intensive care unit, ward, or clinic). Triage then occurs in the preoperative area as decisions are made regarding the sequence in which patients are taken for operation.

Know and Understand the Resources Available

Optimal triage decisions are made with knowledge and understanding of the available resources at each level or stage of patient care. The triage officer must also be immediately aware of changes in resources, whether additional or fewer.

A surgeon is the ideal triage officer for hospital triage positions because he or she understands all components of hospital function, including the operating rooms. This arrangement will not work in situations with limited numbers of surgeons and does not apply to the incident site. The medical incident commander (who may or may not elect to serve as the triage officer) should be the highest-ranking medical professional on the scene who is trained in disaster management.

Planning and Rehearsal

Triage must be planned and rehearsed, as possible. Events that are likely to occur in the local area are a good starting point for mass-casualty planning and rehearsal. For example, simulate a mass-casualty event from an airplane crash if the facility is near a major airport, a chemical spill if near a busy railroad, or an earthquake if in an earthquake zone. Specific rehearsal for each type of possible disaster is not possible, but broad planning and fine-tuning of facility responses based on practice drills is possible and necessary.

Determine Triage Category Types

The title and color markings for each triage category should be determined at a system-wide level as part of planning and rehearsal. Many options are used around the world. One common, simple method is to use tags the colors of a stoplight: red, yellow, and green. Red implies life-threatening injury that requires immediate intervention and/or operation. Yellow implies injuries that may become life- or limb-threatening if care is delayed beyond several hours. Green patients are the walking wounded who have suffered only minor injuries. These patients can sometimes be used to assist with their own care and the care of others. Black is frequently used to mark dead patients. Many systems add another color, such as blue, for "expectant" patients—those who are so severely injured that, given the current number of casualties requiring care, the decision is made to simply give palliative treatment while first caring for red (and perhaps some yellow) patients. Patients who are classified as expectant because of the severity of their injuries would typically be the first priority in situations in which there are only two or three casualties requiring immediate care. However, the rules, protocols, and standards of care change in the face of a mass-casualty event. Remember: "Do the most good for the most patients using available resources."

Triage Is Continuous (Retriage)

Triage should be continuous and repetitive at each level or site where it is required. Constant vigilance and reassessment will identify patients whose circumstances have changed—either because of a change in physiologic status or because of a change in resource availability. As the mass-casualty event continues to unfold, the need for retriage becomes apparent. The physiology of injured patients is not constant or predictable, especially considering the limited rapid assessment required during triage. Some patients will unexpectedly deteriorate and require an "upgrade" in their triage category, perhaps from yellow to red. In others, an open fracture may be discovered after initial triage has been completed, mandating an "upgrade" in triage category from green to yellow. An important group requiring retriage is the expectant category. Although an initial triage categorization decision may label a patient as having nonsurvivable injuries, this may change after all red (or perhaps red and some yellow) patients have been cared for or evacuated (e.g., a young patient with 90% burns may survive if burn center care becomes available).

Triage Scenario I
Gas Explosion in the Gymnasium

SCENARIO: You are summoned to a triage area at a construction site where 5 workers are injured in a gas explosion during the renovation of a gymnasium ceiling. You quickly survey the situation and determine that the patients' conditions are as follows:

PATIENT A—A young male is screaming, "Please help me, my leg is killing me!"

PATIENT B—A young female has cyanosis and tachypnea and is breathing very noisily.

PATIENT C—A 50-year-old male is lying in a pool of blood with his left trouser leg soaked in blood.

PATIENT D—A young male is lying face down and not moving.

PATIENT E—A young male is swearing and shouting that someone should help him or he will call his lawyer.

Questions for Response

1 *For each patient, what is the primary problem requiring treatment?*

PATIENT A—is a young male screaming, "Please help me, my leg is killing me!"

Possible Injury/Problem: _____

_____

PATIENT B—appears to have cyanosis and tachypnea and is breathing very noisily.

Possible Injury/Problem: _____

_____

PATIENT C—is a 50-year-old male lying in a pool of blood with his left trouser leg soaked in blood.

Possible Injury/Problem: _____

_____

PATIENT D—is lying face down and not moving.

Possible Injury/Problem: _____

_____

PATIENT E—is swearing and shouting that someone should help him or he will call his lawyer.

Possible Injury/Problem:_____

_____

2 *Establish your patient priorities for further evaluation by placing a number (1 through 5, with 1 being the highest priority and 5 being the lowest) in the space next to each patient letter.*

_____ Patient A   _____ Patient D

_____ Patient B   _____ Patient F

_____ Patient C

3 *Briefly outline your rationale for prioritizing these patients in this manner.*

Priority 1—Patient _____:

Rationale: _____

_____

_____

_____

(continued)

Triage Scenario I (continued)

Priority 2—Patient _____:

Rationale: _____

_____

_____

_____

_____

_____

Priority 3—Patient _____:

Rationale: _____

_____

_____

_____

_____

_____

Priority 4—Patient _____:

Rationale: _____

_____

_____

_____

_____

_____

Priority 5—Patient _____:

Rationale: _____

_____

_____

_____

_____

_____

4 *Briefly, describe the basic life support maneuvers or additional assessment techniques you would use to further evaluate the problem(s).*

Priority 1—Patient _____:

Basic life support maneuvers or additional assessment techniques: _____

_____

_____

_____

_____

_____

Priority 2—Patient _____:
Basic life support maneuvers or additional assessment techniques: _____

_____

_____

_____

_____

Priority 3—Patient _____:
Basic life support maneuvers or additional assessment techniques: _____

_____

_____

_____

_____

_____

Priority 4—Patient _____:
Basic life support maneuvers or additional assessment techniques: _____

_____

_____

_____

_____

_____

Priority 4—Patient _____:

_____

_____

_____

_____

_____

_____

Priority 5—Patient _____:
Basic life support maneuvers or additional assessment techniques: _____

_____

_____

_____

_____

Triage Scenario II
Gas Explosion in the Gymnasium

Continuation of Scenario I:

1 *Characterize the patients according to who receives basic life support (BLS) or advanced life support (ALS) care and describe what that care would be. (Patients are listed in priority order as identified in Scenario I.)*

PATIENT	BLS	ALS	DESCRIPTION OF CARE
_____	☐	☐	_____
_____	☐	☐	_____
_____	☐	☐	_____
_____	☐	☐	_____
_____	☐	☐	_____

2 *Prioritize patient transfers and identify destinations. Provide a brief rationale for your destination choice.*

PRIORITY	PATIENT	DESTINATION	RATIONALE
1	☐ Trauma center	☐ Nearest hospital	_____
2	☐ Trauma center	☐ Nearest hospital	_____
3	☐ Trauma center	☐ Nearest hospital	_____
4	☐ Trauma center	☐ Nearest hospital	_____
5	☐ Trauma center	☐ Nearest hospital	_____

3 *In situations involving multiple patients, what criteria would you use to identify and prioritize the treatment of these patients?*

_____

_____

_____

_____

4 *What cues can you elicit from any patient that could be of assistance in triage?*

_____

_____

_____

_____

5 *Which patient injuries or symptoms should receive treatment at the scene before prehospital personnel arrive?*

_____

_____

_____

_____

6 *After prehospital personnel arrive, what treatment should be instituted, and what principles govern the order of initiation of such treatment?*

_____

_____

_____

_____

7 *In multiple-patient situations, which patients should be transported? Which should be transported early?*

_____

_____

_____

_____

8 *Which patients may have treatment delayed and be transported later?*

_____

_____

_____

_____

Triage Scenario III
Trailer Home Explosion and Fire

SCENARIO: An explosion and fire, due to a faulty gas line, has involved one trailer home in a nearby trailer park. Because of the close proximity of the incident to the hospital, the prehospital personnel transport the patients directly to the hospital without prior notification. The five patients, all members of the same family, are immobilized on long spine boards when they arrive at your small hospital emergency department. The injured patients are:

PATIENT A—**A 45-year-old male** is coughing and expectorating carbonaceous material. Hairs on his face and head are singed. His voice is clear, and he reports pain in his hands, which have erythema and early blister formation. Vital signs are blood pressure, 120 mm Hg systolic; heart rate, 100 beats per minute, and respiratory rate, 30 breaths per minute.

PATIENT B—**A 6-year-old female** appears frightened and is crying. She reports pain from burns (erythema/blisters) over her back, buttocks, and both legs posteriorly. Vital signs are blood pressure, 110/70 mm Hg; heart rate, 100 beats per minute, and respiratory rate, 25 breaths per minute.

PATIENT C—**A 70-year-old male** is coughing, wheezing, and expectorating carbonaceous material. His voice is hoarse, and he responds only to painful stimuli. There are erythema, blisters, and charred skin on the anterior chest and abdominal walls, and circumferential burns of both thighs. Vital signs are blood pressure, 80/40 mm Hg; heart rate, 140 beats per minute, and respiratory rate, 35 breaths per minute.

PATIENT D—**A 19-year-old female** is obtunded but responds to pain when her right humerus and leg are moved. There is no obvious deformity of the arm, and the thigh is swollen while in a traction splint. Vital signs are blood pressure, 140/90 mm Hg; heart rate, 110 beats per minute, and respiratory rate, 32 breaths per minute.

PATIENT E—**A 45-year-old male** is pale and reports pain in his pelvis. There is clinical evidence of fracture with abdominal distention and tenderness to palpation. There is erythema and blistering of the anterior chest and abdominal walls and thighs. He also has a laceration to the forehead. Vital signs are blood pressure, 130/90 mm Hg; heart rate, 90 beats per minute, and respiratory rate, 25 breaths per minute.

Management priorities in this scenario can be based on information obtained by surveying the injured patients at a distance. Although there may be doubt as to which patient is more severely injured, based on the available information, a decision must be made to proceed with the best information available at the time.

1   ***Identify which patient(s) has associated trauma and/or inhalation injury in addition to body-surface burns.***

☐ Patient A   ☐ Patient B   ☐ Patient C   ☐ Patient D   ☐ Patient E

2   ***Using the table provided below:***

a. Establish priorities of care in your hospital emergency department by placing a number (1 through 5, with 1 being the highest priority and 5 being the lowest) in the space next to each patient letter in the column "Treatment Priority."

b. Identify which patient has associated trauma and/or an airway injury and place a mark in the appropriate column under "Associated."

c. Estimate the percent of body-surface-area (BSA) burn for each patient and enter the percent for each patient letter in the column "% BSA."

d. Identify which patient(s) should be transferred to a burn center and/or a trauma center and place a mark in the appropriate column under "Transfer."

e. Establish your priorities for transfer and enter the priority number under "Transfer Priority."

PATIENT	ASSOCIATED		TREATMENT PRIORITY	%BSA	TRANSFER		TRANSFER PRIORITY
	Trauma	Airway Injury			Burn	Trauma	
A							
B							
C							
D							
E							

Triage Scenario IV
Cold Injury

SCENARIO: You are in your hospital when you receive a call that five members of a doctor's family were snow-mobiling on a lake when the ice broke. Four family members fell into the lake water. The doctor was able to stop in time and left to seek help. The response time of basic and advanced life support assistance was 15 minutes. By the time prehospital care providers arrived, one individual had crawled out of the lake and removed another victim from the water. Two individuals remained submerged; they were found by rescue divers and removed from the lake. Rescuers from the scene provided the following information:

> **PATIENT A—The doctor's 10-year-old grandson** was removed from the lake by rescuers. The ECG monitor shows asystole.
>
> **PATIENT B—The doctor's 65-year-old wife** was removed from the lake by rescuers. The ECG monitor shows asystole.
>
> **PATIENT C—The doctor's 35-year-old daughter,** who was removed from the water by her sister-in-law, has bruises to her anterior chest wall. Her blood pressure is 90 mm Hg systolic.
>
> **PATIENT D—The doctor's 35-year-old daughter-in-law,** who had been submerged and crawled out of the lake, has no obvious signs of trauma. Her blood pressure is 110 mm Hg systolic.
>
> **PATIENT E—The 76-year-old retired doctor,** who never went into the water, reports only cold hands and feet.

1 *Establish the priorities for transport from the scene to your emergency department, and explain your rationale.*

TRANSPORT PRIORITY	PATIENT (IDENTIFY BY LETTER)	RATIONALE
1		
2		
3		
4		
5		

2 *In the emergency department, all patients should have their core temperature measured. Core temperatures for these patients are:*

PATIENT A: 29° C (84.2° F)

PATIENT B: 34° C (93.2° F)

PATIENT C: 33° C (91.4° F)

PATIENT D: 35° C (95° F)

PATIENT E: 36° C (96.8° F)

Briefly outline your rationale for the remainder of the primary assessment, resuscitation, and secondary survey.

PATIENT A: Priority _____ :

_____

_____

_____

_____

_____

PATIENT B: Priority _____ :

_____

_____

_____

_____

_____

PATIENT C: Priority _____ :

_____

_____

_____

_____

PATIENT D: Priority _____ :

_____

_____

_____

_____

PATIENT E: Priority _____ :

_____

_____

_____

_____

_____

Triage Scenario V
Car Crash

SCENARIO: You are the only doctor available in a 100-bed community emergency department. One nurse and a nurse assistant are available to assist you. Ten minutes ago you were notified by radio that ambulances would be arriving with patients from a single motor vehicle crash. No further report is received. Two ambulances arrive with five patients who were occupants in an automobile traveling at 60 mph (96 kph) before it crashed. The injured patients are:

PATIENT A—**A 45-year-old male** was the driver of the car. He apparently was not wearing a seat belt. Upon impact, he was thrown against the windshield. On admission, he is notably in severe respiratory distress. The prehospital personnel provide the following information to you after preliminary assessment: Injuries include (1) severe maxillofacial trauma with bleeding from the nose and mouth, (2) an angulated deformity of the left forearm, and (3) multiple abrasions over the anterior chest wall. The vital signs are blood pressure, 150/80 mm Hg; heart rate, 120 beats per minute; respiratory rate, 40 breaths per minute; and Glasgow Coma Scale (GCS) score, 8.

PATIENT B—**A 38-year-old female** passenger was apparently thrown from the front seat and found 30 feet (9 meters) from the car. On admission she is awake, alert, and reports abdominal and chest pain. The report you are given indicates that, on palpating her hips, she reports pain, and fracture-related crepitus is felt. The vital signs are blood pressure, 110/90 mm Hg; heart rate, 140 beats per minute; and respiratory rate, 25 breaths per minute.

PATIENT C—**A 48-year-old male** passenger was found under the car. You are told that on admission he was confused and responded slowly to verbal stimuli. Injuries include multiple abrasions to his face, chest, and abdomen. Breath sounds are absent on the left, and his abdomen is tender to palpation. The vital signs are blood pressure, 90/50 mm Hg; heart rate, 140 beats per minute; respiratory rate, 35 breaths per minute; and GCS score, 10.

PATIENT D—**A 25-year-old female** was extricated from the back seat of the vehicle. She is 8 months pregnant, behaving hysterically, and reporting abdominal pain. Injuries include multiple abrasions to her face and anterior abdominal wall. You are told that her abdomen is tender to palpation. She is in active labor. The vital signs are blood pressure, 120/80 mm Hg; heart rate, 100 beats per minute; and respiratory rate, 25 breaths per minute

PATIENT E—**A 6-year-old male** was extricated from the floor of the rear seat. At the scene, he was alert and talking. He now responds to painful stimuli only by crying out. Injuries include multiple abrasions and an angulated deformity of the right lower leg. There is dried blood around his nose and mouth. The vital signs are blood pressure, 110/70 mm Hg; heart rate, 180 beats per minute; respiratory rate, 35 breaths per minute.

Questions and Response Key for Students' Response

1 *Outline the steps you would take to triage these five patients.*

_____

_____

_____

_____

_____

_____

_____

_____

2 *Establish your patient priorities by placing a number (1 through 5, with 1 being the highest priority and 5 being the lowest) in the space next to each lettered patient. Then, in the space provided, briefly outline your rationale for prioritizing these patients in this manner.*

Priority _____ **Patient A :** _____

Rationale: _____

_____

_____

_____

_____

Priority _____ **Patient B :** _____

Rationale: _____

_____

_____

_____

_____

_____

Priority _____ **Patient C:** _____

Rationale: _____

_____

_____

_____

_____

_____

Priority _____ **Patient D:** _____

Rationale: _____

_____

_____

_____

_____

_____

Priority _____ **Patient E:** _____

Rationale: _____

_____

_____

_____

_____

Triage Scenario VI
Train Crash Disaster

SCENARIO: Two trains collide head-on at 1800 hours. One train is a commercial tanker carrying eight tanker cars and is driven by an engineer and fireman. No other personnel are on board. The tanks are filled with a highly flammable liquid. The other train is a passenger train traveling on the same track. Weather conditions are mild, and the ambient temperature is 20° C (72° F). Upon arrival at the scene, EMTs and paramedics find:

DECEASED—Two engineers and one fireman

Five passengers, including one infant with a fatal head injury

INJURED—The fireman from the commercial train, ejected 30 feet, with 40% BSA second- and third-degree burns

Forty-seven passengers from the passenger train:

- 12 category Red patients, 8 with extensive (20–50% BSA) second- and third-degree burns
- 8 category Yellow patients, 3 with focal (<10% BSA) second-degree burns
- 22 category Green patients, 10 with painful hand and forearm deformities
- 5 category Blue patients, 3 with catastrophic (>75% BSA) second- and third-degree burns

Two fire companies and two additional ambulances have been called. The local community hospital has 26 beds, 5 primary care providers, and 2 surgeons, 1 of whom is on vacation. The nearest trauma center is 75 miles (120 kilometers) away, and the nearest designated burn center is over 200 miles (320 kilometers) away.

1 *Should community disaster plans be invoked? Why, or why not?*

_____

_____

2 *If a mass-casualty event is declared, who should be the medical incident commander?*

_____

_____

3 *What is the first consideration of the medical incident commander at the scene?*

_____

_____

4 *What considerations should be taken into account in medical operations at the scene?*

_____

_____

5 *What is the second consideration of the medical incident commander at the scene?*

_____

_____

6 *What is the meaning of the red, yellow, green, blue, and black triage categories?*

_____

_____

7 *Given the categories in Question 6, which patients should be evacuated to the hospital, by what transport methods, and in what order?*

_____

_____

8 *What efforts should be taken by the medical incident commander to assist with response and recovery?*

_____

_____

Triage Scenario VII
Suicidal Bomb Blast at a Political Rally

SCENARIO: A suicidal bomb blast has been reported at an evening political rally. The area is 30 minutes away from your level II trauma center. You are summoned to the scene as one of the triage officers. Initial report reveals 12 mortalities and 40 injured. Many rescue teams are busy in evacuation.

You arrive at an area where you find 3 dead bodies and 6 injured patients.

The condition of the 6 injured patients is as follows:

  PATIENT A—A young male, conscious and alert, has a small penetrating wound in the lower neck just to the left side of the trachea, with mild neck swelling, hoarse voice, no active bleeding.

  PATIENT B—A young male is soaked in blood, pale, and lethargic, yet responding to verbal commands. Both legs are deformed and attached only by thin muscular tissue and skin below the knees bilaterally.

  PATIENT C—A young female is complaining of breathlessness, with tachypnea, cyanosis, and multiple, small, penetrating wounds to the left side of her chest.

  PATIENT D—A middle-aged male has multiple penetrating wounds to the left side of the abdomen and left flank, pale looking and complaining of severe abdominal pain. Second- and third-degree burns visible over the lower abdomen.

  PATIENT E—An elderly male, breathless and coughing up bloodstained sputum, is disorientated and has multiple bruises and lacerations over his upper torso.

  PATIENT F—A young male has a large wound on the anterior aspect of the right lower leg with visible bone ends projecting from wound, and is complaining of severe pain. There is no active bleeding.

Questions for Response

1 *Based on the information, describe the potential A, B, C problems for each patient:*

PATIENT A _____

PATIENT B _____

PATIENT C _____

PATIENT D _____

PATIENT E _____

PATIENT F _____

2 *What initial life support maneuvers can be offered before transport to a trauma center (assuming that typical pre-hospital equipment is available at this time)?*

PATIENT A _____

PATIENT B _____

PATIENT C _____

PATIENT D _____

PATIENT E _____

PATIENT F _____

3 *What other considerations do you keep in mind during triage at the scene of this incident?*

_____

_____

_____

_____

(continued)

Triage Scenario VII (continued)

4 *Describe the transfer to trauma center of each patient in order of priority with your rationale (1 being the highest and 6 being the lowest)*

Priority 1   **Patient** _____

Rationale: _____

_____

_____

_____

Priority 2   **Patient** _____

Rationale: _____

_____

_____

_____

Priority 3   **Patient** _____

Rationale: _____

_____

_____

_____

Priority 4   **Patient** _____

Rationale: _____

_____

_____

_____

Priority 5   **Patient** _____

Rationale: _____

_____

_____

_____

Priority 6   **Patient** _____

Rationale: _____

_____

_____

_____

5 *What should be your main management considerations upon arrival of the patients at the trauma center?*

PATIENT A _____

PATIENT B _____

PATIENT C _____

PATIENT D _____

PATIENT E _____

PATIENT F _____

Index